Evidence-Based Practice in Audiology

Brad A. Stach, PhD
Editor-in-Chief for Audiology

Evidence-Based Practice in Audiology

Evaluating Interventions for Children and Adults with Hearing Impairment

Lena Wong, BA, MA, PhD, CCC-A
Associate Professor
Division of Speech and Hearing Sciences
Faculty of Education
University of Hong Kong
Hong Kong

and

Louise Hickson, BSpThy (Hons), MAud, PhD
Professor
School of Health and Rehabilitation Sciences
University of Queensland
Brisbane, Australia

PLURAL PUBLISHING
INC.
SAN DIEGO
OXFORD
MELBOURNE

PLURAL PUBLISHING
INC.

5521 Ruffin Road
San Diego, CA 92123

e-mail: info@pluralpublishing.com
Web site: http://www.pluralpublishing.com

49 Bath Street
Abingdon, Oxfordshire OX14 1EA
United Kingdom

FSC
www.fsc.org
MIX
Paper from responsible sources
FSC® C011935

Typeset in 11/13 Adobe Garamond by Flanagan's Publishing Services, Inc.
Printed in the United States of America by McNaughton & Gunn, Inc.
Second printing in January 2013

Library of Congress Cataloging-in-Publication Data

Evidence-based practice in audiology : evaluating interventions for children and adults with hearing loss / edited by Lena Wong and Louise Hickson.
p. ; cm.
Includes bibliographical references and index.
ISBN-13: 978-1-59756-419-9 (alk. paper)
ISBN-10: 1-59756-419-2 (alk. paper)
I. Wong, Lena. II. Hickson, Louise M.
[DNLM: 1. Hearing Disorders—therapy. 2. Evidence-Based Medicine. WV 270]
LC Classification not assigned
617.8—dc23
2011051391

Contents

Foreword

In 2003, I sat with a small group of friends in a house overlooking a beach. The view was spectacular, but we didn't notice it much. We were engrossed in a discussion of questions about the best ways to provide amplification for hearing-impaired adults and children. The conversation was lively, but attempts to pin down answers always seemed to run into a frustrating dead end. Finally, we admitted that we just didn't know what we knew. We did not have the information needed to identify the trustworthy research or eliminate the flawed efforts. We could not answer our questions in a satisfactory way, or even think about them usefully. It became clear that a formal evaluation of the available evidence about treatments for hearing loss was desperately needed. Based on that conversation, my friends and I undertook an effort that ultimately produced a special issue in the *Journal of the American Academy of Audiology*, which I was given the privilege of guest editing. The special issue included tutorial articles about the process of evidence-based practice (EBP), as well as systematic reviews of several important questions. It was a great success, widely read, and still cited. I think we contributed in a modest way to raising the consciousness of audiology practitioners and researchers about the process and the products of EBP.

The *JAAA* special issue started almost a decade ago, and it was limited. We concentrated mainly on hearing aids, whereas treatments for hearing problems also include cochlear implants and nonamplification rehabilitation. In the past decade, technological advances have produced an amplification landscape that changes at a bewildering rate. At the same time, evidence on the effectiveness of amplification and nonamplification types of treatments has accumulated in numerous venues (peer-reviewed journals, trade magazines, Internet papers, and so on). All this has strongly challenged the abilities of professionals to keep up. In addition, a generation of audiology students, practitioners, and researchers has struggled to grasp the nuances of EBP and to embody the approach in their activities. Meanwhile, the published guidelines that could help support these efforts have been very limited. That's where this book enters the picture. This is the first book to address the application of EBP specifically to the day-to-day enterprises of hearing health care. Between its pages you will find highly accessible chapters on the nitty-gritty details of EBP as well as up-to-date summaries of the latest evidence on many types of treatments for hearing problems.

Lena Wong, Louise Hickson, and I historically intersect at the University of Queensland (my alma mater, fondly remembered). Lena and I began to correspond in 1998 when she set out to apply her skills to creating outcome questionnaires for patients who communicate in Chinese. I first crossed paths with Louise at an international meeting on rehabilitative audiology in 2005. Over the years, Drs. Wong and Hickson have each separately made substantial contributions, with an emphasis on applying scientific principles to helping hearing-impaired persons. Their collaboration on this important book is, therefore, a natural outgrowth of their passions for using science in the service of clinical practice. To further this goal, they have assembled an impressive set of contributing authors that includes many leading lights in hearing rehabilitation.

Evidence-based practice finds its most compelling application when practitioner and patient are face to face. But let's not kid ourselves: it is not easy or quick to independently appraise research to determine the merits of a new treatment or feature. This book will be welcomed by clinicians for its intensive course in the latest evidence about the effectiveness of treatments that they can use. In addition, those who wish to acquire the ability to conduct their own evidence appraisals will find plenty of the practical assistance needed to hone those skills. Also, and this is really important, the book models the whole process of EBP from composing the question that the patient needs answered to checking to see how well the recommended treatment worked. Because EBP is not just about knowing the evidence, it is about knowing how to use it.

However, this book is not only for clinicians whose daily work brings them in contact with individuals who have hearing problems. This book is for everyone who needs to know about the real-world effects of interventions for hearing impairment. This group includes researchers, engineers, and people who allocate public health resources. These individuals make important decisions that can have wide-ranging effects. Presenting up-to-date evidence reviews in one location will facilitate formation of timely research plans and responsible policies. Finally, I am especially delighted to be able to offer this volume to my students. For a decade, I have taught these topics to audiology doctoral students with no textbook to pull the material together. Happily, those days are over.

Robyn Cox, PhD

Acknowledgments

We are very grateful to all those who assisted us to bring this book to fruition—our families and friends, our colleagues at the University of Hong Kong and the University of Queensland, the production team at Plural and, of course, the chapter authors. The authors of each chapter took on a daunting task when they agreed to be part of this first text on Evidence-Based Practice in audiology and we really appreciate the dedication and commitment they showed throughout the process. You never know when you start an endeavor such as this exactly what challenges you will face along the way, but you can guarantee that there will be challenges. We thank all those who contributed to us being able to meet the challenges and to produce a book that represents an enormous collaborative effort.

Contributors

Michelle Arnold, AuD
Research Audiologist
Department of Communication Sciences and Disorders
University of South Florida
WOC Research Associate
James A. Haley Veteran's Health Administration
Tampa, Florida
Chapter 10

Wendy Arnott, PhD
Lecturer in Speech Pathology
School of Health and Rehabilitation Sciences
The University of Queensland
Queensland, Australia
Chapter 12

Lana Britt, AuD
The University of Texas at Dallas
Callier Advanced Hearing Research Center
Dallas, Texas
Chapter 8

Teresa Y. C. Ching, PhD
National Acoustics Laboratories
The Hearing Cooperative Research Centre
Chatswood, Australia
Chapters 5 and 9

Theresa Chisolm, PhD
Department of Communication Sciences and Disorders
University of South Florida
Tampa, Florida
Chapter 10

Laura Czarniak, BS
Doctor of Audiology Student
Program in Audiology and Communication Sciences
Washington University in St. Louis School of Medicine
St. Louis, Missouri
Chapter 2

Richard C. Dowell, PhD
Chair of Audiology and Speech Sciences
The University of Melbourne
Royal Victorian Eye and Ear Hospital
Melbourne, Australia
Chapter 7

Louise Hickson, PhD
Professor
School of Health and Rehabilitation Services
University of Queensland
Queensland, Australia
Chapters 1, 3, and 13

Larry E. Humes, PhD
Distinguished Professor
Department of Speech and Hearing Sciences
Indiana University
Bloomington, Indiana
Chapter 4

Paola Incerti, MAud
Senior Research Audiologist
National Acoustic Laboratories
The Hearing Cooperative Research Centre
Chatswood, Australia
Chapter 9

Gitte Keidser, PhD
Senior Research Scientist
National Acoustic Laboratories
The Hearing Cooperative Research Centre
Sydney, Australia
Chapter 6

Vidya Krull, PhD
Postdoctor Fellow
Department of Speech and Hearing Sciences
Indiana University
Bloomington, Indiana
Chapter 4

Ariane Laplante-Lévesque, PhD
School of Health and Rehabilitation Sciences
University of Queensland, Australia
Postdoctoral Research Fellow
Eriksholm Research Centre, Denmark
Assistant Professor
Linköping University, Sweden
Chapter 3

William Noble, PhD
Professor of Psychology
University of New England
Armidale, Australia
Chapter 11

Olga Peskova
Fullbright Visiting Researcher
The University of Texas at Dallas
Dallas, Texas
Graduate Student
Department of Special Education
Moscow City Pedagogical University
Moscow, Russia
Chapter 8

Kenneth C. Pugh, PhD
Director of Audiology and Clinical Associate Professor
The University of Texas at Dallas
Callier Center for Communication Disorders
Dallas, Texas
Chapter 8

Emily A. Tobey, PhD
Professor and Nelle C. Johnston Chair
The University of Texas at Dallas
Callier Advanced Hearing Research Center
Dallas, Texas
Chapter 8

Maureen Valente, PhD
Associate Professor
Director of Audiology Studies
Program in Audiology and Communication Sciences
Washington University in St. Louis School of Medicine
St. Louis, Missouri
Chapter 2

Michael Valente, PhD
Professor of Clinical Otolaryngology and Director of Adult Audiology
Washington University in St. Louis School of Medicine
St. Louis, Missouri
Chapter 2

Andrea D. Warner-Czyz, PhD
Clinical Assistant Professor
The University of Texas at Dallas
Callier Advanced Hearing Research Center
Dallas, Texas
Chapter 8

Wayne J. Wilson, PhD
Senior Lecturer
School of Health and Rehabilitation Sciences
The University of Queensland
Queensland, Australia
Chapter 12

Lena Wong, PhD
Associate Professor
Division of Speech and Hearing Sciences
Faculty of Education
The University of Hong Kong
Hong Kong
Chapters 1 and 13

Linda Worrall, PhD
Professor
School of Health and Rehabilitation Sciences
University of Queensland
Queensland, Australia
Chapter 3

With thanks to our wonderfully supportive families
Henry, Shannon, and Jaden
Peter, William, Alex, and Robert

PART I

Principles of Evidence-Based Practice (EBP)

CHAPTER 1

Evidence-Based Practice in Audiology

Lena Wong and Louise Hickson

INTRODUCTION

Evidence-Based Practice is a buzz phrase in modern day health care, and audiology is no exception. Many researchers and clinicians stress the importance of this approach but it is not always clear what is understood by the term and what is actually happening to ensure that Evidence-Based Practice occurs in clinical settings. The approach has its roots in medicine and Sackett, Rosenberg, Gray, Haynes, and Richardson (1996) defined Evidence-Based Medicine as, "the conscientious, explicit and judicious use of current best evidence in making decisions about the care of individual patients" (p. 71). Now referred to as Evidence-Based Practice (EBP), incorporating all areas of health care, it involves the integration of the best available research evidence with clinical expertise, the clinical context and the client's preferences and goals (Fig. 1–1). The clinician presents the evidence to the client allowing him/her to make an informed choice about ongoing care. Thus, one of the centre pieces of EBP is shared decision making. It is a process that "requires judgment and artistry, as well as science and logic" (Hoffmann, Bennett, & Del Mar, 2010, p. 4).

EBP can be applied to various clinical areas in audiology, such as the diagnosis or prognosis of particular conditions (e.g., which tests should be used to diagnose central auditory processing disorders in young children? What are the effects of cisplatin on high frequency hearing thresholds long term?); however, the focus of this book is on EBP as it applies to interventions (e.g., what type of amplification is most appropriate for a child with a bilateral severe to profound sensorineural hearing impairment?). This is particularly important in audiology as there are numerous intervention options for children and adults with hearing impairment and it is audiologists' responsibility to provide their clients with the relevant evidence so that an informed choice can be made about what action to take. In this chapter, the process of EBP, as it applies to evaluating interventions, is introduced along with a rationale for its application in audiological rehabilitation. Finally, the structure of the book is described.

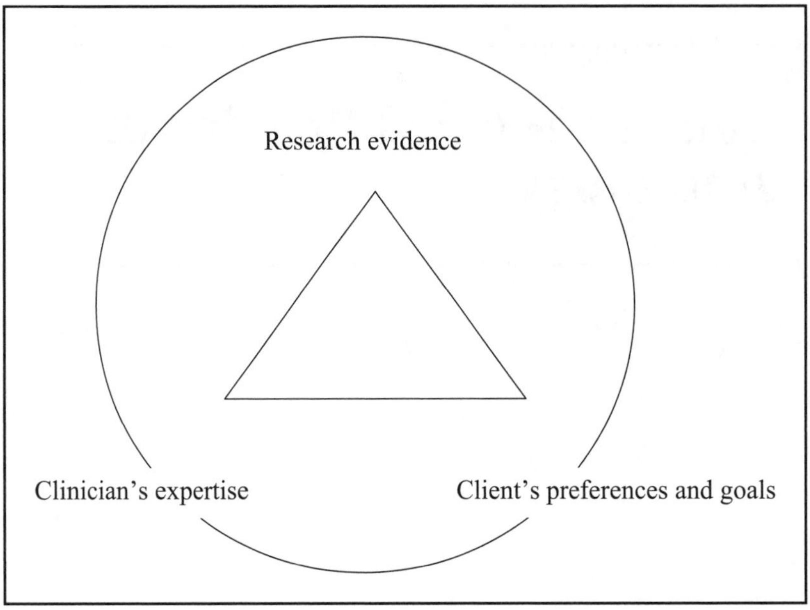

Figure 1–1. *Elements of EBP: Striking a balance between research evidence, clinician's expertise, and client's preferences and goals (the three edges of a triangle) in the clinical context (the large circle in the background).*

WHAT ARE THE STEPS IN EBP?

The process of EBP is typically described as having five steps:

1. defining a clinical question,
2. searching for evidence to address the question,
3. evaluating the available evidence,
4. relating the evidence to the client, and
5. evaluating the outcomes of the EBP process.

This final step highlights the cyclical nature of EBP and how it is essentially a continuous quality improvement process aimed at providing the best possible clinical care to clients. Jackson et al. (2006) described the five EBP steps using A's:

1. Ask a question,
2. Access the information,
3. Appraise the articles,
4. Apply the information, and
5. Audit.

In this section each of the five steps is described with the aim of providing a greater understanding of the process. Emphasis in this chapter is on Steps 1 to 3: Asking a question, Accessing information, and Appraising the articles. Chapter 2 provides more detail about Steps 2 and 3: Accessing the information and Appraising or evaluating the evidence about interventions. Chapter 3 explores the very important Step 4, how to relate the evidence about interventions to clients or Applying the information. Step 5, how outcomes of intervention should be appraised, is discussed in detail in the final chapter of the book.

Step 1: Defining a Clinical Question

The first step in the EBP process is to examine the problem and formulate a clinical question that is well defined and answerable (Rosenthal, 2004). This question should be defined in the context of a client's condition and may not be easily achieved, given the complexity of issues involved. To assist with this, Needleman (2003) recommended breaking down the question into four components indicated by the acronym PICO: Patient/Problem, Intervention, Comparison, and Outcomes. Table 1–1 shows these components along with an example of formulating a question relevant to audiological interventions.

Having a focused question is an important first step. Of course, it may sometimes mean that the literature search that follows reveals little evidence. This is particularly a problem in audiology at times as intervention options, such as the new hearing aid technologies discussed in Chapter 6, may be developed and marketed by industry before the evidence is available in the public domain. Nevertheless, we argue that it is essential for the clinician to know what the evidence is, or is not, for a particular intervention, rather than blindly accepting industry claims about benefits to clients.

Of course, if the research evidence is very limited, it may also be appropriate to broaden the question. In the example given in Table 1–1, it may be necessary to broaden the question to, "What are the outcomes obtained by adults with acquired hearing impairment fitted with frequency transposition hearing aids?" There may be evidence of other outcomes besides speech perception in noise, such as speech perception in quiet or self-reported aid benefit.

The issue of the nature of intervention outcome measures is an important one in audiology. A useful framework for thinking about dimensions of outcome is provided by the World Health Organization International Classification of Functioning, Disability and Health (WHO, 2007). In this framework, the effects of a health condition are described in

Table 1–1. Format for Developing a Structured Question Using the PICO Layout and an Example from Audiology

Patient/problem (P)	What is a concise description of the particular patient (client) or problem?	Adult with acquired severe high frequency sensorineural hearing impairment
Intervention (I)	Which main intervention am I considering?	Frequency transposition hearing aids
Comparison (C)	Am I comparing the treatment against the best alternative or no treatment?	Yes, it will be compared to conventional high frequency amplification
Outcome (O)	What is (are) the main outcome(s) that are of interest to my client and me?	Improved speech perception particularly in noisy situations
Final clinical question:	For clients with acquired severe high frequency sensorineural hearing impairment, do frequency transposition hearing aids provide improved speech perception in noise compared to conventional hearing aids?	

terms of changes to body structure and function, activities, and participation. Impairments refer to changes at the body level (e.g., damage to the outer hair cells of the cochlea, reduced audibility); activity limitations are changes at the level of the person (e.g., inability to hear conversation, problems using the telephone); and participation restrictions are the effects of these on broader aspects of life (e.g., withdrawing from social situations). Effective interventions in audiology would be expected to reduce impairments, limit activity, and restrict participation, subsequently enhancing quality of life for the client. Therefore, it is important to measure outcomes in a comprehensive manner including activity, participation, and quality of life measures. It is not enough to evaluate interventions in terms of tests of impairment alone (Stephens, Jones, & Gianopoulos, 2000; Valente et al., 2006). There are numerous examples of interventions that have positive findings when outcomes are measured in laboratory settings using assessments of impairment (e.g., insertion gain, speech perception tests) but are much less positive when the outcomes are measured in the real world using assessments of activity, participation and quality of life (e.g., self-report questionnaires, observations). A good example of this discrepancy is the evidence surrounding directional microphones. Laboratory-based measures consistently show superior performance that may not be realized in real life situations (Gnewikow, Ricketts, Bratt, & Mutchler, 2009).

Another point to consider when formulating the clinical question initially is that some clients have multiple issues and it may be necessary to prioritize the most important question (Needleman, 2003). For example, the client in Table 1–1 may also have severe tinnitus and may wish to know which hearing aids best alleviate the tinnitus. In this case it would be advisable to talk to the client about what is most important to him or her at this point in time and focus on answering that question or, if both are equally important, then the clinician will need to seek evidence about both questions at the same time.

Step 2: Searching for Research Evidence

After a clinical question has been defined, the next step is to search for evidence. In audiology, there are various sources of evidence, including books, refereed journal articles, trade journals, the Internet, and manufacturer provided information. It is likely that the best research evidence will be found in peer-reviewed journal articles (e.g., *Ear and Hearing*, *International Journal of Audiology*, *Journal of the American Academy of Audiology*, *Audiology and Neurotology*). Many trade journals (e.g., *Hearing Journal*, *ENT News*) are not peer-reviewed and books are not always research based. Searching for evidence from refereed journals can be done on the Internet using database search engines. The most useful ones for audiology are PubMed, PyschINFO, CINAHL, and Scopus. PubMed and PsychINFO are mega search engines that search multiple databases, peer-reviewed journals, books, and/or expert opinions, providing a more comprehensive list of evidence. Other mega search engines include the SumSearch, the Turning Research Into Practice (TRIP) Database, and the National Electronic Library for Health, National Health Services.

University libraries would have access to all of these databases; however, many clinical audiologists may not have access to such systems. If this is the case, then PubMed is the best option as it is available online for free. Within PubMed, select the "Clinical Queries" screen as this is most relevant to intervention studies. Table 1–2 contains a summary of these databases along with their Web addresses.

Table 1–2. Summary of Useful Databases for Searching for Evidence on Audiological Interventions

Database and Web site	*Details*
The Becker Library at the Washington University School of Medicine in St. Louis http://beckerguides.wustl.edu/audiology	Includes major databases, journals and books and other resources in the field of audiology and deaf education
ComDisDome http://www.csa.com/factsheets/cdd-set-c.php or www.comdisdome.com	Includes more than 300,000 records in the communications disorders literature, dated back to 1911.
Cumulative index to nursing and allied health literature (CINAHL) http://www.cinahl.com/	Includes journals, books, audiovisual, pamphlets, software, dissertations, or research instruments.
National Electronic Library for Health, National Health Services (Specialist Library—ENT and Audiology) http://www.library.nhs.uk/ent	The program My Evidence can be used to specify a search and receive updated information. Access to databases that contain systematic reviews as well as common bibliographical databases such as the MEDLINE, books, journals, and guidelines. A specialist section on ENT and audiology is also available.
PubMed http://pubmed.gov	MEDLINE is the largest module of PubMed. The biomedical journal citations and abstracts are created by the U.S. National Library of Medicine (NLM®). Medline cites about 5,400 journals, including journals in the area of audiologic intervention that are published in more than 80 countries. Clinicians may assess the Tutorial at the PubMed Web site to learn how to search in the database and additional information about PubMed can be found at Dollaghn (2007).
PsycINFO http://www.apa.org/psychinfo/	Covers the psychological literature since the 1800s. The database also includes some records from the 1600s and 1700s. Among the 42 million cited references, 80% are from journal articles, 8% are book chapters from authored and edited books and 12% are dissertations and secondary sources from Dissertation Abstracts International. About 99% of 2,450 journal titles covered are peer reviewed.
Scopus http://www.scopus.com/	Contains multidisciplinary journal abstracts and citations, including physics, engineering, life and health sciences, psychology, social sciences, and biological etc. Nearly 18,000 titles are included, of which 16,500 are peer-reviewed journals.

continues

Table 1–2. *continued*

Database and Web site	*Details*
SumSearch http://sumsearch.uthscsa.edu/	Searches Web sites with evidence written by qualified experts, with the majority of links from the NLM, the Database of Abstracts of Reviews of Effectiveness (DARE) and the National Guideline Clearinghouse (NGC) and categorized as textbooks, review articles, practice guidelines, systematic reviews, and original research.
TRIP (Turning Research Into Practice) Database http://www.tripdatabase.com/	Searches more than 75 databases, including PubMed, the DARE and the NGC and other evidence-based materials such as systematic reviews, peer-reviewed journals, guidelines, e-textbooks, expert opinions, patient information.
UK Database of Uncertainties about the Effects of Treatments (UK DUETS), National Health Services, UK http://www.library.nhs.uk/duets/	Publishes uncertainties about the effects of treatment where current and reliable systematic reviews of research evidence are not available. Information sources include questions from clients, carers and clinicians; research recommendations based on systematic reviews and clinical guidelines; and ongoing research such as systematic reviews in preparation and new studies.

Relevant search terms can be found in the clinical question devised in Step 1 of the EBP process. As a starting point, Wilczynski and McKibbon (2010) advocate using the P (patient or problem) and the I (intervention). By way of example, we can consider the clinical question from Table 1–1: For clients with acquired severe high frequency sensorineural hearing impairment, do frequency transposition hearing aids provide improved speech perception in noise compared to conventional hearing aids? Search terms to start with would be: "high frequency hearing loss," "high frequency hearing impairment," "speech perception," and "frequency transposition hearing aids." If searching for these terms yielded limited results then it would be necessary to broaden the search. Sometimes the term (e.g., speech perception) used for the patient or problem may not be inclusive enough and it might be useful to include "speech understanding," "speech intelligibility," and "benefit." Another way to do this is to use what are called truncations and different search engines have different methods for doing this. A common way to do this is by inserting an asterisk after a key word, for example, "hearing*," would search for both hearing loss and hearing impairment. If you are new to searching such databases it is important to read the Help section of the database and/or to speak to a librarian. Chapter 2 provides a more detailed description of how a search could be done and suggests a Web site with links to useful information about search strategies.

Systematic reviews and meta-analyses provide the highest level of evidence in EBP. They systematically locate, appraise, and synthesize research from primary studies (Cook, Mulrow, & Haynes, 1997; Bennett, Leicht-Doyle, & O'Connor, 2010). Meta-analysis is a particular type of systematic review where statistical measures are used to examine and evaluate pooled data from a number of studies. Two examples of meta-analysis are given in Chapter 10 where evidence on aural rehabilitation intervention is discussed. In a systematic review, studies are detailed in terms of their inclusion and exclusion criteria, levels of evidence, participant characteristics, intervention characteristics, and specific outcomes (Chisolm & Portz, 2007). Based on the evidence evaluated, specific conclusions or recommendations are made and as such they are very appealing to busy clinicians with limited time to evaluate the evidence themselves, especially when there are a number of studies to review. Table 1–3 contains examples of systematic review Web sites and examples of systematic reviews can be found in other chapters of this book (e.g., Chapter 8 reviews the evidence about cochlear implants in children). A number of health professions have developed their own discipline specific databases for systematic reviews (e.g., OTseeker for occupational therapists and PEDro for physiotherapists). Although there is no audiology specific site as yet, audiology research is included on the American Speech, Language and Hearing Association (ASHA) site (see Table 1–3) and in speechBITE, a speech pathology database. In Chapter 2, the authors also elucidate the use of a systematized review by clinicians, where a full systematic review may not be possible.

Another way to broaden the search, particularly if no systematic reviews are available, is to search for evidence included in guidelines and position papers from professional organizations such as the (ASHA) and American Academy of Audiology (AAA). ASHA also lists some Web sites of other organizations that contain guidelines of interest to audiologists. It is vital to note, however, that, although most guidelines are written by experts in the field, they are not always evidence based (Irwin, Pannbacker, & Lass, 2007). An example of a good set of guidelines that are evidence based are the "Guidelines for Audiological Management of Adult Hearing Impairment" developed by Valente et al. (2006). These guidelines have applied the techniques used in systematic reviews to evaluate evidence and provide recommendations. A list of Web sites with practice guidelines, position papers, and recommended procedures relevant to the practice of audiology is included in Table 1–4.

The search in Step 2 of the EBP process should result in a list of all relevant information but should not be so broad that there is too much information to evaluate (Rosenthal, 2004). Evidence obtained as a result of the search should then be examined carefully in Step 3.

Step 3: Evaluating the Evidence

Once available evidence has been identified, the next step is to evaluate how well the pieces of evidence have answered the defined question. For each piece, the clinician must: (1) identify the type of evidence, (2) identify its level, and (3) evaluate the quality or grade. In this section, we first introduce a hierarchy of evidence relevant to intervention studies and describe briefly the levels of evidence in the hierarchy. With this hierarchy, the type and level of evidence can be identified. Subsequently, we list three questions that are essential for the appraisal of the quality of evidence and, finally, grades of recommendation for the evidence are discussed. These grades help with the determination of whether the proposed intervention is sufficiently evidence based. More detail on how evidence should be evaluated is provided in Chapter 2.

Table 1–3. Web Sites That Provide Systematic Reviews on Audiological Interventions

Database and Web site	*Details*
ASHA Compendium of EBP Guidelines and Systematic Reviews http://www.asha.org/members/ebp/compendium/	Developed by ASHA's National Center for Evidence-Based Practice in Communication Disorders (N-CEP). Identifies clinical practice guidelines and systematic reviews related to audiology and/or speech-language pathology.
Campbell Collaboration http://www.campbellcolaboration.org	Contains systematic reviews on the effects of social interventions.
Centre for Reviews and Dissemination (CRD) at the University of York, UK. The three databases are the Database of Abstracts of Reviews of Effectiveness (DARE), National Health Services Economic Evaluation Database (NHS EED), and Health Technology Assessment (HTA) http://www.crd.york.ac.uk/crdweb/	The DARE includes 15,000 abstracts of systematic reviews, of which over 6,000 are quality assessed reviews and details of all Cochrane reviews and protocols. The NHS EED includes 24,000 abstracts of health economics papers, focusing on the impacts of interventions used in health and social care. Over 7,000 quality assessed economic evaluations are available. The HTA includes over 8,000 completed and continuing assessments on health technology, such as those conducted by members of the International Network of Agencies for Health Technology Assessment (INAHTA). The abstracts describe the assessments and the reports are not critically appraised.
National Electronic Library for Health, National Health Services http://www.library.nhs.uk/evidence/	The program My Evidence can be used to specify a search and receive updated information. Access to the Cochrane Library, the DARE, the NHS EED, the HTA Database, and the UK DUETS, as well as common bibliographical databases such as MEDLINE, books, journals, and guidelines.
speechBITE http://www.speechbite.com	Provides open access to a catalogue of Best Interventions and Treatment Efficacy in Speech Pathology practice. Evidence related to hearing is also included. This was initiated by the University of Sydney and Speech Pathology Australia to encourage evidence-based practice.
The Cochrane Library http://www.thecochranelibrary.com/	More than 27,000 international contributors of the Cochrane Collaboration produce systematic appraisal of health care interventions, known as Cochrane Reviews.

Table 1–4. Web Sites Where Practice Guidelines, Policy Statements, and Recommended Procedures May Be Found

Database and Web site	*Details*
ASHA Compendium of EBP Guidelines and Systematic Reviews http://www.asha.org/members/ebp/compendium/	Developed by ASHA's National Center for Evidence-Based Practice in Communication Disorders (N-CEP). Includes clinical practice guidelines and systematic reviews related to audiology and/or speech-language pathology.
Canadian Academy of Audiology http://www.canadianaudiology.ca/	Contains position statements and guidelines in Audiology.
National Electronic Library for Health, National Health Services http://www.library.nhs.uk/evidence/	The program My Evidence can be used to specify a search and receive updated information. Access to the Cochrane Library, the DARE, the NHS EED, the HTA Database and the UK DUETS, as well as common bibliographical databases such as the MEDLINE, books, journals, and guidelines.
National Guideline clearinghouse http://www.guideline.gov/	Includes synthesis of some guidelines on selected topic areas, and Expert Commentary on clinical guidelines.
The American Academy of Pediatrics http://aappolicy.aappublications.org/index.dtl	Lists clinical and technical reports, policy, clinical practice guidelines and policy statements from various sources.
The Audiological Society of Australia http://www.audiology.asn.au/	Contains recommended procedures and guidelines for the practice of audiology.
The British Society of Audiology http://www.thebsa.org.uk/	Contains recommended procedures and guidelines for the practice of audiolology.
The National Guideline Clearinghouse http://www.sign.ac.uk/guidelines	Lists guidelines from various sources.
The New Zealand Audiological Society http://www.audiology.org.nz/	Contains recommended procedures and guidelines for the practice of audiology.

Hierarchies of Evidence

Traditionally in EBP, various types of evidence have been classified according to a hierarchy of evidence. There are a number of examples of such hierarchies available in books (e.g., Straus, Richardson, Glasziou, & Haynes, 2005) and online, from sources such as the American Speech-Language and Hearing Association, Oxford Centre for Evidence-based Medicine, the Centre for Health Evidence in the United States, and Australia's National Health and Medical Research Council. Hierarchies are generally quite similar although there are some minor differences. In this text, the hierarchy shown in Table 1–5 is applied.

Table 1–5. Hierarchies of Evidence

Level	*Types of Evidence*
1	Systematic reviews and meta-analyses of studies that are of high level or randomized controlled trials (RCT)
2	Well-designed RCT
3	Treatment studies that are not randomized (e.g., nonequivalent group designs, separate sample pretest/postest design, and time-series designs)
4	Nontreatment studies (e.g., cohort studies, case-control studies, cross-sectional studies, and uncontrolled experiments)
5	Case studies
6	Expert comments

Source: Adapted from "Systematic Reviews: Synthesis of Best Evidence for Clinical Decisions," by R. M. Cox, 2005, *Journal of the American Academy of Audiology, 16*(7), 419–438.

Level 1, evidence from systematic reviews or meta-analyses of randomized controlled trials, is the highest level and Level 6, expert opinion, is the lowest. When the highest level of evidence is not available (which is frequently the case), other individual research studies that address the topic of interest should be evaluated (Mullen, 2007).

What Evidence Is Provided by Different Types of Research Studies?

It can be helpful to think of research as being made up of two major types of studies: descriptive and analytic (Fig. 1–2). Descriptive studies employ surveys, qualitative methods or case reports to *describe* current intervention outcomes. They address questions related to the problem or the person (P) and the outcomes only (O). Analytic studies attempt to *evaluate* the effect of an intervention on an outcome. Therefore, they address all the components of PICO: Problem or person, Intervention, Comparison, and Outcome.

Analytic studies may be further classified into: (1) experimental studies where participants are randomly assigned into groups by the researcher/s and variables are manipulated to address the clinical question/s, and (2) observational analytic studies where the researcher/s do not actively manipulate the intervention or determine the grouping of participants. In observational studies, groups are formed based on some preexisting conditions, not random assignment; therefore, the groups may not be equal or matched. Observational analytic studies are sometimes referred to as quasi-experimental or nonrandomized intervention studies. An example of an experimental analytic study on audiological interventions would be one in which adults with hearing impairment attending a clinic for hearing aid fitting are randomly allocated to a group who receive bilateral digital hearing aids

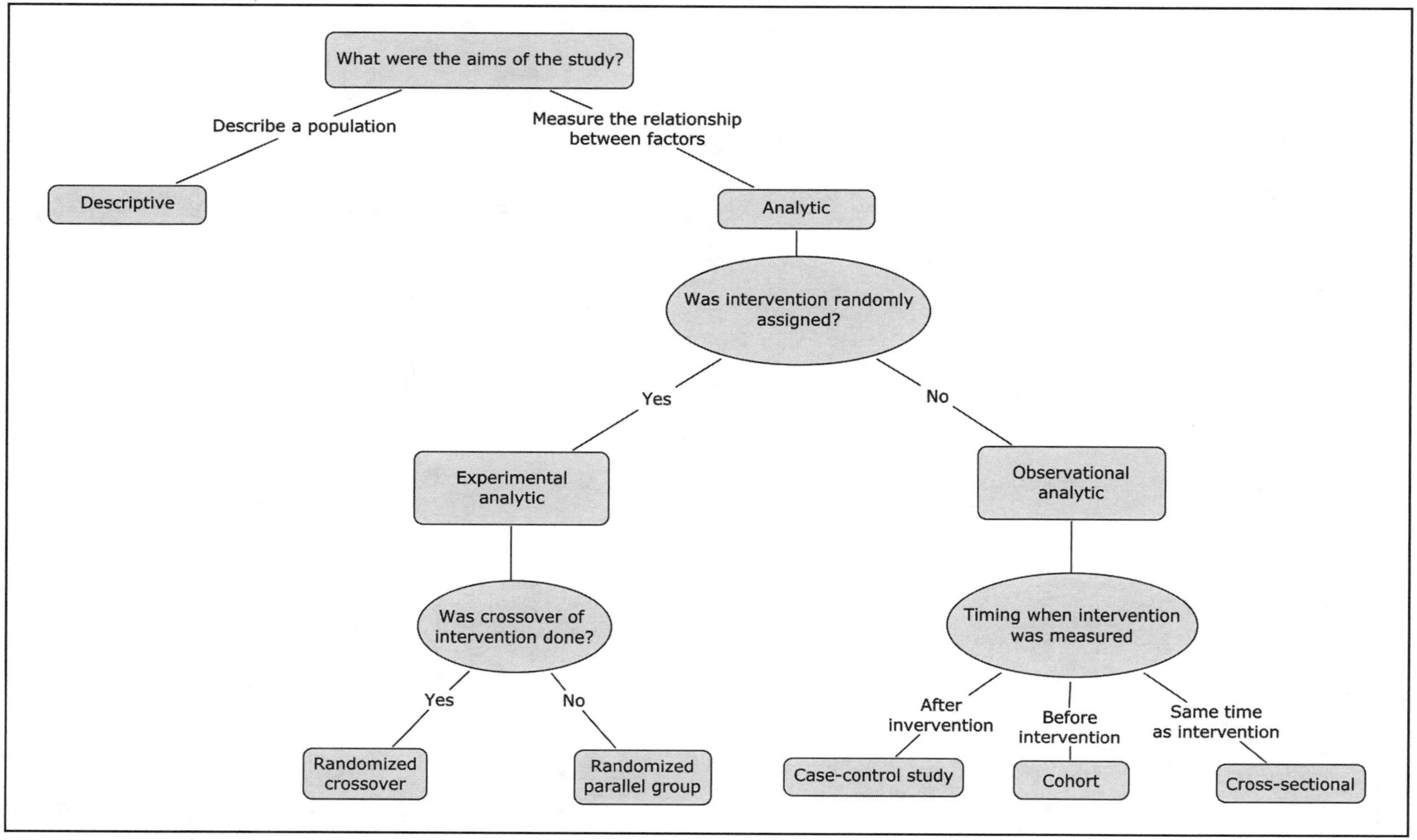

Figure 1–2. *Differentiation of types of research studies. Adapted from the figure of the tree of different studies found on the Centre for Evidence Based Medicine Web site (http://www.c?bm.net/index.aspx?o=1039).*

with omnidirectional microphones and a group who receive bilateral digital hearing aids with directional microphones. Such a study could address the clinical question: Are directional microphones more beneficial than omnidirectional microphones for adults with mild to moderate sensorineural hearing impairment? If sufficiently well-designed it would provide Level 2 evidence as shown in Table 1–5.

An example of an observational analytic study, on the other hand, would be comparing the outcomes obtained in people with hearing impairment who attend a clinic and are fitted with either unilateral or bilateral hearing aids. Research participants are not randomly assigned. Such a study could address the clinical question: What are the differences between benefits obtained with unilateral versus bilateral hearing aids for adults with hearing impairment? This research study could be Level 3 or 4 evidence. Figure 1–2 illustrates questions that may be asked to differentiate different types of studies.

Although RCTs are considered the highest level of evidence for intervention studies, they are not always appropriate. Different types of studies are needed to address different clinical questions and this is summarized in Table 1–6. Therefore, although we have recommended the hierarchy in Table 1–5 for evaluating evidence about audiological interventions, it is important to select the best available evidence within the hierarchy to address specific questions (Del Mar & Hoffmann, 2010a; Harrison & Bickley, 2003). In the chapters of this book, authors examine the highest quality available evidence relevant to different audiological interventions, although RCTs (level 2 evidence) are not common; most evidence is from observational analytic studies (level 4 evidence).

Evaluation of the Quality of Evidence

A particular type of study does not, however, necessarily mean that it will provide quality evidence. Dollaghan (2007) discusses the evaluation of evidence in communication disorders and Mullen (2007) suggests that eight factors should be considered in evaluating evidence for communication sciences and disorders: study design, blinding, sampling, participants, outcomes, significance, precision and intention to treat. In addition, Hoffmann et al. (2010) report on the evaluation of health care evidence and the Journal of the American Medical Association also has a Web site (http://jamaevidence.com/) that addresses all 5 steps in EBP, including how evidence should be evaluated. There are also various critical appraisal checklists (CACs) or critical appraisal tools (CATs) that can be used to assess the internal validity, intervention impact and external validity of evidence. Examples of CACs can be found in Dollaghan (2007), Davis and Crombie (2003), the Critical Appraisal Skills Programme at the UK National Health Service Public Health Resource Unit (http://www.phru.nhs.uk/pages/PHD/resources.htm), and the Critical Appraisal Sheets from Center on Evidence Based Medicine (http://www.cebm.net/index.aspx?o=1157). In the Appendix we provide a CAC that is applicable to the evaluation of research into audiological interventions. Guidelines for the use of the CAC are also provided.

The CAC is divided into three sections that address the key quality questions about each piece of evidence (Del Mar & Hoffmann, 2010b; Guyatt et al., 2000):

1. Is there internal validity? Internal validity refers to whether the evidence is trustworthy and the outcomes are truly attributable to the intervention. It is important to evaluate whether the research has been carried out with sound methodology and the results have been interpreted appropriately.
2. Is the impact large enough? Impact refers to whether the effect of an intervention

Table 1–6. Types of Analytic Studies and Examples from Audiology

Study Type	*What Are They?*	*What Are They Best At Addressing?*	*Example*	*Special Notes*
Randomized controlled trial (RCT) parallel group	Participants are randomly assigned into groups that receive different interventions. Outcomes of these interventions are then measured.	Is the intervention effective? Is one intervention more effective than another?	Hearing aids with omnidirectional and directional microphones are fitted to two groups of participants with matched characteristics. Outcomes are measured and compared.	Researchers and participants are blinded to the group assignment. Withholding intervention may be unethical in some cases.
RCT crossover	Same as RCT but participants are randomly assigned to receive different interventions, followed by another intervention.	Same as RCT	Same as above. As the hearing aids are "swapped" at the end of the first trial, outcomes are measured again and compared.	It takes more time to complete than an RCT parallel group design. Participants serve as own controls and error variance is reduced.
Case-control (mostly retrospective)	A group with a particular outcome is compared to another without those outcomes to see if certain factors would predict that particular outcome.	What are the factors that would predict the desired outcomes?	A group of satisfied users is compared with a group of dissatisfied users to see if directionality of hearing aids fitted would predict degree of satisfaction.	The groups may not be equivalent in other aspects. Confounders are not accounted for. Reliance on recall.
Cohort (mostly prospective)	A group of participants who has been exposed to a factor of interest and a group that has not are examined to determine whether outcomes differ as a result of the factor of interest.	Same as RCT	Outcomes of groups of participants fitted with omnidirectional and directional microphones are compared. The researcher does not assign group membership.	Difficult to control characteristics of the participants to make sure they are equivalent in other factors. Participant drop out could be a problem. Blinding is difficult.
Cross-sectional (same time as intervention)	Participants are measured at a particular point in time to examine their outcomes and the factors associated with the outcomes.	What are the factors that may relate to the intervention outcomes?	A study of the relationship between directionality of hearing aids and self-reported outcomes of benefit, use and satisfaction.	Direct conclusion on causal effects could not be drawn. Recall bias and confounders are not accounted for.

is large enough to reach clinical significance. In research, statistical differences are generally reported and these are not always the same as clinical significance. It is important to consider the size of any differences and what they would mean for individual clients.

3. Is there external validity or does the information apply to my client? This refers to whether the evidence could be applied to a particular client. Effectiveness and feasibility of interventions must be considered here.

For each of the 27 questions in the CAC, the appraiser provides a rating and, after perusing the individual ratings, makes an overall judgment about internal validity, impact, and external validity and then determines an overall clinical bottom line: seriously consider adopting the intervention (evidence is compelling), possibly adopt the intervention (evidence is suggestive) or not adopt the intervention (evidence is equivocal) (Dollaghan, 2007). In general, the introduction, methods and results of a research study contribute to the determination of internal validity. The information provided in the results and discussion sections help to determine the potential impact of the intervention in the clinic and the discussion section contributes to the evaluation of the external validity of the study. The best way to understand how to evaluate or appraise evidence is to select a research study from a peer-reviewed journal and apply the CAC to it, using the guidelines provided in the Appendix.

Evaluating the Grade of Evidence

After the critical appraisal of each piece of evidence, the clinician will draw conclusions about general findings, unanswered questions and limitations, and the level of evidence of each study. Although the highest level of evidence should be used to address each EBP question, it often may be necessary, for example, when working with emerging rehabilitation techniques such as those described in Chapter 6, to rely on evidence that has not been subjected to vigorous scrutiny (e.g., level 5 or 6 evidence from Table 1–5). We may also come across evidence that is not congruent or the evidence may not match the clinical question. Variations in methodologies and/or findings are not uncommon. Valente et al. (2006) and Cox (2005) recommend assigning a grade of recommendation to the overall quality of the evidence related to a specific question about audiological intervention (Table 1–7). This approach is further illustrated in many chapters of this book. Clinicians should continue to evaluate new evidence and determine whether the intervention has been chosen appropriately, especially when C or D grades of recommendation are observed. Similar approaches for grading the strength of recommendation can be found in a report of the United States Preventive Services Task Force (1996) and the Scottish Intercollegiate Guidelines Network (SIGN) (Harbour & Miller, 2001).

Evaluation of Guidelines

Many of the checklists mentioned above are for appraising research studies that are of levels 1 to 5 as listed in Table 1–5. However, as previously mentioned, many practice guidelines are based on nonsystematic reviews of the literature and expert opinions. To properly appraise guidelines of that kind, it may be useful to refer to tools such as the Appraisal of Guidelines Research and Evaluation (AGREE) developed by the European Union. The AGREE has subsequently been endorsed by the U.S. Agency for Health Research and Quality (AHRQ). Six quality domains are evaluated:

1. *Scope and purpose*—What is the general aim of the guideline? What are the particular clinical questions? What is the target client population?

Table 1–7. Grade of Recommendation of Research Quality

Grade	*Description*
A	Mostly Level 1 or 2 studies with conclusions that are consistent across studies
B	Mostly Level 3 or 4 studies *or* Level 1 or 2 studies with findings that are not fully relevant to the population or problem concerned but generalization could be made
C	Mostly Level 5 evidence *or* Mostly Level 3 or 4 studies with findings that are not fully relevant to the population or problem concerned but generalization could be made
D	Mostly Level 6 evidence *or* When most of the evidence lacks consistency or the conclusions are mostly uncertain *or* When most of the evidence exhibits a high chance of bias

Source: Adapted from "Systematic Reviews: Synthesis of Best Evidence for Clinical Decisions," by R. M. Cox, 2005, *Journal of the American Academy of Audiology, 16*(7), 419–438.

Note: Levels of studies are those from Table 1–5.

2. *Stakeholder involvement*—How well represented are the views of the proposed users (e.g., stakeholders, clients)?
3. *Rigor of development*—Was the process used to gather and amalgamate the evidence vigorous? What were the procedures used to reach the recommendation? Are there efforts to revise the guidelines?
4. *Clarity and presentation*—Was the guideline written in a language and format that are easy to comprehend?
5. *Applicability*—How feasible is its application in clinical situations?
6. *Editorial independence*—Were the recommendations made independently? Was probable conflict of interest acknowledged?

In conclusion, when there is a lack of consistent evidence to support the use of an intervention, clinicians may have to rely on their own knowledge of proper research processes (e.g., using appropriate outcome measurement tool and procedures) to address the PICO question in individual cases. That is, the clinician may implement the intervention and evaluate the process and outcomes of the intervention in a "single-case" study. This situation often occurs with the introduction of new amplification technologies. It is important to remember that the critical appraisal of evidence is just one aspect of EBP, as illustrated in Figure 1–1. The next step is to relate the evidence to the client so that a shared decision-making process can be facilitated.

Step 4: Relating the Evidence to the Client

Once it has been determined that the research about a particular question has adequate internal and external validity and impact, then it is time to relate the evidence to the client. At this point it is important to remember the byline from a *British Medical Journal* editorial on EBP in 2002: "Evidence Does Not Make Decisions, People Do" (Haynes, Devereaux, & Guyatt, 2002). Effective communication between client and clinician is the key to integrating client expectations and values with the information about the research evidence. The aim is for shared decision making to occur. The clinician needs to listen very carefully to the client to understand his or her expectations, concerns, experiences, values, and so forth. Information about the research evidence can be presented to clients in a number of different formats: verbal, written, computer-based, DVDs, or any combination of these formats. Specific tools, known as decision aids, are also highly recommended for this process. The evidence about such approaches is evaluated and discussed in Chapter 3.

Step 5: Evaluating Outcomes

In this step, depending on the original purpose of EBP implementation, clinicians may be evaluating: (1) the efficiency and efficacy of steps 1 to 4 and (2) whether the intervention has been properly implemented and whether intended outcomes have been achieved. Two components should be examined: the process and the outcomes. A process evaluation examines the background or the clinical questions, the procedures, the personnel, and the resources that are integral to the implementation of EBP. Here, what actually happened when the intervention was applied is being examined and compared to what was planned. The outcome evaluation examines the impact and effectiveness of an intervention for a particular individual or group of individuals and may include an evaluation of cost-effectiveness. The procedures to evaluate outcomes are discussed in detail in Chapter 13.

WHY USE EBP IN AUDIOLOGY?

EBP has proponents in various areas of health care and was endorsed in a technical report in 2004 and a position statement in 2005 by the American Speech-Language-Hearing Association (Fig. 1–3). EBP is particularly important in audiology where there are various interventions to assist people with hearing impairment (e.g., hearing aids, cochlear implants, hybrid devices, assistive listening devices, auditory training) and a growing body of research evidence that needs to be appraised by clinicians and researchers.

Clinicians are often in a situation where they have to discuss available intervention options with clients, and in the context of EBP the options should be described along with the evidence about their effectiveness, that is, how they perform in real-world conditions and not just in the laboratory setting. Studies that focus on outcomes measured in the laboratory or clinical setting are referred to as studies of efficacy. It is also the case that interventions are costly and clinicians and researchers need to justify intervention decisions to policy makers and third-party payers. EBP can create and provide support for sustaining specific clinical practices. It also allows for explicit acknowledgement of uncertainty and gaps between empirical evidence and clinical practice (Needleman, 2003). For all these reasons, EBP should be an essential mode of practice for those working with audiological interventions for children and adults with hearing impairment.

HOW IS THIS BOOK STRUCTURED?

We hope that this chapter has given the reader a flavor of what EBP is and how EBP relates

In making clinical practice evidence-based, audiologists and speech-language pathologists—

- Recognize the needs, abilities, values, preferences, and interests of individuals and families to whom they provide clinical services, and integrate those factors along with best current research evidence and their clinical expertise in making clinical decisions;
- Acquire and maintain the knowledge and skills that are necessary to provide high quality professional services, including knowledge and skills related to evidence-based practice;
- Evaluate prevention, screening, and diagnostic procedures, protocols, and measures to identify maximally informative and cost-effective diagnostic and screening tools, using recognized appraisal criteria described in the evidence-based practice literatures;
- Evaluate the efficacy, effectiveness, and efficiency of clinical protocols for prevention, treatment, and enhancement using criteria recognized in the evidence-based practice literature;
- Evaluate the quality of evidence appearing in any source or format, including journal articles, textbooks, continuing education offerings, newsletters, advertising, and Web-based products, prior to incorporating such evidence into clinical decision making; and
- Monitor and incorporate new and high quality research evidence having implications for clinical practice

Adapted with permission from *Evidence-Based Practice in Communication Disorders* [Position statement]. Available from http://www.asha.org/policy. Copyright 2005 American Speech-Language-Hearing Association. All rights reserved.

Figure 1–3. *ASHA position statement on EBP.*

to audiological re/habilitation. The remainder of the book describes the principles of EBP as they apply to the evaluation of audiological interventions in children and adults. The reader will learn the process of EBP in Chapters 2 and 3, as well as gain knowledge about the evidence relating to specific interventions (i.e., hearing aids, cochlear implants, aural rehabilitation) and to specific conditions (i.e., tinnitus, central auditory processing disorders) in Chapters 4 to 12.

The book is divided into four sections, with the first section describing principles of EBP, including how to evaluate evidence and how to facilitate evidence-based decisions with clients. The remaining three sections provide a discussion of the best available evidence about hearing aids, cochlear implants, and other interventions. These three sections contain chapters that summarize the best available evidence, highlight areas where further evidence is needed, and discuss how further evidence should be collected and applied in the clinic. The Appendix at the end of the book contains a critical appraisal checklist (CAC) that can be used by clinicians to evaluate whether a piece of evidence has good internal and external validity and impact.

REFERENCES

Bennett, S., Leicht-Doyle, S., & O'Connor, D. (2010). Appraising and understanding systematic reviews and meta analysis. In T. Hoffmann,

S. Bennett, & C. B. Del Mar (Eds.), *Evidence-based practice across the health professions* (1st ed.) (pp. 240–261). Sydney, Australia: Elsevier.

Chisolm, T. H., & Portz, L. J. (2007). Making use of systematic reviews: EBP for the busy clinican. *Audiology Online*. Retrieved March 3, 2010, from http://www.audiologyonline.com/articles/pf_article_detail.asp?article_id=1783

Cook, D. J., Mulrow, C. D., & Haynes, R. B. (1997). Systematic reviews: Synthesis of best evidence for clinical decisions. *Annals of Internal Medicine, 126*, 376–380.

Cox, R. M. (2005). Evidence-based practice in provision of amplification. *Journal of the American Academy of Audiology, 16*(7), 419–438.

Davis, J. P. L., & Creombie, I. K. (2003). The why and how of crtical appraisal. In J. Clarkson, J. E. Harrison, A. I. Ismail, I. Needleman, & H. Worthington (Eds.), *Evidence-based dentistry for effective practice* (pp. 1–18). London, UK: Martin Dunitz.

Del Mar, C., & Hoffmann, T. (2010a). Information needs, asking quesitons and some basics of research studies. In T. Hoffmann, S. Bennett, & C. Del Mar (Eds.), *Evidence-based practice across the health professionals* (pp. 16–37). Chatswood, NSW, Australia: Elsevier.

Dollaghan, C. A. (2007). *The handbook for evidence-based pratice in communication disorders.* Baltimore, MD: Paul H. Brookes.

Gnewikow, D., Ricketts, T., Bratt, G. W., & Mutchler, L. C. (2009). Real-world benefit from directional microphone hearing aids. *Journal of Rehabilitation Research and Development, 46*(5), 603–618.

Guyatt, G. H., Haynes, R. B., Jaeschke, R. Z., Cook, D. J., Green, L., Naylor, C. D., . . . Scott, R. W. (2000). Users' guides to the medical literature: XXV. Evidence-based medicine: Principles for applying the users' guides to patient care. *Journal of the American Medical Association, 284*(10), 1290–1296. doi: 10.1001/jama.284.10.1290

Harrison, J. E., & Bickley, S. R. (2003). Different types of evidence: where and how to find them. In J. Clarkson, J. E. Harrison, A. I. Ismail, I. Needleman, & H. Worthington (Eds.), *Evidence based dentistry for effective practice* (pp. 19–42). London, UK: Martin Dunitz.

Haynes, R. B., Devereaux, P. J., & Guyatt, G. H. (2002). Physicians' and patients' choices in evidence based practice. *British Medical Journal, 324*(7350), 1350.

Harbour, R., & Miller, J. (2001). A new system for grading recommendations in evidence based guidelines. *British Medical Journal, 323*(7308), 334–336.

Hoffmann, T., Bennett, S., & Del Mar, C. (2010). Introduction to evidence-based practice. In T. Hoffmann, S. Bennett, & C. Del Mar (Eds.), *Evidence-based practice across the health professions* (pp. 1–15). Chatswood, NSW, Australia: Elsevier.

Irwin, D., Pannbacker, M., & Lass, N. (2007). Evidence-based practice: Application of research to clinical practice. In *Clinical Research Methods in Speech-Language Pathology and Audiology* (pp. 231–252). San Diego, CA: Plural.

Jackson, R., Ameratunga, S., Broad, J., Connor, J., Lethaby, A., Robb, G., . . . Heneghan, C. (2006). The GATE frame: Critical appraisal with pictures. *Evidence-Based Medicine, 11*(2), 35–38.

Mullen, R. (2007, March 06). The state of the evidence: ASHA develops levels of evidence for communication sciences and disorders. *ASHA Leader*. Retrieved from http://www.asha.org/Publications/leader/2007/070306/f070306b.htm

Needleman, I. (2003). Introduction to evidence based dentistry. In J. Clarkson, J. E. Harrison, A. I. Ismail, I. Needleman, & H. Worthington (Eds.), *Evidence based dentistry for effective practice* (pp. 1–18). London, UK: Martin Dunitz.

Rosenthal, R. N. (2004). Overview of evidence-based practice. In A. R. Roberts & K. R. Yeager (Eds.), *Evidence-based practice manual: Research and outcome measures in health and human services* (pp. 20–29). Oxford, UK: Oxford University Press.

Sackett, D. L., Rosenberg, W. M., Gray, J. A., Haynes, R. B., & Richardson, W. S. (1996). Evidence based medicine: What it is and what it isn't. *Britich Medical Journal, 312*(7023), 71–72.

Stephens, D., Jones, G., & Gianopoulos, I. (2000). The use of outcome measures to formulate intervention strategies. *Ear and Hearing, 21*(4), 15S–23S.

Straus, S. E., Richardson, W. S., Glasziou, P., & Haynes, R. B. (2005). *Evidence-based Medicine: How to practice and teach EBM* (3rd ed.). New York, NY: Elsevier/Churchill Livingstone.

United States Precventive Services Task Force. (1996). The guide to clinical preventive services: Report of the United States Preventive Services Task Force (2nd ed.). Philadelphia, PA: Williams & Wilkins.

Valente, M., Abrams, H. B., Benson, D., Chisolm, T. H., Citron, D., Hampton, D., . . . Sweetow, R. (2006). Guidelines for the audiologic management of adult hearing impairment. *Audiology Today, 18*(5), 32–36.

World Health Organization. (2007). *International Classification of Functioning, Disability and Health (ICF).* Geneva, Switzerland: Author.

Wilczynski, N., & McKibbon, A. (2010). Finding the evidence. In T. Hoffmann, S. Bennett, & C. Del Mar (Eds.), *Evidence-based practice across the health professions* (pp. 38–58). Chatswood, NSW, Australia: Elsevier.

CHAPTER 2

Evaluating the Evidence on Audiological Interventions

Michael Valente, Maureen Valente, and Laura Czarniak

INTRODUCTION

Chapter 1 described the five steps involved in Evidence-Based Practice (EBP). This chapter expands on the second step involving the search for the evidence to answer the clinical question and the third step involving the critical appraisal of the final full-text articles that were retrieved from the search for the evidence. This chapter is intended to help clinicians who want to improve the quality of life of their clients by determining the "best" audiological rehabilitative health care. For example, a clinician may want answers to the following rehabilitative questions:

1. Does a bilateral hearing aid fitting provide better performance than a unilateral fitting?
2. Are feedback management features effective in reducing feedback and providing greater headroom (i.e., additional gain/output)?
3. What is the best fitting option for clients with unilateral hearing loss?
4. Are middle ear implants a viable alternative for clients with moderate-severe to severe sensorineural hearing loss?
5. Is frequency transposition an effective feature for clients with "dead" hair cell regions?
6. Does measuring loudness discomfort levels provide a better fit?
7. What is the difference in the frequency response of a microphone and telecoil? Should the frequency response of the microphone and telecoil be matched for optimum performance when using the telecoil?
8. Does real-ear measurement improve the outcome of a hearing aid fitting?
9. Are adaptive directional microphones more effective than fixed directional microphones?

All too often, when answering these and thousands of other clinical questions, clinicians:

a. Ask what their colleagues may think.
b. Ask what their supervisor may think.
c. Continue to do what has been done within their clinic and never make changes based upon current best evidence.
d. Utilize manufacturer-sponsored continuing education events as a method to gather the "latest information."

What follows is an attempt to convince the clinician that a better way to answer these and other clinical questions is to perform a "systematized" review of the literature followed by a critical appraisal of the final pertinent retrieved references resulting from the systematized review. In this chapter, the authors elected to use the term systematized instead of the more commonly used systematic. The use of systematized is based on the recommendations by Grant and Booth (2009) who define 14 different types of reviews. A systematic review is a method that systematically searches for, appraises, and synthesizes the evidence and is most typically used for the purposes of creating a guideline. Grant and Booth's definition goes further to describe a systematic review as aiming for an exhaustive, comprehensive search with minimal narrative. On the other hand, they define systematized to include elements of a systematic review while stopping short of the comprehensive nature of a systematic review, and typically is conducted as part of a postgraduate student assignment. Thus, the authors believe that the term systematized is more appropriate for the purpose of this textbook and for answering the PICO type clinical questions introduced in Chapter 1. It is hoped to convince the clinician that the best way to answer PICO questions is to search the literature followed by the use of EBP methods to answer these questions. The authors believe this approach is more scientific, scholarly, and professional than answering questions based on hunches, opinions, or simply doing the "same thing."

The primary goal of this chapter is to illustrate to clinicians how to critically appraise each final full-text article retrieved from the systematized search of the literature described in Chapter 1. The critical appraisal of each full-text article is completed by the clinician by asking and answering the appropriate questions reported in the Appendix. To help accomplish this goal, the authors use the example of the following clinical question: "How much additional gain can I obtain from feedback management strategies and which strategy/manufacturer provides the greatest added stable gain?"

STEP 1 OF THE EBP PROCESS: DEFINING A CLINICAL QUESTION

As described in Chapter 1, a quality search of the literature requires an extensive survey of the literature (published and unpublished) on a specific clinical question. After completing a quality search of the literature and critically appraising what has been found, the clinician gains a thorough knowledge base of the topic. In addition, the clinician acquires original concepts to supplement or expand on what has been published on the topic.

Searching the literature for references to answer clinical questions may be made easier for the clinician by using a Patient-Intervention-Comparison-Outcome (PICO) analysis (Heneghan & Badenoch, 2002), reported in Table 1–1. Using the PICO format helps structure clinical-based questions into a framework for formulating search queries to retrieve optimal search results to answer the question (Oxman, Sackett, & Guyatt, 1993). Using the PICO format stems from the concept of EBP which is defined as, "the conscientious, explicit, and judicious use of current best evidence in making decisions about the care of individual clients" (Sackett, Rosenberg, Gray, Haynes, & Richardson, 1996; p. 71).

One example of how PICO is used is reported in Chapter 1. In this chapter, another example is included to further illustrate the process. Most PICOs begin when a clinician experiences a problem or question during his/her clinical experiences. For example, consider the following scenario:

I heard a colleague discuss a recent hearing aid fitting using a relatively new hearing aid. The product was a receiver in-the-canal (RIC) open-fit hearing aid manufactured by a company not typically used by the clinic. This hearing aid was initially selected because the hearing aid reportedly had excellent moisture resistant properties. Without knowing the hearing aid, the clinician familiarized herself with the fitting software and the features of the hearing aid. After the fitting was complete, the client expressed positive reactions about the clarity and "crispness" of the hearing aid and was extremely satisfied. Several days later, however, the client returned. When asked the purpose of the appointment, the client replied, "I enjoy the hearing aids, but I am getting this horrible squealing. Not only is the squealing bothersome to me, but it annoys my husband as well." On observation, each time the client put her hands by her head, the hearing aids would screech continuously. The clinician assured the client that she could easily address this problem and proceeded to connect the hearing aids to the computer. With a click of the mouse, the "feedback management test" within the software was completed. The client left convinced the problem was resolved.

The following week, the client returned still reporting problems with feedback. She reported that when she stood near a wall or solid surface, the hearing aids would once again produce feedback. She demonstrated this in the sound booth by standing near the wall. Feedback began and the clinician was perplexed. The clinician tried several strategies to troubleshoot the problem. First, she tried changing the size of the open-fit domes at the end of the receiver. This failed and then she tried using closed domes. Once again, the feedback reappeared. The length of the receiver was changed and the physical fit of the receiver in the ear canal was adjusted, but the feedback persisted. After contacting the manufacturer and trying several other options, the client decided to return the hearing aids and try a different manufacturer of RIC hearing aids because the feedback from the initial pair of hearing aids was so bothersome.

As exhibited in this brief case report, when a hearing aid user hears feedback, the effects can diminish the benefits provided via amplification. Not only is the sound of feedback bothersome to the listener, it can also degrade important signals being introduced to the hearing aid including speech. Feedback occurs when sound amplified by the hearing aid receiver leaks back to the microphone and is re-processed by the hearing aid. Audible feedback occurs when the leaked signal has a period equal to, or an integer multiple of, the path distance between the microphone and receiver (Ricketts, Johnson, & Federman, 2008). Current digital hearing aids contain complex algorithms to eliminate unwanted feedback. Although the goals of feedback management are the same across manufacturers, the mechanisms and algorithms of reducing the feedback remain diverse.

This clinical interaction caused the clinician to ask: "Was there a physical characteristic of the client's ear canal that caused such disruptive feedback or was the feedback reduction method used by this hearing aid inferior to other manufacturers?" The use of different feedback reduction methods by different manufacturers will produce variations in the amount of feedback cancellation. The most common question regarding feedback is how much additional gain in the frequency response can be achieved when a feedback suppression technique is enabled compared to when the suppression technique is disabled. This measurement is termed added stable gain (ASG) or additional gain before feedback (AGBF). Measurements of ASG and AGBF are most commonly used to describe the effectiveness of a feedback suppression method. A wealth of literature describing the intricacies of various feedback cancellation algorithms is present. Studies investigating feedback cancellation strategies use many methods to illustrate the efficacy of the algorithms, including using human subjects, artificial manikins, and computer simulations. The following example provides the results of a systematized review investigating various feedback suppression methods and the measures used to assess the efficacy of an algorithm. A broad range of findings are reported and critiqued, and concluding remarks are provided.

When viewing a client and trying to provide the best possible care, the clinician may want to know all the hearing aids available for his/her client and which hearing aid(s) provide the greatest amount of added stable gain (ASG). That is, how much more gain can be achieved with the hearing aid with and without the feedback management feature turned off and on? To place this question into the PICO format the clinician might consider:

Patient: any client who is a candidate for hearing aids (amplification)

Intervention: feedback management (feedback; suppression; cancellation; algorithm)

Comparison: feedback management is not available or turned off

Outcome: added stable gain (ASG); added stable gain before feedback (AGBF); maximum stable gain (MSG); speech recognition; sound quality judgment.

STEP 2 OF THE EBP PROCESS: SEARCHING FOR THE EVIDENCE USING A SYSTEMATIZED REVIEW

The authors do not discuss in great detail how to complete a systematized review because this was covered extremely well in Chapter 1. A few important points, however, are made to either reinforce the information provided in Chapter 1 or add a few additional thoughts. As a reminder, the question is, "How much greater gain/output can be achieved in a hearing aid with and without the feedback management feature turned off and on?" As illustrated above, the first stage is to organize the clinical question into the PICO format to separate each component of the clinical question into each of the PICO elements. The second stage is to identify all known "keywords" and "search strings" including synonyms, relating to each PICO concept. The third stage is a priori to create "limits" of the search before executing a literature search. Establishment of limits reduces the magnitude of the search and reduces any bias and subjective selection of works retrieved during the search. For the example about the PICO on feedback management in this chapter, the following limits were applied:

- *Language:* English-only references.
- *Date of publication:* 1990 to present. Clinicians, in their database search, can set any preferred limits on the range of the date of publication. The limits for the date of publication are arbitrary, but typically begin from when the question was thought to originate to the present. During the search, the clinician can change the date of publication based on the findings from the previous search.
- *Publication type:* peer-reviewed journal references. Often, there is an assumption that information obtained from peer-reviewed journals is of sufficient quality to exclude non-peer-reviewed journals from the search. It is the opinion of the authors, however, that valuable clinical information can often be obtained from non-peer-reviewed journals. Limiting the search to peer-reviewed journals may be excessively limiting, especially for new and emerging

technologies as discussed in Chapter 6. Clearly, when critically appraising non-peer-reviewed journals, the level of scrutiny on the part of the clinician needs to be raised significantly.

- *Level of evidence:* The clinician should determine the level of evidence each article provides and grade the evidence for the PICO question, using the information in Tables 1–5 and 1–7 provided in Chapter 1. When completing the systematized review, search engines do not allow clinicians to limit the search based on the targeted desired level and grade of evidence (1–3; A–B in this example). This "filtering" of the retrieved articles for acceptance or rejection for further review is exclusively the responsibility of the clinician after reading the Structured Abstract and/or the Methods section of the retrieved articles. It is in the Structured Abstract and/or Methods section that investigators describe the experimental design of the investigation. After reading these sections, the clinician will decide if the description of the investigation achieves the target level of evidence (see Table 1–5 and Figure 1–2 for detailed descriptions of the numerous types of studies). If the criteria are not achieved then the retrieved reference is excluded. If the criteria are achieved then the retrieved reference is included and a critical appraisal of the full-text article is completed followed by assignment of the overall grade of evidence for the articles.

The fourth stage is to create "search queries" using the keywords and search strings identified earlier in the PICO. The fifth stage is to select the appropriate database(s) to locate the best evidence to answer the clinical question (see Tables 1–2, 1–3, and 1–4). There is no correct or incorrect method to begin the process of formulating search queries. Many databases allow for flexibility of combining multiple single keyword queries into a single search string. The idea is to experiment and "get your feet wet" with various queries on different databases, using keywords from controlled vocabularies and natural language. Review the list of keywords identified for each PICO element and think about ways to combine some keywords into a search query ("search strings"). Experiment with a search using keywords from each PICO concept or limit your search to one keyword from a PICO element. Another strategy is to search for controlled vocabulary keywords based on keywords identified. Typically, it is recommended that the clinician use more than one database to search the literature for the relevant articles. For our example of searching the literature for the PICO question on feedback management, the authors used Scopus (http://www.scopus.com/), Inspec (http://www.theiet.org/publishing/inspec/), and Google Scholar (http://scholar.google.com/). Other popular search engines that could be used include Agency for Healthcare Research and Quality (AHRQ) http://www.ahrq.gov/, Cumulative Index to Nursing and Allied Health Literature (CINAHL) http://www.ebscohost.com/cinahl/, or PubMed/MEDLINE http://www.ncbi.nlm.nih.gov/.

Using the PICO question about feedback management as an example, for each of the three database queries (Table 2–1), the authors documented:

1. The number of queries for each database (five in this example, but can be more or less than this, based on the discretion of the clinician).
2. The keywords or search string(s) used in each query for each of the three databases. Again, the number of keywords and combinations of keywords to create search strings can be more or less than illustrated in Table 2–1 depending on the discretion of the clinician.

Table 2–1. Summary of Database Review for Scopus, Inspec, and Google Scholar

Inclusion Criteria	*Exclusion Criteria*
English language 1990 to Present	Conference proceedings
Peer-reviewed	Non-peer-reviewed or conference paper
Evidence level 1–3	Evidence level lower than 3

SCOPUS

Query	*Search string*	*Hits*	*Results excluded by title*	*Results excluded by abstract*	*Results excluded by full text*	*Results excluded by duplicates*	*Accepted for review*
#1	Topic = (feedback) AND Topic = (hearing aid)	78	58	3	2	N/A	15
#2	Topic = (feedback cancellation) AND Topic = (hearing aid)	36	18	—	—	16	2
#3	Topic = (feedback algorithm) AND Topic = (hearing aid)	37	17	—	—	16	1
#4	Topic = (feedback suppression) AND Topic = (hearing aid)	14	6	—	—	—	1
#5	Topic = (stable gain) AND Topic = (hearing aid)	13	8	—	—	5	0

INSPEC

Query	*Search string*	*Hits*	*Results excluded by title*	*Results excluded by abstract*	*Results excluded by full text*	*Results excluded by duplicates*	*Accepted for review*
#1	Topic = (feedback) AND Topic = (hearing aid)	65	45	3	1	12	4
#2	Topic = (feedback cancellation) AND Topic = (hearing aid)	11	6	—	1	4	0
#3	Topic = (feedback algorithm) AND Topic = (hearing aid)	11	—	—	—	11	0
#4	Topic = (feedback suppression) AND Topic = (hearing aid)	25	15	—	—	10	0
#5	Topic = (stable gain) AND Topic = (hearing aid)	20	14	—	—	6	0

GOOGLE SCHOLAR

Query	*Search string*	*Hits*	*Results excluded by title*	*Results excluded by abstract*	*Results excluded by full text*	*Results excluded by duplicates*	*Accepted for review*
#1	Topic = (feedback) AND Topic = (hearing aid)	19	16	—	—	3	0
#2	Topic = (acoustic feedback) AND Topic = (hearing aid)	28	8	—	—	18	2
#3	Topic = (feedback algorithm) AND Topic = (hearing aid)	9	5	—	—	4	0
#4	Topic = (feedback suppression) AND Topic = (hearing aid)	5	2	—	—	3	0
#5	Topic = (stable gain) AND Topic = (hearing aid)	0	—	—	—	—	0

Note: All search strings were automatically limited to journal articles. Conference papers and medically based articles were excluded.

3. The total number of references found (Hits) for keyword and/or search string used in the database (0 to 78).
4. The number of references eliminated from the initial total list of references based exclusively on the title (0 to 58). That is, a large number of initial hits were excluded for critical appraisal because it was clear from the title that the content of the reference was not adequately related to the clinical question.
5. The number of references eliminated from the remaining list of references based exclusively on the abstract (0 to 3). That is, some of the remaining initial hits were excluded for critical appraisal because it was clear from the abstract that the content of the reference was not adequately related to the clinical question.
6. The number of references excluded from the initial total list of references based exclusively on the fact that the reference was a duplicate (0 to 18). That is, several initial hits were excluded for critical appraisal because it was clear from the title that it was a duplicate of a previously cited reference.
7. The number of references eliminated from the remaining list of references after reading the remaining full-text article (0 to 2). That is, some of the initial hits were excluded for critical appraisal because it was clear after reading the full-text article that the content of the reference was not adequately related to the clinical question.
8. Finally, there were 25 remaining references accepted for critical appraisal after going through the four stages of elimination described above. The final references meeting the requirements of the limits were used as evidence to answer the clinical question and a critical appraisal of these final references was performed.

It is not uncommon to have very few references remaining after this process of eliminating references that are not relevant to the PICO question. Although the above search resulted in 25 references, Chisolm et al. (2007) initially found 171 references about the quality of life outcomes for adults fitted with hearing aids, but this number was reduced to 16 after completing a similar process. It was these 16 full-text references that Chisolm et al. (2007) critically appraised to find the best evidence using many of the same questions raised in the Appendix. The next challenging stage is to critically appraise the final remaining references after completing the process of elimination outlined above and the procedures are described in the next section of this chapter.

Searching the literature is a skill that is best learned through trial and error. The clinician must:

1. Practice with various databases to learn more about the nuances of each database.
2. Experiment with different keywords to discover how various databases interpret the query.
3. Review the keywords as noted for each work.
4. Note that author keywords, controlled vocabularies and natural language keywords are helpful to understand how databases map keywords to selected works.

The clinician should not become discouraged if results are not relevant to the query. Points to consider are:

- Can the query be paraphrased or reworded?
- Can the number of keywords be reduced?
- Are the Boolean operators (e.g., "AND"/ "OR"/"NOT") being used correctly?
- Was correct spelling used for all the queries? One misspelling can produce negative results.

- Were keywords from a controlled vocabulary used (i.e., Medical Subject Headings or MeSH)? Databases (e.g., PubMed/MEDLINE at http://www.ncbi.nlm.nih.gov) that index using controlled vocabulary keywords usually offer a tool to search the keywords in the controlled vocabulary.
- Are there any other keywords based on natural language to consider for the query?
- Was more than one database used? One database will not contain all references to the literature.
- Were the features and functions of each database utilized for the search?

Putting It All Together in One Web Site

Recently, Cathy Sarli, MLS, AHIP, Scholarly Communications Specialist at Washington University School of Medicine in St. Louis, created a new homepage within the Becker Library at Washington University School of Medicine in St. Louis (http://beckerguides.wustl.edu/audiology) to include:

a. All the major databases for Audiology and Deaf Education
b. Journals and books for Audiology and Deaf Education
c. Other resources (professional organizations) for Audiology and Deaf Education
d. News feeds into one centralized Web site.

The authors urge the interested reader to use this Web site. Furthermore, the authors believe this Web site is a generous gift to the scientific and educational community. The Scope of Audiology Practice has expanded rapidly. It is time for all practitioners to critically read the literature in a scholarly and "lifelong learning" manner. Furthermore, it is critical for the clinician to develop critical analysis skills for optimum application of current research to daily practice.

STEP 3 OF THE EBP PROCESS: CRITICALLY APPRAISE THE REMAINING FULL-TEXT ARTICLES

The most difficult part of finding the best evidence is for the clinician to critically appraise the final full-text articles found during the search of the literature. This requires the clinician not to simply read the articles, but to critically analyze the articles to evaluate the strength and weaknesses of the evidence contained within each article. This is not an easy task for the unseasoned and untrained clinician. By untrained, the authors believe that most clinicians are not sufficiently trained in research methodology, experimental design, and statistical analysis to adequately complete the process of critically appraising the literature. However, textbooks such as this and the increasing number of programs at the Masters and Doctoral level that include experimental design and statistical analysis in the core curriculum may change this over time. The process of completing a systematized search and the follow-up critical appraisal can be time consuming and requires patience and experience. In order to successfully complete the critical appraisal of the full-text articles, the clinician must take on a skeptical persona by asking and answering some very important, but critical, questions while carefully reading each reference.

Critical questions a clinician must ask when reading each final reference retrieved from the systematized review should include many of the 26 questions raised in the Appendix. In addition to the questions raised in the

Appendix, the authors would add the following important questions:

When reading the Methods section:

1. Did the author(s) complete a power analysis to ensure an appropriate sample size was implemented for the study? Documenting that a power analysis was performed is becoming increasingly more common in professional journals and is becoming a requirement for many Institutional Review Boards (IRB) or Human Ethics Review Committees.
2. Did the author(s) report counterbalancing and/or randomization as part of the experimental protocol? Was experimental bias on the part of the researcher or client identified and controlled? Was single or double blinding used? Was the research funded by a commercial entity and would there be concomitant bias or conflict of interest concerns?
3. Was the research protocol submitted to the Institutional Review Board (IRB) or Human Ethics Review Committees at the author(s) affiliation?
4. Were subjects provided an Informed Consent and was there documentation that the Informed Consent was signed prior to entering the study?
5. Did the author(s) report using a control or experimental group?
6. Did the author(s) provide adequate specification of subject recruitment as well as inclusion and exclusion criteria?
7. Were the subjects homogenous or heterogeneous? If heterogeneous, to what degree and how might this have affected outcomes?
8. If the content of the manuscript was related to fitting of hearing aids, did the author(s) document verification and validation procedures?
9. Was this section clearly written such that the reader could replicate the study?
10. Did the author(s) state how and when equipment calibration took place?

When reading the Results section:

1. Did the author(s) report the subject age (mean and standard deviation) and gender (number of male and female)? If appropriate, did the authors designate experienced or inexperienced users of amplification as well as years of experience?
2. Did the author(s) report "dropouts" and explain why subjects dropped out from the study? The clinician may consider how such attrition may affect the results of the study.
3. Did the author(s) use appropriate statistical analysis and explain this process well?
4. Were the conclusions from the statistical analysis appropriate?
5. Did the figures and/or tables correctly report the results of the study and were they clear? Were the abscissa and ordinate appropriately labeled and was the range along the ordinate consistent across figures reporting on the same dependent variable? When the figure or table reported mean data was the standard deviation also reported? Did the figures and/or tables coincide with the findings reported in the body of the text?
6. Did the author(s) calculate and report effect size (Cohen's *d*)?
7. Did the author(s) report the 95% confidence interval of the difference between the means?
8. Did the author(s) demonstrate that procedures were held constant during the course of the study and that adequate procedures were in place to ensure that the equipment maintained its calibration?

9. Were confounding variables identified and controlled?
10. Were the outcome measures valid and reliable? Were there any data provided on test-retest measures?

When reading the Discussion section:

1. Did the author(s) report any weaknesses in their study?
2. Did the author(s) discuss how the results compared with what was reported in the past? If the results did not agree with what was reported in the past was a suitable explanation provided?
3. Did the author(s) point out how the results from the current study could be used to raise questions for future research?
4. Did the author(s) answer the experimental questions that were raised in the Introduction?

At this point, it may be helpful to point out that the process described above for critically appraising an article is precisely the same level of critical thinking a journal editor will seek when he/she contacts an "expert" to review a manuscript submitted for consideration for publication. This is the peer-review process. During this process, the editor seeks three experts who are willing to independently review the manuscript using specific instructions from the editor. In the end, the editor will ask each reviewer to recommend acceptance, acceptance with minor revisions, acceptance with major revisions, major revisions followed by a re-review, or rejection. When the reviewer makes his/her recommendation, the reviewer submits a detailed report of the scientific quality of the submitted manuscript with very detailed comments why the submitted manuscript should be accepted or rejected. During the review process, the reviewer will ask many of the questions raised above as "proof" as to what the reviewer considers is the scientific quality of the submitted manuscript. The reader should keep in mind that the vast majority of manuscripts submitted for consideration for publication are rejected because the content of the submission does not meet the standards of excellence of the journal.

Example of a Critical Appraisal

Table 2–2 summarizes the experimental design, number of subjects (many of the articles utilized computer simulation or KEMAR), outcome measures, and whether or not power analysis was performed for the 25 articles that were selected for critical appraisal based on their relevance to the PICO question. These variables are important for determination of internal validity, as stated in Chapter 1. From the critical appraisal, the following observations were drawn about the nature of the evidence on this topic:

1. Studies examining feedback management use various sound stimuli which makes comparison of results across the studies difficult. Clinicians should consider how types of sound stimuli may affect the outcomes of the studies.
2. Several studies used complex computer simulations to describe the feedback path and proposed algorithms to eliminate feedback. Studies falling into this category can be extremely difficult for most clinicians to understand due to complex mathematical algorithms that weredescribed. It would be helpful if reviewers and editors would keep this in mind when the submitted manuscript is intended for clinicians or other readers who may have limited background in engineering.
3. Studies involving feedback management are generally descriptive in nature. The

Table 2–2. Summary of Articles on Feedback Management for Full Review

Study	*Design*	*Human Subjects*	*KEMAR*	*Computer Simulation*	*Outcome Measures*	*Power Analysis*
Boukis et al. (2006)	Descriptive	*N* = 17	N	N	Sound quality	N
Dyrlund et al. (1994)	Descriptive	*N* = 29	N	N	FB margin	N
Engebretson et al. (1993)	Descriptive	—	Y	Y	ASG	N
Freed (2006)	Descriptive	—	N	Y	ASG; error level	N
Freed & Soli (2006)	Descriptive	—	Y	Y	ASG	N
French-St. George et al. (1993)	Descriptive	*N* = 9	N	N	Word Recognition; ASG	N
Greenberg et al. (2000)	Descriptive	*N* = 7	N	N	MSG; sound quality	N
Grimm et al. (2009)	Descriptive	*N* = 10	N	N	MSG; ASG	N
Johnson et al. (2007)	Descriptive	*N* = 16	N	N	Sound quality	N
Joson et al. (1993)	Descriptive	—	N	Y	Howling margin (ASG)	N
Kates (1991)	Descriptive	—	Y	Y	FB cancellation	N
Kates (1999)	Descriptive	—	Y	Y	FB path frequency response	N
Kates (2001)	Descriptive	—	Y	Y	MSG	N
Lee et al. (2007)	Descriptive	—	N	Y	Misalignment of FB pathway	N
Maxwell et al. (1995)	Descriptive	*N* = 2	N	N	ASG; sound quality	N
Merks et al. (2006)	Descriptive	—	Y	Y	ASG; entrainment	N
Rafaely et al. (2000)	Descriptive	*N* = 4	N	N	FB variability	N

Table 2–2. *continued*

Study	*Design*	*Human Subjects*	*KEMAR*	*Computer Simulation*	*Outcome Measures*	*Power Analysis*
Ricketts et al. (2008)	Descriptive	*N* = 16	N	N	AGBF	N
Rombouts et al. (2006)	Descriptive	—	N	Y	Error norm	N
Shusina et al. (2006)	Descriptive	—	N	Y	FB path estimation	N
Siqueira et al. (1996)	Descriptive	*N* = 6	Y	N	Sound quality	N
Siqueira et al. (2000)	Descriptive	—	N	Y	FB path bias	N
Spriet et al. (2005)	Descriptive	—	N	Y	Misalignment of FB pathway	N
Spriet et al. (2007)	Descriptive	—	N	Y	MSG	N
Vicen-Bueno et al. (2009)	Descriptive	*N* = 10	N	N	Limit gain; ASG	N

Note: FB = feedback, ASG = added stable gain, MSG = maximum stable gain, AGBF = added gain before feedback, Entrainment = difference between the short-term spectra with the FB cancellation enabled and disabled, converted to a perceptual correlate.

primary outcome of the studies typically described the magnitude of ASG achieved when an antifeedback algorithm was enabled or reported the results of a computer simulation of a feedback algorithm. It takes extra effort to create an analytical investigation that randomly assigns an intervention or examines differences between case subjects and controls.

4. Sample sizes were generally small. When human subjects were used, sample sizes ranged from three to 16 participants. Large-scale studies could take more time and effort to complete and therefore may not address new technologies that are already on the market. None of the studies completed a power analysis based on a priori assumption of effect size.
5. For many studies, statistical analyses of mean data were not completed. Many authors made general comments about the findings of their studies, yet statistical significance was not calculated. It is difficult for a clinician to draw conclusions from the authors' findings when no mention is made as to whether or not the results reached statistical significance. Furthermore, it is difficult for a clinician to determine whether the studied algorithms provide clinical benefit to hearing aid users. In other words, although some conclusions were made by the

authors about *efficacy*, none addressed the *effectiveness* of these technologies. Therefore, clinicians should collect their own real world client data and make decisions about whether or not to adopt the technology.

6. As reported earlier, much of the literature regarding feedback management involved studies that were computationally difficult and required a background in engineering. The authors drew conclusions about the efficacy of various feedback cancellation techniques, but these results are very difficult to interpret from a clinician standpoint. In fact, very few studies used "stand-alone" hearing aid circuitry to assess the benefits of the feedback reduction algorithms. Computer-driven simulations were often used as were manikin simulations. This resulted in two potential biases. First, the physical characteristics of the median ear canal of a manikin may be different from the individual ear canal in a human subject. Although this point seems obvious, measurements that are highly dependent on ear canal characteristics can be greatly affected by the properties of the ear being tested. The second bias lies in simulations that are entirely computer driven. Computer driven simulations allow for complex computations to occur within the algorithm with little effect on power consumption. A feedback reduction algorithm may appear successful when simulated, but recreating the same technology within the microprocessor of a hearing aid may produce different results.
7. Comparisons of feedback reduction techniques across manufacturers were rare. Three articles described ASG that can be expected with feedback reduction; however, the manufacturers were not specified. One article was funded by a hearing aid manufacturer and the authors reported that the feedback management of "their company" outperformed the other feedback management algorithms used in the study. It is important to consider possible biases when interpreting the results of experiments of this nature.

The following are key findings related to ASG that may be expected from feedback management methods from the evidence to date:

- Ricketts et al. (2008) reported statistically significant differences between the feedback management algorithms in commercial products. The ASG before feedback ranged from 0 to 15 dB. A large degree of variability was reported.
- Freed and Soli (2006) reported a wide range of performance, with ASG ranging from 0 to 18 dB across the nine feedback algorithms tested.
- Merks, Banerjee, and Trine (2006) reported that the Starkey Destiny 1200 outperformed five other commercial behind-the-ear hearing aids, although there is potential for author bias here as previously discussed.
- Engebretson and French-St. George (1993) reported the adaptive equalization algorithm provided 20 dB of ASG.
- Freed (2006) reported clipping in the cancellation path provided increased ASG.
- Greenberg, Zurek, and Brantley (2000) reported that a continuous noise reduction algorithm performed best by providing 8.5 dB of ASG.

Conclusions related to the "best" feedback management algorithm remain ambiguous. As previously discussed, many of the articles pertaining to feedback algorithm testing were computationally difficult to comprehend. It is clear there are many feedback processing strategies that hold promise.

However, the findings of the reviewed studies would be more clinically applicable if the feedback management strategies were tested under more realistic settings, that is, if studies of effectiveness were carried out. The following is a summary of key findings on the efficacy of feedback management algorithms:

1. Feedback cancellation appears to be the most prominent algorithm used by commercial hearing aid manufacturers.
2. Feedback cancellation requires proper estimation of the feedback pathway because improper estimation leads to bias in the pathway.
3. If bias is present in the feedback pathway, the feedback canceller may degrade the desired signal by inadvertently canceling the signal.
4. Feedback algorithms that continuously adapt to the acoustic scene provide better feedback reduction than stationary algorithms.

It is important for the clinician to familiarize himself/herself with the feedback management strategies used by each manufacturer and remain current about novel feedback management techniques. Unfortunately, the literature in this area does not provide the manufacturer names of the various hearing aids for which feedback algorithms were tested. Thus, the clinician must rely on experience and familiarization with the manufacturers' feedback reduction strategies to provide the best fit possible for hearing aid users.

SUMMARY

We hope that a clinician reading this chapter will obtain a greater appreciation of the process required to provide the highest level of care to clients. First, clinicians should be able to develop greater skills in creating PICO questions based on daily interactions with clients. Second, clinicians should be able to develop the skills required to convert these questions into "keywords" and "search strings" to search databases to find the best evidence to answer the questions. Third, clinicians should develop greater comfort in critically appraising the evidence and judge if the results from the evidence answer the PICO questions. Fourth, clinicians should have greater comfort in their ability to apply the evidence to a particular client so that the care of the client will have the best possible outcome. Finally, hopefully clinicians will remember that the EBP is a lifelong endeavor that will get easier as experience in using the process improves over time.

REFERENCES

Boukis, C., Mandic, D. P., & Constantinides, A. G. (2006). Toward bias minimization in acoustic feedback cancellation systems. *Journal of the Acoustical Society of America. 121*(3), 1529–1537.

Chisolm, T., Johnson, C., Danhauer, J., Portz, L., Abrams, H., Lesner, S., . . . Newman, C. (2007). A systematic review of health-related quality of life and hearing aids: final report of the American Academy of Audiology task force on the health-related quality of life benefits of amplification in adults. *Journal of the American Academy of Audiology, 18*, 151–183.

Dyrlund, O., Henningsen, L. B., Bisgaard, N., & Jensen, J. H. (1994). Digital feedback management (DFS). Characterization of feedback margin improvements in a DFS hearing instrument. *Scandinavian Audioliology, 23*, 135–138.

Engebretson, A. M., & French-St. George, M. (1993). Properties of an adaptive feedback equalization algorithm. *Journal of Rehabilitation and Research Development, 30*(1), 8–16.

Freed, D. J. (2006). Adaptive feedback cancellation in hearing aids with clipping in the feedback path. *Journal of the Acoustical Society of America, 123*(3), 1618–1626.

Freed, D. J., & Soli, S. D. (2006). An objective procedure for evaluation of adaptive antifeedback algorithms in hearing aids. *Ear and Hearing, 27*, 383–398.

French-St. George, M., Wood, D. J., & Engebretson, A. M. (1993). Behavioral assessment of adaptive feedback equalization in a digital hearing aid. *Journal of Rehabilitation and Research Development, 20*(1), 17–25.

Grant, M., & Booth, A. (2009). A typology of reviews: An analysis of 14 review types and associated methodologies. *Health Information and Libraries Journal, 26*, 91–108.

Greenberg, J. E., Zurek, P. M., & Brantley, M. (2000). Evaluation of feedback-reduction algorithms for hearing aids. *Journal of the Acoustical Society of America, 108*(5), 2366–2376.

Grimm, G., Hohmann, V., & Kollmeier, B. (2009). Increase and subjective evaluation of feedback stability in hearing aids by a binaural coherence-based noise reduction scheme. *IEEE Translation of Audiology Speech Language Proceedings, 17*(7), 1408–1419.

Heneghan, C., & Badenoch, D. (2002). *Evidence-based medicine toolkit.* London, UK: BMJ Publishing Group.

Johnson, E. E., Ricketts, T. A., & Hornsby, B.W.Y. (2007). The effect of digital phase cancellation feedback reduction systems on amplified sound quality. *Journal of the American Academy of Audiology, 18*, 404–416.

Joson, H., Asano, F., Suzuki, Y., & Stone, T. (1993). Adaptive feedback cancellation with frequency compression for hearing aids. *Journal of the Acoustical Society of America, 94*(5), 3248–3254.

Kates, J. M. (1991). Feedback cancellation in hearing aids: Results from a computer simulation. *IEE Translation of Signal Processing, 39*(3), 553–562.

Kates, J. M. (1999). Constrained adaptation for feedback cancellation in hearing aids. *Journal of the Acoustical Society of America, 106*(2), 1010–1019.

Kates, J. M. (2001). Room reverberation effects in hearing aid feedback cancellation. *Journal of the Acoustical Society of America, 109*(1), 367–378.

Lee, S., Kim, I. Y., & Park, Y.C. (2007). Approximated affine projection algorithm for feedback cancellation in hearing aids. *Computer Methods and Programs in Biomedicine, 87*, 254–261.

Maxwell, J. A., & Zurek, P. M. (1995). Reducing acoustic feedback in hearing aids. *IEEE Translation of Speech Audiology Proceeding, 3*(4), 304–313.

Merks, I., Banerjee, S., & Trine, T. (2006). Assessing the effectiveness of feedback cancellers in hearing aids. *Hearing Review, 13*(4), 54–59.

Oxman, A., Sackett, D., & Guyatt, G. (1993) Users' guides to the medical literature. How to get started. The Evidence-Based Medicine Working Group. *Journal of the American Medical Association, 270*(17), 2093–2095.

Rafaely, B., Roccasalva-Firenze, M., & Payne, E. (2000). Feedback path variability modeling for robust hearing aids. *Journal of the Acoustical Society of America, 107*(5), 2665–2673.

Ricketts, T., Johnson, E., & Federman, J. (2008). Individual differences within and across feedback management hearing aids. *Journal of the American Academy of Audiology, 19*, 748–757.

Rombouts, G., van Waterschoot, T., Struyve, K., & Moonen, M. (2006). Acoustic feedback cancellation for long acoustic paths using a nonstationary source model. *IEEE Translation of Signal Processing, 54*(9), 3426–3434.

Sackett, D., Rosenberg, W., Gray, J., Haynes, R., & Richardson, W. (1996) Evidence based medicine: What it is and what it isn't. *British Medical Journal, 13*(1), 71–72.

Shusina, N. A., & Rafaely, B. (2006). Unbiased adaptive feedback cancellation in hearing aids by closed-loop identification. *IEEE Translation of Audiology and Speech Language Proceedings, 14*(2), 658–665.

Siqueira, M. G., & Alwan, A. (2000). Steady-state analysis of continuous adaptation in acoustic feedback reduction systems for hearing-aids. *IEEE Translation of Speech and Audiology Proceedings, 8*(4), 443–453.

Siqueira, M. G., Speece, R., Petsalis, E., & Alwan, A. (1996). Subband adaptive filtering applied to acoustic feedback reduction in hearing aids. *Proceedings of the Asilomar Conference on Signals, Systems, and Computers.*

Spriet, A., Proudler, I., Moonen., M., & Wouters, J. (2005). An instrumental variable method for adaptive feedback cancellation in hearing aids.

IEEE International Conference on Acoustics, Speech and Signal Processing, 3, 129–132.

Spriet, A., Rombouts, G., Moonen, M., & Wouters, J. (2007). Combined feedback and noise management in hearing aids. *IEEE Trans Audiology Speech Language Proceedings, 15(*6), 1777–1790.

Vicen-Bueno, R., Martinez-Leira, A., Gil-Pita, R., & Rosa-Zurera, M. (2009). Modified LMS-based feedback-reduction subsystems in digital hearing aids based on WOLA filter bank. *IEEE Translation of Instrument Measurements, 58*(9), 3177–3190.

CHAPTER 3

Matching Evidence with Client Preferences

Ariane Laplante-Lévesque, Louise Hickson, and Linda Worrall

INTRODUCTION

As described in Chapter 1, Evidence-Based Practice (EBP) is "the conscientious, explicit, and judicious use of current best evidence in making decisions about the care of individual patients" (Sackett, Rosenberg, Gray, Haynes, & Richardson, 1996, p. 71). Chapters 4 to 13 of this book focus on the first part of EBP's definition, which is the evidence. In contrast, this chapter aims to cover the second part of EBP's definition, which is how to come to the best intervention decisions for individual clients. Therefore, the specific objectives of this chapter are: (1) to highlight the importance of involving clients in EBP, (2) to describe three approaches and tools to help involving clients in EBP (joint goal setting, shared decision making, and decision aids); and (3) to provide practical tips regarding the use of these approaches and tools.

EBP is sometimes applied in clinical practice by only considering the research and not including the other important elements of client and clinician preferences as well as the clinical context (see Figure 1–1 in Chapter 1). This leads to EBP being wrongly applied as a "cookbook" or disease-oriented approach, where, solely based on the health condition and the evidence, one intervention is determined to be best for all clients. Sackett and colleagues warn against this kind of health standardization and stress that EBP should combine evidence with clinical expertise and the client's "clinical state, predicament and preferences" (Sackett, Richardson, Rosenberg, & Haynes, 1997, p. 4). An example of this in audiology would be the fitting of hearing aids with multiple manually selectable listening programs to all adult clients with hearing impairment irrespective of the client's communication needs and preferences. Although there is high level evidence for multiple listening programs and they have been found to be beneficial for some clients (Keidser, Dillon, & Byrne, 1995), some others are unable to manage different listening programs or do not wish to wear their hearing aids in different acoustic environments.

In this chapter, client preferences are defined broadly to include any client factor that influences the five steps of the EBP process as described in Chapter 1. These steps are: (1) defining a clinical question; (2) searching for evidence to answer the question; (3) evaluating the available evidence; (4) relating the evidence to the client; and (5) evaluating the outcomes of the EBP process. For example, rehabilitation goals, reasons for help-seeking, and perspectives of communication partners may influence Step 1 (defining the clinical question) as well as Step 5 (evaluating the outcomes of the EBP process).

The three approaches and tools this chapter focuses on (joint goal setting, shared decision making, and decision aids) are in line with modern approaches in all health areas that stress the importance of client involvement. We have chosen to focus on these three approaches and tools but we acknowledge that many others may also facilitate the matching of the evidence with client preferences. Clinicians wishing to practice EBP need to know that the evidence for including client preferences is strong. Although the evidence for joint goal setting, shared decision making, and decision aids is reviewed later in this chapter, collectively the take home message is that client involvement in EBP improves intervention outcomes. A meta-analysis of 35 studies showed that interventions taking client preferences into account result in improved intervention adherence and outcomes (Swift, Callahan, & Vollmer, 2011). A systematic review found that client-centeredness, where the clinician recognizes that each client is different, impacts positively on client satisfaction with the health services they received (Lewin, Skea, Entwistle, Zwarenstein, & Dick, 2009). Those who believe that client-centeredness is inherent to a clinician's personal style and that it is impossible to teach old dogs new tricks need to reconsider these misconceptions as the systematic review found that training can improve the extent to which clinicians use client-centeredness. Furthermore, from an ethical standpoint EBP must respect the client's autonomy and informed consent (Slowther, Ford, & Schofield, 2004) and this cannot occur without matching the evidence with the client preferences.

In this chapter the evidence about involving clients in audiological rehabilitation is first described, followed by descriptions of the three approaches and tools that can promote client involvement: joint goal setting, shared decision making, and decision aids. For each of these three, the approach or tool is first described, then the evidence about its use presented, followed by a "how to" guide for clinical use and, finally, two case examples.

WHAT IS THE EVIDENCE FOR INVOLVING CLIENTS IN AUDIOLOGICAL REHABILITATION?

Audiological rehabilitation has been described as a sequence of decisions (Hyde & Riko, 1994). Clients and their significant others face many choices on the road to successful audiological rehabilitation. They must decide to seek help, to pursue an intervention, and to follow all the steps to successful implementation and maintenance of the intervention (Milhinch & Doyle, 1990). Little empirical evidence on the nature of audiological rehabilitation decision making is currently available. A paternalistic approach to decision making (clinician making the decision) has dominated historically; however, for Stephens, the decision-making step is "a vital stage in the rehabilitative process in which key decisions are made jointly between the professionals and the hearing impaired people together with an input from Significant Others (author's own capitalization)" (1996, p. 61). Table 3–1 summarizes three examples of research reports that described audiological intervention decision making from the client's perspective. The first study described how caregivers of children with hearing impairment made decisions regarding pediatric cochlear implantation (Okubo, Takahashi, & Kai, 2008), the second study reported how adults with cochlear

Table 3–1. Examples of Research on Audiological Rehabilitation Decision Making

	Cochlear implantation for children with hearing impairment (Okubo et al., 2008)	*Choice of device by cochlear implant candidates (Migirov et al., 2009)*	*Hearing aids and communication programs for adults with acquired hearing impairment (Laplante-Lévesque et al., 2010b)*
Research methodology	Qualitative (grounded theory of interviews)	Quantitative (univariate analysis of surveys)	Qualitative (content analysis of interviews)
Participants	Caregivers of 23 children with hearing impairment (21 mothers, 4 fathers, 1 grandmother)	184 people with cochlear implants	22 adults with acquired hearing impairment seeking help for the first time
Intervention options	Cochlear implant or no cochlear implant	Nucleus cochlear implant, MED-EL cochlear implant, or Advanced Bionics cochlear implant	Hearing aids, communication programs, or no intervention
Examples of factors considered	Expected auditory and speech benefits, medical complica tions, cost of cochlear implant upgrades, etc.	Device quality/ reliability, device size, color, and shape, battery life, etc.	Expected adherence and outcomes, financial costs, convenience, other people's experiences, recommenda-tions, and support, etc.
Involvement of significant others in decisions, e.g., family members	Yes	Yes	Yes

implants chose which type of device to receive (Migirov, Taitelbaum-Swead, Hildesheimer, Wolf, & Kronenberg, 2009), and the third study described how adults with acquired hearing impairment made decisions regarding hearing aids and communication programs (Laplante-Lévesque, Hickson, & Worrall, 2010b). Decision making in the context of pediatric cochlear implantation has also been investigated by another research team (Johnston et al., 2008). Overall, Table 3–1 highlights how people involved in audiological rehabilitation face various decisions.

JOINT GOAL SETTING

Joint goal setting typically is used at the start of a rehabilitation process. This is a critical point for EBP, as it is when Step 1, defining the clinical question, typically occurs. Understanding what clients want to achieve assists clinicians in focusing on the most relevant research evidence to examine in subsequent EBP steps.

What Is Joint Goal Setting?

Joint goal setting in health refers to the client and the clinician discussing together meaningful objectives or desired outcomes, events, or processes, either relating to the client's current health status or relating to broader life goals (Austin & Vancouver, 1996; Naik, Schulman-Green, McCorkle, Bradley, & Bogardus, 2005). It is a collaborative process shared between client and clinician and typically occurs early in the rehabilitation process, such as at an assessment appointment. Goal setting in the rehabilitation or health context can have many aims, such as to: (1) enhance client autonomy; (2) improve outcomes; (3) assess individualized rehabilitation outcomes; and (4) provide information to stakeholders such as health service funders, quality auditors, accreditation agencies, and professional bodies (Levack, Dean, Siegert, & McPherson, 2006).

Historically, the potential benefits of goal setting in rehabilitative audiology were highlighted over 20 years ago (McKenna, 1987). Roberts and Bryant (1992) identified three functions of goal setting in audiological rehabilitation: (1) to motivate the client to take an active role in their rehabilitation; (2) to educate the client to continue seeking information; and (3) to evaluate progress toward goal achievement. Research reports on behavioral communication education interventions for adults with hearing impairment mentioned the use of individualized intervention goals (Andersson, Melin, Scott, & Lindberg, 1995; Lindberg, Scott, Andersson, & Melin, 1993). Stephens (1996) also described how goal setting could be used in adult audiological rehabilitation. There are also examples of goal setting tools for use with children (Palmer & Mormer, 1998; Ullauri, Crofts, Wilson, & Titley, 2007).

What Is the Evidence for Joint Goal Setting?

This section focuses on the adult population as the evidence in pediatrics is limited. Goal setting can affect client behaviors (Locke & Latham, 2002) and joint goal setting can enhance quality of care (Bogardus et al., 2004), with much of the evidence in this field coming from other areas of health outside audiology. Goal setting has been used successfully in the management of chronic health conditions, for example, when helping diabetic clients achieve healthy behaviors (DeWalt et al., 2009). Brown, Bartholomew, and Naik (2007) reported that joint goal setting for older men with hypertension improved the likelihood of these goals supporting effective self-management of a health condition. Likewise, it has been reported that adult occupational therapy clients who were involved in joint goal setting reported greater perceived confidence in self-management following rehabilitation than a control group who did not set goals (Wressle, Eeg-Olofsson, Marcusson, & Henriksson, 2002). Clients attending neurological rehabilitation who actively participated in goal setting also reported increased satisfaction with the rehabilitation process (Holliday, Cano, Freeman, & Playford, 2007). Overall, the research presented above is of high quality, with large sample sizes and controlled designs. For example, the Bogardus et al. (2004) and the Holliday, Cano, Freeman, and Playford (2007) studies both included at least 200 participants, whereas the Wressle, Eeg-Olofsson, Marcusson, and Henriksson (2002) and the Holliday et al. (2007) studies both used a block design controlled study. However, blinding of the clinician and of the client is of course not possible when the intervention tested involves their participation in goal setting. Although joint goal setting has been applied in audiological rehabilitation we are not aware of any research evidence about the relationship between goal setting and outcomes for people with hearing impairment. Our recommendation to use this approach when applying EBP in the clinic is based on the positive evidence about its benefits for clients with other health conditions. Furthermore, goal setting techniques used in audiology are similar to those in other fields of health and therefore their outcomes are likely to be transferable. Goal Attainment Scaling (GAS) is a popular method of scoring the extent to which individual goals are achieved in the course of intervention, with goals set along with quantifiable attainment levels (Turner-Stokes, 2009). As described below, GAS has inspired goal setting in audiology (Dillon, James, & Ginis, 1997).

How Can Joint Goal Setting Be Implemented in Audiological Rehabilitation?

The Client-Oriented Scale of Improvement (COSI; Dillon, Birtles, & Lovegrove, 1999; Dillon et al., 1997) asks clients to nominate up to five rehabilitation goals and to rate their perceived reduction in disability and resulting ability to communicate in these specific goal situations at the conclusion of rehabilitation. The COSI was the first goal setting tool that clinicians working with adults with hearing impairment widely integrated into practice. The individualized nature of the COSI has been generally appreciated by clients, as described by an audiologist: "it gives the client some ownership over the rehabilitation program" (Dillon & So, 2000, p. 3).

The use of the COSI is well established for joint hearing aid goal setting and it has also been used for audiological interventions other than hearing aids (see, for example, Hickson, Worrall, & Scarinici, 2007). The COSI has also been adapted for the pediatric population: the COSI-C is available online (National Acoustic Laboratories, 2004b). In a pilot study, the COSI-C was found to be the most reliable tool to collect feedback from parents of children who wore a cochlear implant and a hearing aid in the other ear (Ullauri, Crofts, Wilson, & Titley, 2007).

Although the COSI appears to be the most popular goal setting tool, others have been developed and applied. For example, the Glasgow Hearing Aid Benefit Profile (GHABP; Gatehouse, 1999, 2000, 2001), although designed more specifically as an outcome measure tool, can also be used for goal setting with adults with hearing impairment. More recently, Jennings (2009) successfully used GAS with 46 adults with hearing impairment participating in a group-based rehabilitation program. The goals were set individually prior to rehabilitation. The participants described each of their goals in terms of the environment in which they occurred, the people involved, and how participants currently addressed them. Participants also identified the extent to which they wanted the goals improved. Goal attainment was reviewed after rehabilitation completion and 6 months later and GAS was found useful, not only to measure outcomes, but also to organize the rehabilitation process.

Likewise, in pediatric rehabilitation, a number of the tools designed for outcomes measurement could be effectively used to set goals. The Parents' Evaluation of Aural/Oral Performance of Children (PEACH; Ching

& Hill, 2007), for example, evaluates the effectiveness of amplification for infants and school-age children with mild to profound hearing impairment. The measure is based on parents' observations of the functional performance of their child in everyday life in a range of listening situations (e.g., responding to name in quiet, participating in conversation in noise, conversing on the phone). The child receives a score based on their parents' observations of performance for each behavior over a 1-week period. Goals could be set to improve performance for particular behaviors in subsequent rehabilitation.

In summary, there are a number of clinical tools available for joint goal setting in adults and children and these would assist the clinician to understand the particular needs of each client and focus intervention (and therefore EBP) accordingly. The psychometric properties of these tools have not been fully reported and therefore further research is required. Nonetheless, these tools all have the advantage of being individualized and short measures suitable for clinical practice. Of course, adopting a measure or a tool is just one step towards effective collaborative goal setting and Table 3–2 provides some suggestions for how to apply such tools in the clinic.

SHARED DECISION MAKING

Although joint goal setting typically occurs at the commencement of rehabilitation, shared decision making can happen at various stages of the rehabilitation process and is central to EBP. We focus here on the consideration of shared decision making as it occurs at the point in the rehabilitation process when decisions are made about interventions to pursue.

Table 3–2. Tips for Successful Joint Goal Setting

Familiarize yourself with the measure. The COSI (for adults) and the COSI-C (for children) and instructions for administration are available on line at http://www.nal.gov.au/pdf/COSI-administration-instructions.pdf and http://www.nal.gov.au/pdf/COSI-C-Administration%20Instructions.pdf .
Clients value clinicians who will listen to their story and whom they trust (Laplante-Lévesque et al., 2010a) hence take the time to hear each clients' individual story and develop a relationship that engenders trust. A good 'working alliance' between client and clinician is associated with better treatment outcomes for clients (Horvath & Symonds, 1991).
Work toward "SMARTER" goals: Specific, Measurable, Agreed upon, Realistic, Timely, Ethical, and Recorded (Wade, 2009).
Clients' goals change over time. There is a need to frequently review goals and their outcomes so that the ongoing needs of the clients can be addressed (Stephens & Kramer, 2010).
Set collaborative goals with family members for young children with hearing impairment (Roush & Kamo, 2008).
Engage teenagers with hearing impairment in their own goal setting (English, 2008).
Involve communication partners of adult clients as they may influence goals (Laplante-Lévesque et al., 2010a).

What Is Shared Decision Making?

Decision making is best represented on a continuum, from sole clinician participation at one end to total client participation at the other end. Three main approaches to intervention decision making have been identified on this continuum: paternalistic, shared, and informed (Charles, Gafni, & Whelan, 1997, 1999). Shared decision making occupies the middle of the decision-making continuum: paternalistic decision making (clinician making the decision with little client participation) is at one end and informed decision making (client making the decision with little clinician participation) is at the other end. In shared decision making, or the middle position on the continuum, the information exchange, deliberation, decision making, and intervention action are performed together by the client and the clinician (Charles et al., 1997, 1999). It signifies involving clients in decision making "to the extent that they desire" (Edwards & Elwyn, 2006, p. 317). Some of the other terms used in the literature to describe client participation in intervention decision are informed decision making, client-clinician partnership, concordance, evidence-based client choice, client autonomy, client self-determination, active client participation, and client participation.

What Is the Evidence for Shared Decision Making?

Again the focus of evidence in this area has been with the adult population and client participation in intervention decisions has been found to have two main advantages. First, it respects the client's right to autonomy and informed consent (Emanuel & Emanuel, 1992; Lidz, Appelbaum, & Meisel, 1988) as client involvement is central to shared decision making. Second, in a similar fashion to joint goal setting, it achieves better intervention adherence and outcomes than other approaches (e.g., paternalistic decision making, where the clinician makes the decision with little client participation). A comprehensive systematic review (Level 1 evidence as described in Table 1–5 in Chapter 1) reported the results of 11 randomized controlled trials and found shared decision making to be particularly suitable for people with chronic health conditions, when more than one intervention is available, and when the interventions require more than one session (Joosten et al., 2008). This is clearly the case for audiological rehabilitation: hearing impairment is most often chronic in nature, there are a number of different intervention options (e.g., hearing aids, cochlear implants, counseling, or hearing assistive technology), and interventions almost always require ongoing sessions.

Research evidence indicates that shared decision making leads to better outcomes for people with chronic health conditions. For example, clients with myocardial infarction who chose between group cardiac rehabilitation and individual cardiac rehabilitation were more likely to complete their rehabilitation program than clients who were randomly assigned to one of the two rehabilitation programs (Wingham, Dalal, Sweeney, & Evans, 2006). Similarly, clinically depressed clients who chose to pursue counseling achieved better outcomes than their counterparts who were randomized to the same intervention (Chilvers et al., 2001). The literature on diabetes also signals favorable outcomes when clients are offered their preferred decision-making role (Michie, Miles, & Weinman, 2003; van Dam, van der Horst, van den Borne, Ryckman, & Crebolder, 2003).

In summary, research evidence from other fields of health indicates that shared decision making could well be very beneficial for people with hearing impairment. It is likely to lead to improved intervention adherence and improved outcomes of rehabilitation; however further research in audiology is necessary to determine if this is the case.

How Can Shared Decision Making Be Implemented in Audiological Rehabilitation?

Although we argue that clients should be offered a role in any audiological rehabilitation decision, we also acknowledge that not all clients want to be involved to the same extent. In general, younger clients, clients with more years of formal education, and female clients are more likely to prefer participation in health decisions (for a review, see Say, Murtagh, & Thomson, 2006). It is still unclear whether the influence of age is indeed an age effect or rather a cohort effect, with the new generation of older adults expected to prefer more participation than their predecessors.

Understandably, clients want to be adequately prepared before participating in health decision making and Table 3–3 contains some tips for effectively implementing shared decision making. Prerequisites to shared decision making include knowledge (for example, of the health condition and of the benefits and limitations of the interventions available), explicit encouragement of client participation by the clinician, appreciation of the client's rights and responsibilities to play an active role in decision making, awareness of choice, and sufficient time (Fraenkel & McGraw, 2007). Clients having access to information is a fundamental part of shared decision making. Good communication skills are required

Table 3–3. Tips for Successful Shared Decision Making

Prepare clients for shared decision making by stating early that they will be invited to be involved in decisions.
Try to understand the client's experience and expectations, e.g., ask the client what they expected would happen at the clinic.
Communicate information at a level appropriate to clients. Be prepared to simplify explanations, use nontechnical language, convey quantitative information in a qualitative way and use diagrams to aid comprehension.
Communicate the values of your workplace to your clients.
Ensure that clients feel comfortable to ask questions.
Build a partnership with the client.
Describe the evidence about interventions to the client, including any uncertainties.
Take into account the values and preferences of your clients when discussing the options.
Check that clients understand the information provided and the options available to them.
Give clients time to go away and think about options. Many will want to involve their communication partners too.

Source: Based on Epstein et al. (2004).

to adequately describe the evidence to clients so that shared decision making can occur (Epstein, Alper, & Quill, 2004; Ford, Schofield, & Hope, 2003).

In a recent study, we explored the shared decision making experiences of adults with acquired hearing impairment presenting for rehabilitation for the first time (Laplante-Lévesque, Hickson, & Worrall, 2010a). Participants were presented with four intervention options (hearing aid fitting, a group communication program, an individual home-based communication program, and no intervention) in a context of shared decision making. We used a structured format for the presentation of the options—specifically, we used a decision aid, which is described in more detail in the following section of the chapter. After the participants had made a decision, 22 of them were interviewed about their experiences. According to the evidence from the interview data, the results were organized into a model of audiological rehabilitation shared decision making, which is presented in Figure 3–1. The participants described their decision making by its actors (i.e., who is involved in decision making), processes (i.e., what are the decision-making steps), and dimensions (i.e., what influences decision making). The dimensions refer to clients' experiences and preferences for decision making. This includes their decision-making style, their health care preferences, and their perceptions of the specific decision they were facing.

Two recurrent themes in the interviews, "my story" and "trust," highlight the importance of a client-centered and ethical approach to shared decision making in audiological rehabilitation. The first theme, "my story," reflected the fact that adults with acquired hearing impairment wished their clinicians to hear their experiences and preferences. In other words, they viewed client-centeredness as a prerequisite to audiological rehabilitation shared decision making and were not comfortable with a prescriptive approach that does not allow for individual differences. The second theme, "trust," was also central to the participants' experiences with shared decision making. Participants only wanted to engage in shared decision making with clinicians they perceived as motivated to improve their well-being and this has also been reported when shared decision making occurred with general medical practitioners (Edwards & Elwyn, 2006; Lown, Hanson, & Clark, 2009). In the medical literature, trust can either refer to the profession as a whole or to a particular medical practitioner (McKinstry, Ashcroft, Car, Freeman, & Sheikh, 2009). This distinction was also made by adults with acquired hearing impairment describing their level of trust either towards the general profession of audiology or toward specific audiologists. Therefore in order for shared decision making to be effective in audiology, trust in both the profession and the individual audiologist are important. Given the high importance that this study's participants gave to trust as a theme, it appears that lack of trust may be a barrier to shared decision making in audiology.

DECISION AIDS

We focus here on decision aids as a means to assist clinicians with the important EBP step that is relaying evidence to clients.

What Are Decision Aids?

Decision aids provide information on intervention options and their benefits and limitations. They are "tools designed to prepare clients to participate in making specific and deliberated choices among health care options

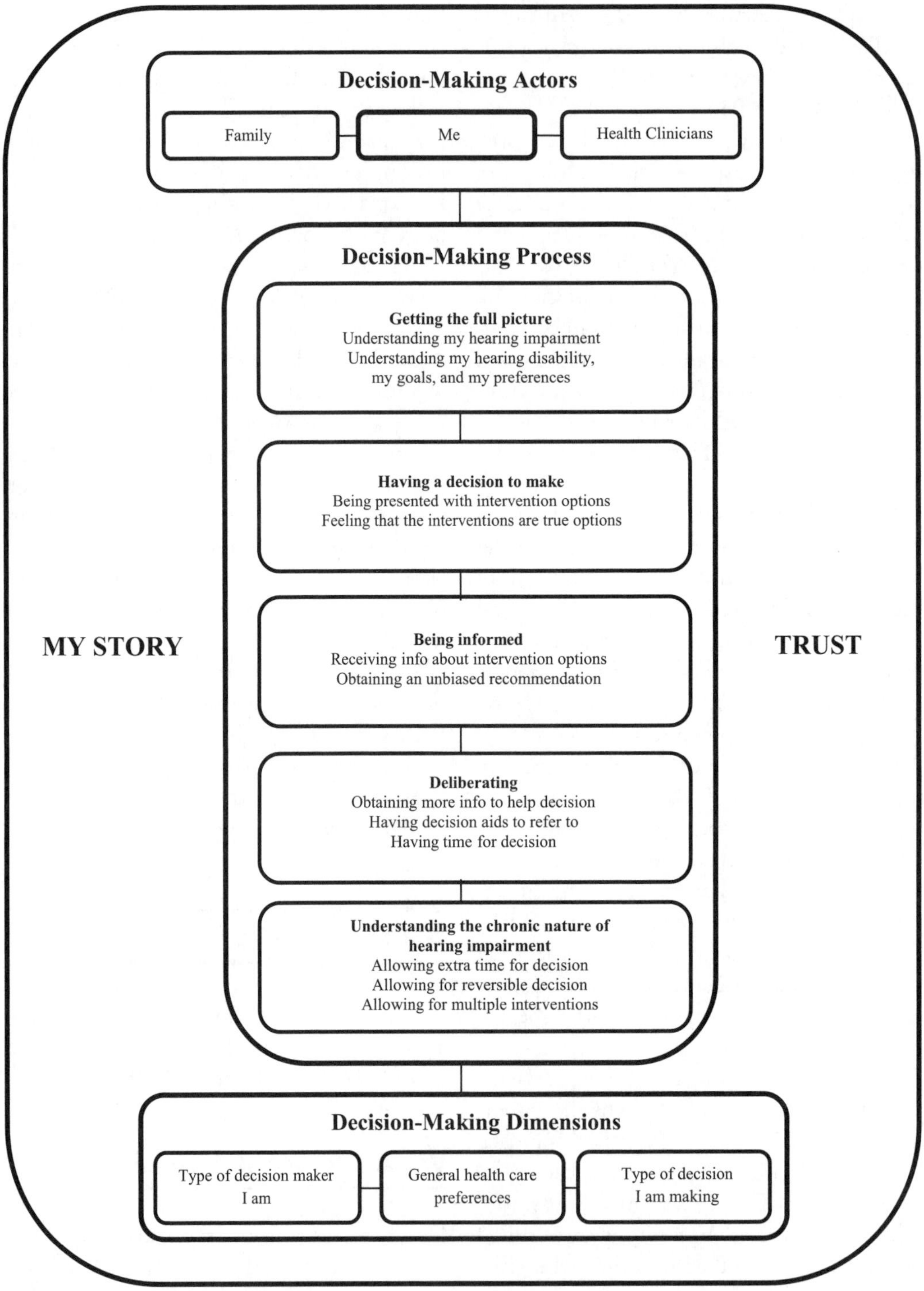

Figure 3–1. *Model of audiological rehabilitation shared intervention decision making according to adults with acquired hearing impairment.*

in ways they prefer. Patient decision aids supplement (rather than replace) clinician's counseling about options" (O'Connor et al., 2009, p. 3). Decision aids describe the evidence surrounding a health condition, the intervention options, their associated benefits and limitations. As they are evidence-based, they should be updated as new evidence becomes available. A decision aid can take various forms such as a leaflet, a board, a poster, an audio or audiovisual recording, or an interactive computer-based presentation. Decision aids are used by the client and the clinician to enable a systematic, consistent, and unbiased presentation of the intervention options. They provide information on the evidence about the benefits and limitations of the available interventions and help clients clarify their goals and values relevant to the health condition and the intervention options so that their intervention decision is compatible with those. Decision aids have great potential to be used in step 4 of the EBP process, that is, relating evidence to the client.

What Is the Evidence for Using Decision Aids?

A systematic literature review on decision aid outcomes in health revealed that they improve client knowledge of intervention options, facilitate decisions, and increase client participation in decision making (O'Connor et al., 2009). Decision aids are important as a means of giving clients consistent and unbiased information about the evidence related to a particular intervention. Inconsistencies in the presentation of intervention options (e.g., introducing a bias in the option presentation or omitting to tell clients about uncertainties in the evidence) can intentionally or unintentionally direct the client toward a specific intervention (Ashcroft, Hope, & Parker, 2001; Elwyn, Edwards, Gwyn, & Grol, 1999; Wills & Holmes-Rovner, 2003).

How Can Decision Aids Be Implemented in Audiological Rehabilitation?

Based on the clients' needs and the evidence about possible interventions, different clients require different options to be presented to them. For example, parents may need to consider if their baby should be fitted with a cochlear implant or a hearing aid and an adult client may need to consider surgical or a bone-anchored hearing aid fitting intervention for a middle ear condition. The quality of decision aids fluctuates greatly and a decision aid quality criteria framework has been published (Elwyn et al., 2006). The framework, available online, promotes the systematic development and study of decision aids that provide adequate and appropriate content. Decision aids should provide accurate yet parsimonious information and individualized decision aids that adapt to each client's situation have been advocated.

A decision aid for parents considering sequential bilateral cochlear implantation for their child with hearing impairment was designed and piloted by a group of audiologists and experts in decision aids (Johnston et al., 2009). The decision aid was found to successfully increase parents' knowledge regarding bilateral cochlear implantation, including its benefits and risks. The decision aid is available as an appendix to the article published by Johnston and colleagues (2009).

A decision aid summarizing the intervention options available to adults with acquired hearing impairment is also available (Laplante-Lévesque et al., 2010b). Although the decision aid itself has not yet been evaluated, the 153 adults with acquired hearing impairment who used it found it useful. For example, they reported that the decision aid "was well laid out, the fors and againsts, simple and explanatory." According to the clients, it included "good, well presented information" and "it's short enough to give the information at a glance, but it's not too short." Clients used the decision aids "to show people what was available," especially with their significant others in the comfort of their own home: "I sat down, went through it with my wife, and talked about it." Table 3–4 presents tips for developing successful decision aids, which, as described above, are strongly supported by research evidence. It summarizes the International Patient Decision Aid Standards instrument (IPDASi), a decision aid quality framework. It also provides a link to the Ottawa Personal Decision Guide (OPDG), a generic decision aid designed for use in any health decision. The OPDG is available in several versions and languages.

CASE STUDIES

In this section two case examples of best practice in relating evidence to clients are presented.

Case Study 1—Ron

This first case study is based on interview excerpts with adults with hearing impairment seeking help for the first time who were involved in shared decision-making research

Table 3–4. Tips for Successful Decision Aids

Consult the Ottawa Personal Decision Guide (OPDG), a generic decision aid designed for use in any health decision. It is available in several versions and languages (http://decisionaid.ohri.ca/decguide.html). Familiarize yourself with the International Patient Decision Aid Standards instrument (IPDASi), a quality framework for decision aids put together by a group of world experts (Elwyn et al., 2006). The IPDASi covers 10 dimensions:

1. Information (e.g., does the decision aid describe the options available?)
2. Probabilities (e.g., does the decision aid compare outcome probabilities across options?)
3. Values (e.g., does the decision aid help imagine what it is like to experience the social effects of the options?)
4. Decision guidance (e.g., does the decision aid provide a step-by-step way to make the decision?)
5. Development (e.g., has the decision aid been field tested?)
6. Evidence (e.g., does the decision aid provide a production or publication date?)
7. Disclosure (e.g., does the decision aid provide information about the funding used for its development?)
8. Plain language (e.g., is the readability level of the decision aid known?)
9. Evaluation (e.g., does the decision aid improve client knowledge?)
10. Test—for decision aids directed at screenings or assessments (e.g., does the decision aid describe the chances that the health condition is detected with and without the test?)

mentioned above (Laplante-Lévesque et al., 2010a, 2010b). Direct quotes of research interviews are presented here. Ron, a 62-year-old retired plumber, is a keen musician. He plays guitar in a band with friends and enjoys regular outings with his partner, Jillian. Ron was initially reluctant to make an appointment with an audiologist as he had heard that hearing aids could not cure his noise-induced hearing impairment. Ron eventually made an appointment with Anne, an audiologist.

Ron attended the appointment by himself even though Jillian played a big part in him seeking help. As part of the case history, Anne asked Ron about his main hearing-related activity limitations and participation restrictions and also learnt that Ron noticed his first hearing difficulties 10 years ago. After the hearing assessment, Anne described the results by relating them to Ron's hearing experiences. She prompted Ron to discuss his rehabilitation goals and these were recorded with the COSI. Ron's top priority goals were to be able to hear better when out at social events with Jillian and to be able to hear his grandchildren more clearly. Ron said, "I want to do the best of what's available at the moment." Anne then described the intervention options available to Ron: both those she offered (i.e., hearing aids, hearing assistive technology) and those available through other sources (i.e., group communication programs offered by the local association of people with hearing impairment, computer-based speech-reading classes to be completed at home). Anne outlined the benefits and limitations of these intervention options using a decision aid and she discussed each option in light of Ron's rehabilitation goals. Ron liked Anne's informative approach and he said, "You cut to the chase. You provided the exact amount of information I needed." Anne gave Ron a copy of the decision aid with the summary of the intervention options and suggested he discuss this with his partner Jillian and perhaps a few other family members and friends.

A week later, Anne called Ron, who told Anne that he would like to acquire hearing aids and to complete computer-based speech-reading classes from home. He said he made his decision easily: "I can't think of any aspect of my hearing or my problem or my approach to it that you haven't covered. So that helped me tremendously in making my decision. The other deciding factor was when you explained the pros and the cons." Ron is now a successful hearing aid user who also completed speech-reading classes from home. He has built a strong ongoing relationship with his audiologist Anne.

Case Study 2—Liam

Liam was born at a hospital where a universal newborn hearing screening program was in place. Liam was only 6 weeks old when his parents learnt he had a profound bilateral hearing impairment. They were devastated by the news as they had no experience of hearing impairment and were extremely concerned about what lay ahead for Liam and for them. The audiologist, Michael, who diagnosed Liam's hearing impairment, explained the initial options available to Liam and the need for the earliest possible intervention. He did this in extended sessions with the parents and grandparents by describing the options (i.e., hearing aids, cochlear implants), the evidence about outcomes for children with profound hearing loss using these options (see Chapters 5 and 8), and by showing them the devices and answering their many questions. Michael tried not to direct the conversation too much and used open-ended questions to help the family explore the options and their own feelings. For example, he began by asking the parents, "What do you know about hearing aids?" This allowed Michael to tailor his discussions with them appropriately.

During and after each session he provided the family with written material, including decision aids, and encouraged them to read this further at home. The information focused on hearing impairment, its effects on children, and the evidence about the effectiveness of interventions, including the evidence that the earlier the intervention the greater the benefits. Liam's parents expressed concern that they could not understand some of the information but still wanted to take it, saying, "We have a friend who's a doctor and we'd like to show this to her." Liam was fitted with hearing aids at 3 months of age and the family is going through a decision-making process regarding subsequent cochlear implant fitting. A team of people around them, including the audiologist, ear, nose, and throat specialist, speech pathologist, and social worker, are supporting them using a shared decision-making approach.

SUMMARY

In this chapter, we have highlighted the importance of involving clients in EBP, have described three approaches and tools to help involve clients in EBP (joint goal setting, shared decision making, and decision aids), and have provided practical tips about the use of these approaches and tools, including two case examples. We hope that both clinicians and researchers will continue to view EBP as not only a technique that focuses on scientific evidence but also as an approach that facilitates the best intervention decisions for individual clients.

This step in the EBP process, relating the evidence to the client, is wide open for future research. As highlighted throughout the chapter, although there is evidence from other fields, there is little evidence about the relationship between the three approaches described here and the outcomes of audiological rehabilitation. Some debate and consensus about the most appropriate outcome measures for audiological rehabilitation needs to take place. For example, whether these approaches improve rates of help-seeking and intervention uptake, adherence, benefits, and satisfaction in audiology should be investigated. To assess shared decision making, one could compare intervention outcomes in people involved in the intervention decision with people randomly assigned to the same intervention. This research design is called a randomized controlled trial with preference arms (Brewin & Bradley, 1989; Lambert & Wood, 2000). In this research design, each participant is asked a priori for intervention preference. Participants with a preference for an intervention are not randomized and complete their intervention of choice whilst participants without a preference for an intervention complete the intervention to which they are randomized (Brewin & Bradley, 1989). This design isolates the effect of preferences on intervention uptake and outcomes. According to a systematic review, the magnitude of the effect of client preferences as measured in randomized controlled trials in fact are smaller than initially predicted (King et al., 2005), but it would be interesting to determine whether this is true for hearing rehabilitation. Each participant's degree of preference for an intervention (from no preference to strong preference) can also be assessed and linked back to the preference effect. Randomized controlled trials with preference arms are an insightful combination of evidence-based practices and client-centeredness (Bensing, 2000). In addition, research on all approaches is especially scarce for the pediatric population. In an era where parents and children have increasing choices about interventions, such research must be a high priority.

REFERENCES

Andersson, G., Melin, L., Scott, B., & Lindberg, P. (1995). An evaluation of a behavioural treatment approach to hearing impairment. *Behavioural Research and Therapy, 33*, 283–292.

Ashcroft, R., Hope, T., & Parker, M. (2001). Ethical issues and evidence-based patient choice. In A. Edwards & G. Elwyn (Eds.), *Evidence-based patient choice: Inevitable or impossible?* (pp. 53–65). Oxford, UK: Oxford University Press.

Austin, J. T., & Vancouver, J. B. (1996). Goal constructs in psychology: Structure, process, and content. *Psychological Bulletin, 120*, 338–375.

Bensing, J. (2000). Bridging the gap. The separate worlds of evidence-based medicine and patient-centered medicine. *Patient Education and Counseling, 39*, 17–25.

Bogardus, S. T., Bradley, E. H., Williams, C. S., Maciejewski, P. K., Gallo, W. T., & Inouye, S. K. (2004). Achieving goals in geriatric assessment: Role of caregiver agreement and adherence to recommendations. *Journal of the American Geriatrics Society, 52*, 99–105.

Brewin, C. R., & Bradley, C. (1989). Patient preferences and randomised clinical trials. *British Medical Journal, 299*, 313–315.

Brown, V. A., Bartholomew, L. K., & Naik, A. D. (2007). Management of chronic hypertension in older men: An exploration of patient goal-setting. *Patient Education and Counseling, 69*, 93–99.

Charles, C., Gafni, A., & Whelan, T. (1997). Shared decision-making in the medical encounter: What does it mean? (Or it takes two to tango). *Social Science and Medicine, 44*, 681–692.

Charles, C., Gafni, A., & Whelan, T. (1999). Decision-making in the physician-patient encounter: Revisiting the shared treatment decision-making model. *Social Science and Medicine, 49*, 651–661.

Chilvers, C., Dewey, M., Fielding, K., Gretton, V., Miller, P., Palmer, B., . . . Harrison, G. (2001). Antidepressant drugs and generic counselling for treatment of major depression in primary care: Randomised trial with patient preference arms. *British Medical Journal, 322*, 772–775.

Ching, T. Y. C., & Hill, M. (2007). The Parents' Evaluation of Aural/Oral Performance of Children (PEACH) Scale: Normative data. *Journal of the American Academy of Audiology, 18*, 220–235.

DeWalt, D. A., Davis, T. C., Wallace, A. S., Seligman, H. K., Bryant-Shilliday, B., Arnold, C. L., . . . Schillinger, D.(2009). Goal setting in diabetes self-management: Taking the baby steps to success. *Patient Education and Counseling, 77*, 218–223.

Dillon, H., Birtles, G., & Lovegrove, R. (1999). Measuring the outcomes of a national rehabilitation program: Normative data for the Client Oriented Scale of Improvement (COSI) and the Hearing Aid User's Questionnaire (HAUQ). *Journal of the American Academy of Audiology, 10*, 67–79.

Dillon, H., James, A., & Ginis, J. (1997). Client oriented scale of improvement (COSI) and its relationship to several other measures of benefit and satisfaction provided by hearing aids. *Journal of the American Academy of Audiology, 8*, 27–43.

Dillon, H., & So, M. (2000). Incentives and obstacles to the routine use of outcomes measures by clinicians. *Ear and Hearing, 21*(Suppl. 4), 2–6.

Edwards, A., & Elwyn, G. (2006). Inside the black box of shared decision making: Distinguishing between the process of involvement and who makes the decision. *Health Expectations, 9*, 307–320.

Elwyn, G., Edwards, A., Gwyn, R., & Grol, R. (1999). Towards a feasible model for shared decision making: Focus group study with general practice registrars. *British Medical Journal, 319*, 753–756.

Elwyn, G., O'Connor, A., Stacey, D., Volk, R., Edwards, A., Coulter, A., . . . Whelan, T. (2006). Developing a quality criteria framework for patient decision aids: Online international Delphi consensus process. *British Medical Journal, 333*, 417–419.

Emanuel, E. J., & Emanuel, L. L. (1992). Four models of the physician-patient relationship. *Journal of the American Medical Association, 267*, 2221–2226.

English, K. (2008). Educating and couseling children and teens with hearing loss. In J. R. Madell, & G. Flexer (Eds.), *Pediatric audiology: Diagnosis, technology and management* (pp. 278–282). New York, NY: Thieme.

Epstein, R. M., Alper, B. S., & Quill, T. E. (2004). Communicating evidence for participatory decision making. *Journal of the American Medical Association, 291*, 2359–2366.

Ford, S., Schofield, T., & Hope, T. (2003). What are the ingredients for a successful evidence-based patient choice consultation?: A qualitative study. *Social Science and Medicine, 56*, 17–25.

Fraenkel, L., & McGraw, S. (2007). What are the essential elements to enable patient participation in medical decision making? *Journal of General Internal Medicine, 22*, 614–618.

Gatehouse, S. (1999). Glasgow Hearing Aid Benefit Profile: Derivation and validation of a client-centred outcome measure for hearing aid services. *Journal of the American Academy of Audiology, 10*, 80–103.

Gatehouse, S. (2000). The Glasgow Hearing Aid Benefit Profile: What it measures and how to use it. *Hearing Journal, 53*(3), 10, 12, 14, 16, 18.

Gatehouse, S. (2001). Self-report outcome measures for adult hearing aid services: Some uses, users, and options. *Trends in Amplification, 5*, 91–110.

Hickson, L., Worrall, L., & Scarinci, N. (2007). A randomized controlled trial evaluating the Active Communication Education program for older people with hearing impairment. *Ear and Hearing*, 28, 212–230.

Holliday, R. C., Cano, S., Freeman, J. A., & Playford, E. D. (2007). Should patients participate in clinical decision making? An optimised balance block design controlled study of goal setting in a rehabilitation unit. *Journal of Neurology, Neurosurgery and Psychiatry, 78*, 576–580.

Horvath, A.O., & Symonds, B.D. (1991). Relation between working alliance and outcome in psychotherapy: A meta-analysis. *Journal of Counseling Psychology, 38*, 139–149.

Hyde, M. L., & Riko, K. (1994). A decision-analytic approach to audiological rehabilitation. In J.-P. Gagné & N. Tye-Murray (Eds.), *Research in audiological rehabilitation: Current trends and future directions* (pp. 337–374). Gainesville, FL: *Journal of the Academy of Rehabilitative Audiology*: Monograph supplement.

Jennings, M. B. (2009). Evaluating the efficacy of a group audiological rehabilitation program for adults with hearing loss using a goal attainment scaling approach. *Canadian Journal of Speech-Language Pathology and Audiology, 33*, 146–153.

Johnston, J. C., Durieux-Smith, A., Fitzpatrick, E., O'Connor, A., Benzies, K., & Angus, D. (2008). An assessment of parents' decision-making regarding paediatric cochlear implants. *Canadian Journal of Speech-Language Pathology and Audiology, 32*, 169–182.

Johnston, J. C., Durieux-Smith, A., O'Connor, A., Benzies, K., Fitzpatrick, E. M., & Angus, D. (2009). The development and piloting of a decision aid for parents considering sequential bilateral cochlear implantation for their child with hearing loss. *Volta Review, 109*, 121–141.

Joosten, E. A. G., DeFuentes-Merillas, L., de Weert, G. H., Sensky, T., van der Staak, C. P. F., & de Jong, C. A. J. (2008). Systematic review of the effects of shared decision-making on patient satisfaction, treatment adherence and health status. *Psychotherapy and Psychosomatics, 77*, 219–226.

Keidser, G., Dillon, H., & Byrne, D. (1995). Candidates for multiple frequency response characteristics. *Ear and Hearing, 16*, 562–574.

King, M., Nazareth, I., Lampe, F., Bower, P., Chandler, M., Morou, M., . . . Lai, R. (2005). Conceptual framework and systematic review of the effects of participants' and professionals' preferences in randomized controlled trials. *Health Technology Assessment, 9*(35), 1–186.

Lambert, M. F., & Wood, J. (2000). Incorporating patient preferences into randomized trials. *Journal of Clinical Epidemiology, 53*, 163–166.

Laplante-Lévesque, A., Hickson, L., & Worrall, L. (2010a). A qualitative study of shared decision making in rehabilitative audiology. *Journal of the Academy of Rehabilitative Audiology, 43*, 27–43.

Laplante-Lévesque, A., Hickson, L., & Worrall, L. (2010b). Factors influencing rehabilitation decisions of adults with acquired hearing impairment. *International Journal of Audiology, 49*, 497–507.

Levack, W. M. M., Dean, S. G., Siegert, R. J., & McPherson, K. M. (2006). Purposes and mechanisms of goal planning in rehabilitation: The need for a critical distinction. *Disability and Rehabilitation, 28*, 741–749.

Lewin, S., Skea, Z. C., Entwistle, V. A., Zwarenstein, M., & Dick, J. (2001). Interventions for providers to promote a patient-centred approach in clinical consultations. *Cochrane Database of Systematic Reviews*, (4). doi: 10.1002/14651858.CD003267.

Lidz, C. W., Appelbaum, P. S., & Meisel, J. D. (1988). Two models of implementing informed consent. *Archives of Internal Medicine, 148*, 1385–1389.

Lindberg, P., Scott, B., Andersson, G., & Melin, L. (1993). A behavioural approach to individually designed hearing tactics training. *British Journal of Audiology, 27*, 299–301.

Locke, E. A., & Latham, G. P. (2002). Building a practically useful theory of goal setting and task motivation: A 35-year odyssey. *American Psychologist, 57*, 705–717.

Lown, B. A., Hanson, J. L., & Clark, W. D. (2009). Mutual influence in shared decision making: A collaborative study of patients and physicians. *Health Expectations, 12*, 160–174.

McKenna, L. (1987). Goal planning in audiological rehabilitation. *British Journal of Audiology, 21*, 5–11.

McKinstry, B., Ashcroft, R., Car, J., Freeman, G. K., & Sheikh, A. (2006). Interventions for improving patients' trust in doctors and groups of doctors. *Cochrane Database of Systematic Reviews*, (3). doi: 10.1002/14651858.CD004134.pub2 .

Michie, S., Miles, J., & Weinman, J. (2003). Patient-centredness in chronic illness: What is it and does it matter? *Patient Education and Counseling, 51*, 197–206.

Migirov, L., Taitelbaum-Swead, R., Hildesheimer, M., Wolf, M., & Kronenberg, J. (2009). Factors affecting choice of device by cochlear implant candidates. *Otology and Neurotology, 30*, 743–746.

Milhinch, J. C., & Doyle, J. (1990). Clients' decision-making: Choosing a hearing health care service. *Australian Journal of Audiology, 12*, 45–53.

Naik, A. D., Schulman-Green, D., McCorkle, R., Bradley, E. H., & Bogardus, S. T., Jr. (2005). Will older persons and their clinicians use a shared decision-making instrument? *Journal of General Internal Medicine, 20*, 640–643.

National Acoustic Laboratories. (2004a). *Client Orientated Scale of Improvement.* Retrieved July 2nd, 2010, from http://www.nal.gov.au/pdf/COSI-Questionnaire.pdf

National Acoustic Laboratories. (2004b). *Client Orientated Scale of Improvement for Children.* Retrieved July 2nd, 2010, from http://www.nal.gov.au/pdf/COSI-C-Questionnaire.pdf

O'Connor, A. M., Bennett, C. L., Stacey, D., Barry, M., Col, N. F., Eden, K. B., . . . Jones, J. (2001). Decision aids for people facing health treatment or screening decisions. *Cochrane Database of Systematic Reviews*, (3). CD001431.

Okubo, S., Takahashi, M., & Kai, I. (2008). How Japanese parents of deaf children arrive at decisions regarding pediatric cochlear implantation surgery: A qualitative study. *Social Science and Medicine, 66*, 2436–2447.

Palmer, C.V., & Mormer, E.A. (1998). Defining the children's and parents' expectations of the hearing aid fitting. *Hearing Journal, 51*(9), 80.

Roberts, S. D., & Bryant, J. D. (1992). Establishing counseling goals in rehabilitative audiology. *Journal of the Academy of Rehabilitative Audiology, 25*, 81–97.

Roush, J., & Kamo, G. (2008). Counseling and collaboration with parents of children with hearing loss. In J.R. Madell & G. Flexer (Eds.), *Pediatric audiology: Diagnosis, technology and management* (pp. 269–277). New York, NY: Thieme.

Sackett, D. L., Richardson, W. S., Rosenberg, W., & Haynes, R. B. (1997). *Evidence-based medicine: How to practice and teach EBM.* New York, NY: Churchill Livingstone.

Sackett, D. L., Rosenberg, W. M., Gray, J. A., Haynes, R. B., & Richardson, W. S. (1996). Evidence based medicine: What it is and what it isn't. *British Medical Journal, 312*, 71–72.

Say, R., Murtagh, M., & Thomson, R. (2006). Patients' preference for involvement in medical decision making: A narrative review. *Patient Education and Counseling, 60,* 102–114.

Slowther, A., Ford, S., & Schofield, T. (2004). Ethics of evidence based medicine in the primary care setting. *Journal of Medical Ethics, 30,* 151–155.

Stephens, D. (1996). Hearing rehabilitation in a psychosocial framework. *Scandinavian Audiology, 25*(Suppl. 43), 57–66.

Stephens, D., & Kramer, S. E. (2010). *Living with hearing difficulties: The process of enablement.* Chichester, UK: Wiley-Blackwell.

Swift, J. K., Callahan, J. L., & Vollmer, B. M. (2011). Preferences. *Journal of Clinical Psychology: In Session, 67,* 155–165.

Turner-Stokes, L. (2009). Goal attainment scaling (GAS) in rehabilitation: A practical guide. *Clinical Rehabilitation, 23,* 362–370.

Ullauri, A., Crofts, H., Wilson, K., & Titley, S. (2007). Bimodal benefits of cochlear implant and hearing aid (on the non-implanted ear): A pilot study to develop a protocol and a test battery. *Cochlear Implants International, 8,* 29–37.

van Dam, H. A., van der Horst, F., van den Borne, B., Ryckman, R., & Crebolder, H. (2003). Provider-patient interaction in diabetes care: Effects on patient self-care and outcomes. A systematic review. *Patient Education and Counseling, 51,* 17–28.

Wade, D. T. (2009). Goal setting in rehabilitation: An overview of what, why and how. *Clinical Rehabilitation, 23,* 291–295.

Wills, C. E., & Holmes-Rovner, M. (2003). Patient comprehension of information for shared treatment decision making: State of the art and future directions. *Patient Education and Counseling, 50,* 285–290.

Wingham, J., Dalal, H. M., Sweeney, K. G., & Evans, P. H. (2006). Listening to patients: Choice in cardiac rehabilitation. *European Journal of Cardiovascular Nursing, 5,* 289–294.

Wressle, E., Eeg-Olofsson, A.-M., Marcusson, J., & Henriksson, C. (2002). Improved client participation in the rehabilitation process using a client-centred goal formulation structure. *Journal of Rehabilitation Medicine, 34,* 5–11.

PART II

Hearing Aids

CHAPTER 4

Hearing Aids for Adults

Larry E. Humes and Vidya Krull

EVIDENCE ABOUT THE EFFECTIVENESS OF HEARING AIDS FOR ADULTS

In the United States, approximately two-thirds of the hearing aids sold are purchased by adults over the age of 60 years (e.g., Strom, 2006). This is most likely the case elsewhere around the world as well. As a result, a chapter in this book devoted to the review of the evidence on the effectiveness of hearing aids in adults is very appropriate. As discussed in Chapter 1, effectiveness refers to the impact of an intervention applied to an average population under average conditions, that is, in the "real world." A separate chapter (Chapter 5) is devoted to a similar topic, but for children wearing hearing aids. In addition, the focus here is on the overall effectiveness of hearing aids, relative to communication without hearing aids, rather than comparisons of technologies, such as omnidirectional versus directional microphones. The evidence underlying various technology comparisons is the subject of Chapter 6.

How does one document the effectiveness of hearing aids in adults? Most would probably answer this question very generally by indicating that one needs to obtain measures of the helpfulness or benefit of hearing aids. Others might argue that one should measure things like "satisfaction" or hearing aid "usage" to study effectiveness. Still others might define this in terms of the hearing aid wearer's ability to overcome activity limitations and participation restrictions imposed by the hearing loss. Even if there were consensus with regard to the types of measures to be obtained, there still may not be agreement among researchers or clinicians as to what actually should be measured and how it should be measured. For example, for measures of helpfulness or benefit, should these be so-called "objective" measures of benefit, based on the perception of standardized lists of words or sentences with and without the hearing aid, or "subjective" self-report measures of benefit obtained using a variety of standardized questionnaires? Thus, to study the effectiveness of hearing aids, most might argue for the use of some type of outcome measure to demonstrate effectiveness, but there is considerable uncertainty regarding which measures to include, as well as the number and type of such measures.

Another central issue to the study of hearing aid effectiveness is the need for knowledge regarding when to obtain outcome measures. Although this has probably received less attention than the issue of what to measure, several studies have focused on when such outcome measures should be obtained.

The first portion of this chapter overviews several critical measurement issues that must be addressed when assessing the effectiveness of hearing aids in older adults. First, we summarize a series of research studies from our laboratory at Indiana University that has focused specifically on the issues of *what* to measure regarding hearing aid outcomes and *when* to obtain those measures. With regard to what should be measured, there are often several choices as to *how* those outcomes should be measured and this is discussed as well. After this brief review, the results of a thorough review of the existing evidence regarding the effectiveness of hearing aids in adults is presented.

WHAT TO MEASURE

Research at Indiana University conducted over the past 15 years on outcome measures has been updated, reviewed, and summarized on various occasions, the most recent being a comparison of technologies by Humes, Ahlstrom, Bratt, and Peek (2009a) and Humes, Wilson, and Thompson (2009b). A hallmark of each of the studies conducted at Indiana University was that each made use of a reasonably sized sample of older adults wearing hearing aids and multiple outcome measures were obtained from each participant. In some early studies, for example, as many as 20 outcome measures were obtained (Humes, 2001; Humes, Garner, Wilson, & Barlow, 2001). Across all of these studies (Humes, 2001, 2003, 2007; Humes et al., 2001, 2002a, 2002b, 2004, 2009a), although additional supplemental outcome measures may have been incorporated in some studies and not others, a standard core test battery of outcome was shared across all of these studies. These 11 outcome measures included the four scales of the Hearing Aid Performance Inventory (HAPI; Walden, Demorest, & Hepler, 1984), three of the scales of the Glasgow Hearing Aid Benefit Profile (Gatehouse, 1999), a very slight modification of the MarkeTrak V hearing aid satisfaction survey (HASS) (Humes et al., 2001; Kochkin, 2000), a measure of hearing aid usage obtained from daily entries into a hearing aid diary, and aided and unaided measures of speech understanding obtained via the Connected Speech Test (CST; Cox, Alexander, & Gilmore, 1987) with the speech signal presented at 65 dB SPL from a loudspeaker at 0-degrees azimuth and the multitalker babble competition presented at 57dB SPL from a loudspeaker at 180-degrees azimuth.

This common battery of outcome measures was employed across several different studies at Indiana University in recent years, each with a different hearing aid technology, and the analysis of matched groups of at least 50 hearing aid wearers selected for across-technology comparisons failed to reveal significant group differences in outcome (Humes et al., 2004, 2009a). We recently extended such comparisons of group performance across technologies to 35 adults fitted with open-fit, six-channel, directional behind-the-ear devices (Humes et al., 2009b). The primary difference between this group of 35 participants and each of the groups of about 50 participants fitted with other technologies and described in Humes et al. (2009a) was that the open-fit group had about 4 to 10 dB better hearing thresholds in the higher frequencies (2000–8000 Hz) than the other groups (consistent with fitting guidelines). Except for aided speech-recognition performance, there were no group differences in outcome for the additional group of 35 open-fit hearing aid wearers compared to the other four groups fit with different technologies. Moreover, given the incorporation of directional microphones into the open-fit behind-the-ear devices and the spatial arrangement of the speech and competing babble, differences in aided speech recognition were expected.

Given the minimal differences in outcome observed across technologies for this series of Indiana University studies, the data were pooled across studies. All told, the dataset available by pooling the data from these four Indiana University studies results in a total sample of N = 368 participants, each with the same core battery of 11 outcome measures available for analysis. Of the 368 participants, 67% were male and 66% were first-time hearing aid users, both of which appear to be typical of the US population of hearing aid purchasers over a comparable time period (Kochkin, 2009). In addition, they ranged in age from 60 to 89 years with a mean age of 73.9 years, had high-frequency (1000, 2000, and 4000 Hz) pure-tone averages of 49.8 dB HL when averaged for the right and left ears combined, and scored 64.7% unaided on the CST for the standard test condition (speech at 65 dB SPL, signal-to-noise ratio of +8 dB).

It also should be noted that, in addition to a common core battery of outcome measures, several other aspects of the test protocols in each of the Indiana University studies were shared across studies. For example, all hearing aid fittings were bilateral, which is also typical of hearing aid fittings in the United States over this same time period (Kochkin, 2009). In addition, in every study, real-ear measurements were used to adjust the frequency-gain characteristics to targets, within typical clinical tolerances (typical root-mean-square error between target and obtained real-ear gain of 4 to 8 dB; Humes et al., 2004). Furthermore, all of the outcome measures were obtained at 4 to 6 weeks postfit (plus other postfit intervals beyond this in some studies, as noted below). Following the initial fitting and delivery of the devices to the wearer, including an initial hearing aid orientation, participants returned for one additional session about midway between the fitting session and the measurement of outcomes 4 to 6 weeks postfit. This intermediate session included additional hearing aid counseling and the collection of some baseline measures for hearing aid outcomes. Finally, in all of the Indiana University studies, the hearing aid wearer purchased the devices from the Indiana University clinic at the normal clinic price and in accordance with normal clinical policies, but then was paid for his or her participation in the subsequent follow-up sessions.

Factor analysis was used to reduce the redundancy in this set of outcome measures and to identify various dimensions of hearing aid outcome (Humes, 1999, 2003). Given the high subjects-to-variables ratio (368:11), an excellent factor solution was obtained with three oblique (correlated) principal components accounting for 74.6% of the variance, KMO measure of sampling adequacy = 0.87, and communalities all above 0.7, except for the CST benefit measure (communality = 0.59) (Gorsuch, 1983). The component weights resulted in easily interpreted factors.

The component weights (from the pattern matrix) for each of the three factors identified in the solution and each of the 11 outcome measures are shown in Figure 4–1. All of the "helpfulness" ratings and satisfaction ratings were weighted heavily on the first factor and this has been interpreted as "benefaction," a combination of self-reported benefit and satisfaction. The second factor identified was interpreted as hearing aid usage because both measures of usage were weighted heavily on this factor (component weights less than 0.35 are not shown in Figure 4–1 for clarity). Interestingly, the measure of objective benefit, or the difference in aided and unaided

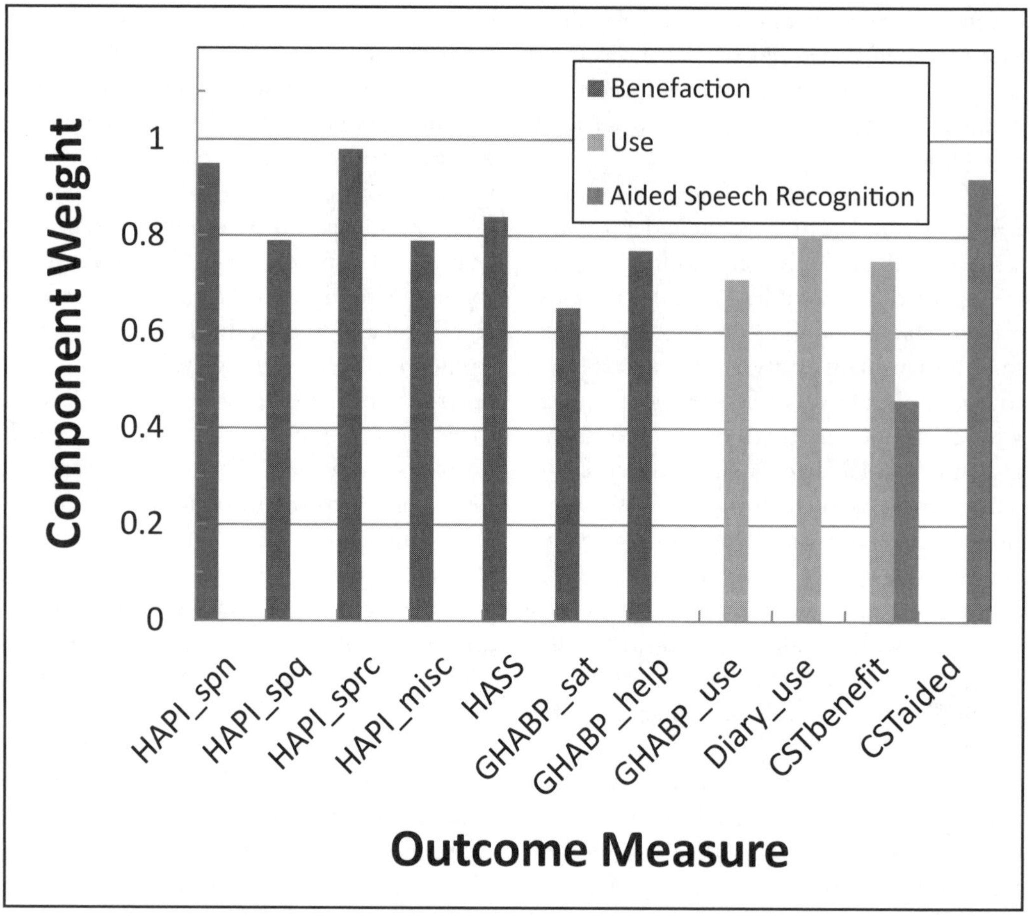

Figure 4–1. *Component weights for each of the 11 hearing aid outcome measures on each of the resulting three factors in the best-fitting principal-components factor analysis for the pooled data set from several Indiana University studies (N = 368). HAPI_spn = speech-in-noise subscale of HAPI; HAPI_spq = speech-in-quiet subscale of HAPI; HAPI_sprc = speech with reduced cues subscale of HAPI; HAPI_misc = miscellaneous subscale of HAPI; GHABP_sat = satisfaction subscale of GHABP; GHABP_help = helpfulness subscale of GHABP; GHABP_use = usage subscale of GHABP; Diary_use = hours of usage recorded in daily diary or log; CST_benefit = aided CST score minus unaided CST score; CST_aided = aided CST score.*

CST scores, is also weighted most heavily on this factor, as well as the third factor. Also, it should be noted that the correlation between the first two factors was $r = 0.47$, which suggests a moderate association between benefaction and usage. Finally, the third component or dimension of hearing aid outcome is interpreted as aided speech-recognition performance as the aided CST score is the most heavily weighted outcome variable for this factor, with moderate weighting of the CST benefit measure on this factor as well. The correlation of this factor with the other two factors was below $r = 0.12$ in both cases, suggesting that this outcome dimension is largely independent of the other two.

The foregoing factor analyses of the outcome measures from 368 older hearing aid wearers with mild to moderate hearing loss collected across a wide range of hearing aid technologies are important in that three separate and somewhat independent dimensions of hearing aid outcome were identified. Thus, the most complete evaluation of the effectiveness of hearing aids in older adults should include at least three types of measures: (1) self-reported benefit or satisfaction (but both unnecessary); (2) self-reported usage; and (3) aided speech understanding for representative listening conditions. It is quite possible, for example, to demonstrate effectiveness in one outcome domain without necessarily demonstrating it in the other two domains. In that sense, studies with multiple outcome measures tapping each of these three dimensions offer the most complete assessment of hearing aid effectiveness.

HOW TO MEASURE OUTCOME

The brief overview of research on what to measure with regard to hearing aid outcomes identified three key dimensions, but makes no statement as to how performance on each dimension should be measured. This issue concerns not only which specific test or tests should be used to measure performance for each of the three outcome dimensions, but also the nature of the tests to be used. Of course, at a minimum, the tests to be used must be both reliable and valid measures of the desired outcome dimension. For each outcome dimension to be measured, there are several such measures available. For benefaction, the choices include not only those already noted when describing the core battery in the Indiana University studies (HAPI; GHABP; MarkeTrak/HASS), but also measures of satisfaction, such as Satisfaction with Amplification in Daily Living (SADL; Cox & Alexander, 1999), and benefit, such as the Abbreviated Profile of Hearing Aid Benefit (APHAB; Cox & Alexander, 1995) or the Client-Oriented Scale of Improvement (COSI; Dillon, James, & Ginis, 1997). With regard to usage, the GHABP contains an item on the portion of each day the hearing aid is used and we have made use of daily diaries to log the number of hours of usage as well. Such self-report measures of usage have been validated via objective measures of usage, such as those available in the data-logging feature of hearing aids (e.g., Humes et al., 1996). Finally, another outcome-assessment tool that has emerged more recently, and has been translated into several different languages, is the International Outcome Inventory for Hearing Aids (IOI-HA; Cox, Stephens, & Kramer, 2002; Cox, Alexander, & Beyer, 2003). This 7-item survey assesses helpfulness and usage, as well as other dimensions not typically included in other outcome measures for hearing aids, such as impact on one's enjoyment of life. Factor analyses of IOI-HA data have typically identified two factors underlying survey responses (wearer's introspection about hearing aids and influence of hearing aids on wearer's interactions with outside world; Cox & Alexander, 2002).

Regardless of the particular tool selected to quantify the dimensions of benefaction and usage via self-report surveys, one of the challenges is the interpretation of those scores. Although some of the measures are designed to be administered pre- and postfit, this is often not the case. Rather, the hearing aid wearer is asked to think back in time, considering their earlier unaided experiences, then judge whether the hearing aid has improved or helped performance relative to the earlier unaided experiences. Gatehouse (1994) and Dillon et al. (1997) have reviewed the pros and cons regarding various options for the administration of self-report hearing aid outcome measures. For the many self-report surveys of hearing aid outcome that have been used in a postfit only administration format, the results are often interpreted relative to normative data from a large sample of (presumably) similar hearing aid wearers. One can then compare the performance of another individual or group of individuals to those normative data to determine if the person or group is performing "better than average," "worse than average," and so forth. The challenge, however, is in translating such comparisons to normative data into either positive or negative outcomes. For example, assume that average helpfulness and satisfaction ratings for hearing aid performance in background noise are quite low in the normative sample, if the wearer or group of wearers yields "typical" or "average" performance, is that a positive outcome? What if even "above average" ratings, but still relatively low helpfulness and satisfaction ratings, are observed, is that a positive outcome?

Assessing benefaction and usage using a pre- and postfitting assessment would at least permit the possibility of examining improvement within participants. Here, however, as in other repeated-measures designs, there are issues of learning, practice, familiarization, fatigue, and boredom that may bias the second assessment relative to the first. Equivalent forms must often be developed and evaluated. This approach makes most sense when using scales that assess communication or handicap pre- and postfit, rather than surveys specifically designed for the evaluation of hearing aids. For example, the use of the Hearing Handicap Inventory for the Elderly (HHIE) (Ventry & Weinstein, 1982) enables a general assessment of hearing handicap and instructions can request that the patient base his or her responses on the recent past: unaided function for the prefit assessment and aided function for the postfit assessment. Likewise, the APHAB tabulates the "frequency of problems" for auditory experiences and can be completed both before and after the hearing aid fit. Use of control groups, who receive the same schedule of repeated assessment, but no intervention, are recommended for studies relying on self-report measures as the occurrence of "response shifts" can occur between test and retest (Joore, Potjewijd, Timmerman, & Anteunis, 2002; Schwartz & Sprangers, 1999). It is not always possible or realistic, however, to test control groups on many of the outcome measures of interest. For example, it makes no sense for a control group, not fitted with hearing aids, to complete assessments of hearing aid benefit or helpfulness, such as the HAPI or GHABP, or to complete measures of hearing aid satisfaction, such as MarkeTrak/HASS or SADL, or to complete measures of hearing aid usage, if they are not actually fitted with hearing aids.

Interpretation of aided speech-understanding alone is also problematic. As a result, most commonly, prefit and postfit measures of speech understanding are obtained and the change in performance is evaluated. Although this measure is "objective" in the sense that responses to various standardized tests of speech understanding can be scored as correct or incorrect, the use of a prefit/postfit design introduces all of the same potential confounding factors noted for the self-report measures. Thus, availability of equivalent forms and the use of a control group are also important factors to consider with regard to how outcomes should be obtained. Another important factor here, however, has to do with the validity of the test conditions. Walden (1997) provided a nice review and discussion of some of the choices to consider here. Basically, one needs to use stimuli, both the speech signal and the competition, that are representative of everyday listening while still yielding reliable scores. As noted by Walden (1997), there often is a lack of consensus with regard to the single set of test conditions that would be most representative, which then necessitates the use of multiple test conditions. Walden (1997), for example, suggests speech levels of 50, 60, and 70 dBA, paired with background conditions of +10 dB, +5 dB, and +2 dB signal-to-noise ratio, respectively; spanning a range of expected everyday listening conditions. He also recommends the use of the CST, as this test makes use of passages, each composed of a series of sentences with key words to be scored, with each sentence in a given passage tied to the same common topic (gloves, umbrellas, etc.). The test is administered in a background of multitalker babble as well. Again, the notion is to construct a reliable and standardized assessment of aided speech understanding that is believed to be representative of many everyday listening situations for the hearing aid wearer.

In addition to the use of control groups without hearing aids to assess the effects of repeated administrations of the outcome measures, another effective design in other health-related intervention studies has been the use of placebo groups. Given the reliance on a number of self-report measures to document at least two of the three dimensions of outcome (benefaction and usage), the need for a placebo group is critical (e.g., Beecher, 1955; Roberts, Kewman, Mercier, & Hovell, 1993). What is envisioned here with regard to a placebo device would be a fully functional and physically identical hearing aid, but programmed to provide 0 dB insertion gain from 250 through 6000 Hz; that is, restoring the lost pinna and ear canal resonances only. Alternatively, an open-fit device modeled after a placebo tinnitus masker used in an ongoing clinical trial in the United States (Formby & Hawley-Kaczka, 2009) would appear to be a feasible option for hearing aid research as well. Although it would appear to be relatively easy to implement placebo groups in studies of hearing aid efficacy and effectiveness, our review of the literature was unable to discover a single study that made use of a placebo group.

In summary, even if there is consensus regarding what should be measured to document the effectiveness of hearing aids in adults, there are still many choices and potential factors that can influence outcome with regard to how performance is quantified in each of these dimensions. For the most part, in the review to follow, most studies made use of postfit only self-report measures without the inclusion of control or placebo groups.

WHEN TO MEASURE OUTCOME

Aside from *what* should be measured with regard to hearing aid outcome and *how* it should be measured, another important practical issue regarding hearing aid outcome measures is *when* they should be obtained from the wearer. The research conducted at Indiana University represents, to our knowledge, both the largest data set available on the longitudinal changes in hearing aid outcome, with multiple measurement intervals over a period of 1 year (N = 134) and 2 years (N = 47), and also the longest postfit period of examination (3 years, N = 9) (Humes et al., 2002a, 2002b; Humes & Wilson, 2003). From these and other data (e.g., Saunders & Cienkowski, 1997; Surr, Cord, & Walden, 1998; Turner, Humes, Bentler, & Cox, 1996), it can be concluded that valid and reliable communication-related hearing aid outcome measures, such as aided speech understanding, can be obtained at 4 to 6 weeks postfit. However, other types of measures, such as some measures of self-reported benefit and satisfaction, may require 3 to 6 months for outcomes to stabilize (e.g., Humes et al., 2002b; Mulrow, Tuley, & Aguilar, 1992). Thus, for these measures, a postfit interval of at least 6 months may be desirable for the examination of "long-term" outcomes. As a result, as noted in the review of existing evidence, the majority of data available on the effectiveness of hearing aids in adults concern the measurement of short-term outcomes, rather than long term. Importantly, however, all evidence reviewed below was obtained at least 4 weeks postfit.

THE EVIDENCE BASE

Methods

A systematized review (see Chapter 2) was undertaken to examine the evidence base with regard to hearing aid effectiveness in adults. This began with an online search on the Medline subset of PubMed using the keywords: hearing aid, outcome, and adults. Limits were placed on the search to restrict results to journal articles that were published since 1990 in English and dealt with humans, specifically adults (defined by PubMed as those at or above the age of 19 years). This initial search yielded a total of 783 articles. The titles of these articles were reviewed by the second author. Those that were not related to hearing aid outcomes in adults or that dealt with special clinical populations were removed, resulting in a total of 165 articles. The abstracts of the remaining articles were examined further by both authors and those articles that did not measure subjective (self-report) or objective (speech-understanding) outcomes for hearing aids wearers were removed. As the focus here was on aided versus unaided effects, those articles that specifically dealt with technology comparisons with limited publication of unaided baseline measures were sorted into a separate group not considered here, leaving 33 articles of interest that dealt with subjective and or objective measures of hearing aid outcomes relating to hearing aid benefit, satisfaction, or usage. Original articles subsequently were downloaded and reviewed in detail.

Review of the Evidence

Five of the 33 articles were noted by the chapter's authors to have a randomized controlled trial design (Level 2 evidence, Table 1–5) and were categorized as such. Two were randomized controlled studies that were not blinded, two made use of double blinding, and a third was a randomized single-blind study. However, for two of the three randomized controlled studies, it was not the treatment that was randomized. In one case (Larson et al., 2000), it was the treatment sequence in a crossover design that was randomized, but there were no control or placebo groups incorporated with random assignment to these groups. This was because the focus in that study was on the comparison of aided benefits across technologies more than the effectiveness of any of the technologies. Likewise, another randomized controlled study (Metselaar et al., 2009) randomized the prescription or fitting process received by the patients, but not the treatment (hearing aids vs. no hearing aids or placebo devices). Only one study (Yueh et al., 2001) truly pursued a randomized controlled trial (Level 2 evidence, Table 1–5; Grade A research quality, Table 1–6) of hearing aid intervention, including the use of a control group, although no placebo group was incorporated. Most of the remaining 30 articles were classified as "nonrandomized intervention" studies (Level 3 evidence, Table 1–5; Grade B research quality, Table 1–6).

The review of the evidence from these 33 articles on hearing aid effectiveness is organized below according to the outcome dimension investigated. In some cases, the same study appears in multiple tables as multiple outcomes were obtained in that study. As noted previously, three primary dimensions of hearing aid outcome have emerged from existing research: benefaction, usage, and aided speech understanding. Evidence from the literature regarding the effectiveness of hearing aids for each of these dimensions of outcome are reviewed separately. However, as indicated below, one particular outcome measure, the IOI-HA, has received considerable attention in recent years and is difficult to categorize along any of the three dimensions of outcome. Although it includes measures of benefaction and usage, it also includes other measures not encompassed by these dimensions. As a result, it was decided to review the evidence with regard to the effectiveness of hearing aids in adults separately for this outcome measure. We begin, however, with review of the outcome dimension for which there is the greatest volume of evidence: benefaction.

Benefaction

Table 4–1 provides brief summaries of the 27 studies of hearing aid effectiveness, listed in chronological order, that made use of self-report measures of satisfaction, benefit, or both. This is the largest volume of evidence for any one of the outcome dimensions and no doubt reflects both a fundamental interest in the "helpfulness" of hearing aids and the users' satisfaction with those devices. It also is a likely outcome of pooling studies of satisfaction and benefit; dimensions probably believed to be independent at the time of study. Although there were many procedural differences across studies and a wide range of outcome measures employed, when and how benefaction was measured was appropriate, based on the considerations reviewed earlier in this chapter. The results obtained are very similar across studies. If a pre- and postfitting outcome measure was employed, such as the HHIE, the COSI, the Profile of Hearing Aid Benefit (PHAB), or the APHAB, significant improvements were noted from unaided to aided listening. If norm-based outcome measures were used, such as the HAPI, GHABP, Marke Trak/HASS, or SADL, then mean ratings consistent with "helpful" and "satisfied" were observed. These generally positive findings, however, must be qualified by noting that the majority of the data are from older adults with mild to moderate or mild to severe sloping hearing loss fitted with bilateral hearing aids that were adjusted to gain targets via real-ear measurements. Thus, similar conclusions may not apply to other populations or protocols.

Usage

Table 4–2 summarizes 12 studies of hearing aid effectiveness with hearing aid usage as the outcome measure. All of the studies only provide descriptive, self-report ratings obtained from the hearing aid wearers. In general, the studies indicate that most of the wearers in these studies wore their hearing aids at least 4 hours/day, with many wearing their hearing aids 8 hours/day. For several studies that made use of the GHABP, the typical rating for usage reflected hearing aid use corresponding to "about three-quarters of the time." As was the case for benefaction, these observations must be qualified by noting that the majority of the data are from older adults with mild to moderate or mild to severe sloping hearing loss fitted with bilateral hearing aids that were adjusted to gain targets via real-ear measurements.

Table 4–1. Summaries of 27 Studies of Hearing Aid Effectiveness that Made Use of Benefit, Satisfaction, or Both as Outcome Measures

Author(s)	*N*	*Mean Age*	*Degree and Configuration of Hearing Loss*	*Unilateral/ Bilateral Fits*	*Real-Ear Verification*	*Research Design*	*Outcome Measures*	*Overall Results*
Mulrow et al. (1992)	192	72	Mean HFPTA = 52 dB HL	97% Unilateral	Not reported	Nonrandomized intervention study	HHIE, QDS, GDS, SPMSQ	HHIE and all QOL measures improved significantly from prefit to 4 months postfit and benefits were sustained through 12 months for all but the cognitive measure (SPMSQ).
Bentler et al. (1993)	65	64	Various: Mild flat to mild to profound steeply sloping	85% Unilateral; 15% Bilateral	Yes	Nonrandomized intervention study	HPI, satisfaction questionnaire	HPI: Mean data indicate "frequently" could understand speech, music, etc. Satisfaction questionnaire: Mean data suggest "moderately satisfied" to "very satisfied" with hearing aids.
Humes et al. (1996)	20	72	Mild to severe sloping	Bilateral	Yes	Nonrandomized intervention study	HHIE, HAPI, satisfaction survey	Significant reduction in hearing handicap (HHIE) with hearing aids. HAPI: overall, "helpful" to "very helpful" ratings. Satisfaction survey: overall, "satisfied."

Author(s)	*N*	*Mean Age*	*Degree and Configuration of Hearing Loss*	*Unilateral/ Bilateral Fits*	*Real-Ear Verification*	*Research Design*	*Outcome Measures*	*Overall Results*
Humes et al. (1997)	110	25–90	Various: Mild to moderate gently sloping to moderately-severe gently sloping	Bilateral	Yes	Randomized double-blind study	MELE, HAPI	No significant differences in aided performance between the two processing schemes; aided performance in both cases were better than unaided scores.
Jerram & Purdy (1997)	197	70	Not reported	51% Unilateral	Not reported	Nonrandomized intervention study	SHAPI	Overall mean rating higher than comparable studies, indicating lower hearing aid benefit level; mean rating positively correlated with subject age but not with weekly hours of use.
Dillon et al. (1997)	98	71	Median better-ear PTA = ~30 dB HL	Mix	Yes	Nonrandomized intervention study	COSI, HHIE, MPHAB, SHAPIE, HAUQ, satisfaction scales	COSI: Overall mean change score consistent with "better" or "much better" response. Significant changes in HHIE from unaided to aided. Most of remaining analyses correlational among outcome measures.
Walden et al. (1998)	40	66	Mild to moderately severe sloping	Bilateral	Yes	Nonrandomized intervention study	PHAB	Aided PHAB ratings significantly better than unaided for all PHAB subscales.

continues

Table 4–1. *continued*

Author(s)	*N*	*Mean Age*	*Degree and Configuration of Hearing Loss*	*Unilateral/ Bilateral Fits*	*Real-Ear Verification*	*Research Design*	*Outcome Measures*	*Overall Results*
Dillon et al. (1999)	4,421	76	Median better-ear PTA = ~30 dB HL	Not reported	Not reported	Retrospective analysis	COSI, HAUQ (including satisfaction & usage)	COSI: Overall mean change score consistent with "better" or "much better" response—89% with mean improvement of "better" and 40% with mean improvement of "much better." Residual hearing midway between hearing "most of the time" and "all of the time." HAUQ: average of "helpful" and "satisfied" ratings.
Humes et al. (1999)	55	>18	Various: Mild to moderate gently sloping to moderately severe gently sloping	Bilateral	Yes	Nonrandomized intervention study	HAPI	Mean ratings of "helpful" on HAPI for both hearing aid circuits.
Walden et al. (1999)	40	66	Mild to moderate sloping	Bilateral	Yes	Nonrandomized intervention study	PHAB	Aided PHAB ratings significantly better than unaided for all PHAB subscales

Author(s)	*N*	*Mean Age*	*Degree and Configuration of Hearing Loss*	*Unilateral/ Bilateral Fits*	*Real-Ear Verification*	*Research Design*	*Outcome Measures*	*Overall Results*
Hosford-Dunn & Halpern (2000)	361	76	Mild to severe sloping	64% Bilateral	Most cases, at follow-up	Nonrandomized intervention study	SADL	Psychometric properties of SADL are verified; PCA identified 4 main domains: Benefit/Value, followed by Service/Cost domains. Telephone use accounted for most of the variance in the data and was also item with lowest satisfaction rating
Larson et al. (2000)	360	67	Mild to severe sloping	Bilateral	Yes	Randomized double-blind study	PHAP/ PHAB	Each of three hearing aid circuits significantly reduced the frequency of problems on 6 of the 7 PHAB subscales.
Humes et al. (2001)	173	73	Mild to severe sloping	Bilateral	Yes	Nonrandomized intervention study	HAPI, HHIE, MarkeTrak-IV, HASS, GHABP, precursor to GHABP	Significant reduction in hearing handicap (HHIE) with hearing aids. Average ratings of "satisfied" for satisfaction scales and "helpful" for benefit scales.

continues

Table 4–1. *continued*

Author(s)	*N*	*Mean Age*	*Degree and Configuration of Hearing Loss*	*Unilateral/ Bilateral Fits*	*Real-Ear Verification*	*Research Design*	*Outcome Measures*	*Overall Results*
Yueh et al. (2001)	60	4 groups of 15; means 67–72	Mild to moderate sloping	Bilateral	Yes	Randomized controlled study	HHIE, APHAB	Significant reduction in hearing handicap (HHIE) with hearing aids. Significant reduction in frequency of problems on several APHAB subscales with hearing aids. No differences on these measures for control group or ALD group (except for background noise subscale for ALD group).
Cox & Alexander (2001)	196	70	Mild to severe sloping	Bilateral	Not reported	Nonrandomized intervention study	SADL, separate satisfaction rating	SADL and satisfaction rating consistent with average responses of "satisfied." True for SADL global and subscale scores, except for the Negative Features subscale which equated to "neutral" or "dissatisfied."

Author(s)	*N*	*Mean Age*	*Degree and Configuration of Hearing Loss*	*Unilateral/ Bilateral Fits*	*Real-Ear Verification*	*Research Design*	*Outcome Measures*	*Overall Results*
Humes et al. (2002)	134	73	Mild to severe sloping	Bilateral	Yes	Nonrandomized intervention study	HASS, GHABP, HADBI	Mean data support overall rating of "satisfied" on satisfaction measures and "helpful" for benefit measures. Some small, but statistically significant decreases were noted over first 6 months.
Humes et al. (2004)	53	74	Mild to severe sloping	Bilateral	Yes	Nonrandomized intervention study	HAPI, HHIE, HASS, GHABP, HDABI	Both devices provided significant benefit to wearers; no significant differences in benefits provided by either device at 1- or 6-month postfit intervals.
Stark & Hickson (2004)	93 hearing impaired; 78 significant others	72 hearing impaired; 64 significant others	Various: 81% with PTA from mild to moderate; 19% with mild loss	55% Unilateral	Yes	Nonrandomized intervention study	HHIE and SF-36; significant others completed Quantified Denver Scale and SF-36	Significant reduction in hearing handicap (HHIE) with amplification. With one exception for hearing-impaired person, no significant improvements in health-related QOL (SFS-36) were noted for either hearing-impaired or significant other.

continues

Table 4–1. *continued*

Author(s)	*N*	*Mean Age*	*Degree and Configuration of Hearing Loss*	*Unilateral/ Bilateral Fits*	*Real-Ear Verification*	*Research Design*	*Outcome Measures*	*Overall Results*
McArdle et al. (2005)	380	69	Mild to severe sloping	Bilateral	Yes	Randomized controlled study	WHO-DAS II, APHAB, HHIE	Significant effects of hearing aids on WHO-DAS II, APHAB and HHIE; larger for latter two hearing-specific measures.
McPherson & Wong (2005)	19	73	Mild to moderate; configuration not reported	Unilateral	Yes	Nonrandomized intervention study	COSI, PHAP-C	COSI results showed that hearing difficulty for participants was "better" or "slightly better" with trial device than in unaided condition. PHAP-C results showed that participants infrequently experienced difficulty in everyday listening situations when wearing their device.
Uriarte et al. (2005)	1,014	75	40 dB HL PTA in better ear	55% Bilateral	Yes	Nonrandomized intervention study	SADL and CSS (Client Satisfaction Survey)	Global SADL = 5.27 (out of 7). From CSS, ~75% reported at least "moderate help" from hearing aid.

Author(s)	*N*	*Mean Age*	*Degree and Configuration of Hearing Loss*	*Unilateral/ Bilateral Fits*	*Real-Ear Verification*	*Research Design*	*Outcome Measures*	*Overall Results*
Cox et al. (2005)	151 VA; 79 PP	72 (VA); 75 (PP)	Mild to severe sloping in both groups	VA: 99% Bilateral; PP: 85% Bilateral	Unclear	Nonrandomized intervention study	HHIE, SHAPIE, SADL	Significant benefit, unaided to aided, for both groups on HHIE and APHAB. SHAPIE shows mean scores of "helpful" for both groups. Overall, "satisfaction" with hearing aids reported for both groups.
Noble and Gatehouse (2006)	274	67	Moderate to severe; configuration not reported	74% Unilateral	Presumably yes; equipment and protocol in place, but no records	Nonrandomized intervention study	SSQ	Significant improvements on the SSQ for one aid, two aids, or both on a total of 80% of the 50 listening situations included.
Takahashi et al. (2007)	164	73	Mild to severe sloping	Bilateral	Yes	Nonrandomized intervention study	PHAP/ PHAB, GHABP, SADL	Significant improvement from unaided to aided for PHAP, GHABP; ~70% indicated hearing aid at least "quite helpful," ~90% were at least "reasonably satisfied." Global SADL ~ 5.5 on 7-point scale.

continues

Table 4–1. *continued*

Author(s)	*N*	*Mean Age*	*Degree and Configuration of Hearing Loss*	*Unilateral/ Bilateral Fits*	*Real-Ear Verification*	*Research Design*	*Outcome Measures*	*Overall Results*
Smith et al. (2008)	304	4 groups; Means range from 63 to 73	Mild to moderate PTA	~50% Bilateral	"Whenever possible"	Nonrandomized intervention study	GHABP	Corrected GHABP benefit scores of 60–70% on a 0–100% scale. Significantly greater benefit noted for bilateral fitting than for those fitted unilaterally.
Metselaar et al. (2009)	254	71	31–102 dB HL; Mean HFPTA = 58 dB HL	77% Bilateral	Yes	Randomized double-blind study	HHDI, GDS, EQ-5D, APHAB	Hearing aid fitting had positive impact on self-reported disability and handicap associated with hearing loss.
Johnson et al. (2010)	154	74	Self-report only; moderate to moderately severe	Not reported	Not reported	Nonrandomized intervention study	APHAB	Significant benefit, unaided to aided.

List of Abbreviations and Acronyms: ALD = Assistive Listening Device; APHAB = Abbreviated Profile of Hearing Aid Benefit; COSI = Client Oriented Scale of Improvement; CSS = Client Satisfaction Survey (Uriarte et al., 2005); EQ-5D = European Quality of Life-5-dimensions; GDS = Geriatric Depression Scale (Yesavage, Brink, & Rose, 1983); GHABP = Glasgow Hearing Aid Benefit Profile; HADBI = Hearing Aid Disability and Benefit Inventory; HAPI = Hearing Aid Performance Inventory; HASS = Hearing Aid Satisfaction Survey; HAUQ = Hearing Aid Users' Questionnaire (Forster & Tomlin, 1988); HFPTA = High-Frequency Pure-Tone Average (1, 2, & 4 kHz); HHDI = Hearing Handicap and Disability Inventory (WHO, 2001); HHIE = Hearing Handicap Inventory for the Elderly; HPI = Hearing Performance Inventory (Giolas, Owens, Lamb, & Schubert, 1979); MELE = Magnitude Estimation of Listening Effort; MPHAB = Modified Profile of Hearing Aid Benefit (Dillon, James, & Ginis, 1997); PCA = Principal Component Analysis; PHAB = Profile of Hearing Aid Benefit (Cox & Gilmore, 1990); PHAP/PHAB = Profile of Hearing Aid Performance/ Profile of Hearing Aid Benefit; PHAP-C = Profile of Hearing Aid Performance—Chinese version; PP = Private Practice; PTA = Pure-Tone Average (0.5,1, & 2 kHz); QD S= Quantified Denver Scale of Communication Function (Alpiner, 1982; Tuley et al., 1990); SADL = Satisfaction with Amplification in Daily Life; SF-36 = Quality of Life (Short Form-36); SHAPI = Shortened Hearing Aid Performance Inventory (Schum, 1992); SHAPIE = Shortened Hearing Aid Performance Inventory for the Elderly (Dillon, 1994); SPMSQ = Short Portable Mental Status Questionnaire (Pfeiffer, 1975); SSQ = Speech, Spatial and Qualities of Hearing Scale (Gatehouse & Noble, 2004); VA = Veterans Affairs; WHO-DAS II = World Health Organization's Disability Assessment Scale II (WHO, 2001).

Table 4–2. Summaries of 12 Studies of Hearing Aid Effectiveness with Hearing Aid Usage as the Outcome Measure

Author(s)	*N*	*Mean Age*	*Degree and Configuration of Hearing Loss*	*Unilateral/ Bilateral Fit*	*Real-Ear Verification*	*Research Design*	*Outcome Measures*	*Overall Results*
Bentler et al. (1993)	65	64	Various: Mild flat to mild to profound steeply sloping	85% Unilateral; 15% Bilateral	Yes	Nonrandomized intervention study	Use-time questionnaire	Mean use-time exceeded 6 hours/day at 12 months postfit.
Humes et al. (1996)	20	72	Mild to severe sloping	Bilateral	Yes	Nonrandomized intervention study	Datalogging and daily diary	Diary: about 11 hours/day; Datalogger: about 8 hours/day.
Humes et al. (1997)	110	25–90; No additional details	Various: Mild to moderate gently sloping to moderately severe gently sloping	Bilateral	Yes	Randomized double-blind study	Daily logs	Mean use of 7.7 hours/day. Severe group about 9 hours/day. Mild and moderate groups about 7 hours/day.
Humes et al. (1999)	55	>18; No additional details	Various: Mild to moderate gently sloping to moderately severe gently sloping	Bilateral	Yes	Nonrandomized intervention study	Daily logs	Mean use of 7.5 hours/day.

continues

Table 4–2. *continued*

Author(s)	*N*	*Mean Age*	*Degree and Configuration of Hearing Loss*	*Unilateral/ Bilateral Fit*	*Real-Ear Verification*	*Research Design*	*Outcome Measures*	*Overall Results*
Dillon et al. (1999)	4,421	76	Median better-ear PTA = ~30 dB HL	Not reported	Not reported	Retrospective analysis	Usage question from HAUQ	~60% wore aids at least 4 hrs/day.
Humes et al. (2001)	173	73	Mild to severe sloping	Bilateral	Yes	Nonrandomized intervention study	GHABP, daily diary	Diary: Mean use time of 9 hours/day in both groups. GHABP: Used hearing aid "about 3/4 of the time."
Humes et al. (2002)	134	73	Mild to severe sloping	Bilateral	Yes	Nonrandomized intervention study	GHABP, daily diary	Diary: Mean use time of about 9.5 hours/day in both groups. GHABP: Used hearing aid "about 3/4 of the time."
Humes et al. (2004)	2 groups of 53	74	Mild to severe sloping	Bilateral	Yes	Nonrandomized intervention study	GHABP, daily diary	Diary: Mean use time of about 8 hours/day in both groups. GHABP: Used hearing aid "about 3/4 of the time."
Uriarte et al. (2005)	1,014	75	40.2 dB HL PTA in better ear	55% Bilateral	Yes	Nonrandomized intervention study	SADL and CSS (Client Satisfaction Survey)	91% used their hearing aids at least 1 hour/day and ~56% at least 5 hours/day.

Author(s)	*N*	*Mean Age*	*Degree and Configuration of Hearing Loss*	*Unilateral/ Bilateral Fit*	*Real-Ear Verification*	*Research Design*	*Outcome Measures*	*Overall Results*
Cox et al. (2005)	151 VA; 79 PP	72 (VA); 75 (PP)	Mild to severe sloping; both groups	VA: 99% Bilateral; PP: 85% Bilateral	Unclear	Nonrandomized intervention study	Usage question	~80% in each group wore aids at least 4 hrs/day; average usage in each group about 8 hrs/day.
Takahashi et al. (2007)	164	73	Mild to severe sloping	Bilateral	Yes	Nonrandomized intervention study	GHABP	~60–65% wear their hearing aids at least "3/4 of the time."
Smith et al. (2008)	304	4 groups; Means range from 63–73	Mild to moderate PTA	~50% Bilateral	"Whenever possible"	Nonrandomized intervention study	Self-reported usage	About 75% of subjects use hearing aids 4 or more hours per day.

List of Abbreviations and Acronyms: CSS = Client Satisfaction Survey (Uriarte et al., 2005); GHABP = Glasgow Hearing Aid Benefit Profile; HAUQ = Hearing Aid Users' Questionnaire (Forster & Tomlin, 1988); HFPTA = High-Frequency Pure-Tone Average (1, 2, & 4 kHz); PP = Private Practice; PTA = Pure-Tone Average (0.5, 1, & 2 kHz); SADL = Satisfaction with Amplification in Daily Life; VA = Veterans Affairs.

IOI-HA

A total of 8 studies, each making use of the IOI-HA as the outcome measure, are summarized in Table 4–3. The results of most of these studies have been summarized in Figure 4–2, with the results grouped by the severity of hearing loss (mild to moderate in the top panel and moderate to severe in the bottom panel). From Figure 4–2, it is apparent that mean scores across studies are generally in the range of 3 to 4 on this 5-point scale, with differences across studies in mean ratings of 0.5 to 1 scale unit quite common. From comparisons of mean data in the top and bottom panels, it is also apparent that the ratings vary with the severity of hearing loss, as noted originally by Cox et al. (2003) and confirmed recently by Smith, Noe, and Alexander (2009). In particular, those older adults with moderate to severe hearing loss typically report greater usage and benefit than those with mild to moderate hearing loss, as well as lower scores for residual activity limitations, residual participation restrictions, and impact on others. Again, these conclusions must be tempered by the fact that these data are from fairly homogeneous subject groups, similar in age (older adults), hearing loss (mild to moderate or moderate to severe sloping), and hearing aid fitting (bilateral). This is advantageous for comparisons across studies or for pooling data, but is disadvantageous in terms of establishing the generality of these findings for adult hearing aid wearers.

Aided Speech Understanding

Table 4–4 provides brief summaries of 9 studies of aided speech understanding pertaining to the effectiveness of hearing aids in adults. To be included here, data for both unaided and aided performance had to be available. Although an assortment of speech materials was employed, the CST has been used most frequently over the past couple of decades. Subject samples were again comprised of older adults with sloping sensorineural hearing loss fitted bilaterally with real-ear verification of target gain. Although not noted in Table 4–4, various versions of the National Acoustic Laboratories (NAL) prescriptive targets were incorporated most frequently in these studies (which was also the case for the studies addressing the other outcome dimensions as well). The general pattern that emerges across these studies is that aided speech-understanding performance was found to be significantly greater than unaided performance in every study and for most conditions tested, except for test conditions employing higher speech levels (≥74 dB SPL) and low signal-to-noise ratios (<+3 dB). In the case of these (exceptional) test conditions, it was often observed that there were no significant differences between aided and unaided performance.

Table 4–3. Summaries of Studies of Hearing Aid Effectiveness that Used the IOI-HA as the Outcome Measures

Author(s)	*N*	*Mean Age*	*Degree and Configuration of Hearing Loss*	*Unilateral/ Bilateral Fit*	*Real-Ear Verification*	*Research Design*	*Overall Results*
Kramer et al. (2002)	505	64	Various: Mild to profound high frequency (1, 2, 4 kHz) hearing loss; Mean HFPTA = 67 dB HL	58% Bilateral	Not reported	Nonrandomized intervention study	See Figure 4–2.
Cox et al. (2003)	154	77	Moderate to severe sloping	79% Bilateral	Not reported	Nonrandomized intervention study	See Figure 4–2.
Olusanya (2004)	99	46 (16–89)	~1/3 profound; 1/3 severe; 1/3 moderate or moderately severe based on PTA at .5, 1, 2, & 4 kHz in better ear	Bilateral	Not reported	Nonrandomized intervention study	See Figure 4–2.
McPherson and Wong (2005)	19	73	Mild to moderate; configuration not reported	Unilateral	Yes	Nonrandomized intervention study	See Figure 4–2.
Takahashi et al. (2007)	164	73	Mild to severe sloping	Bilateral	Yes	Nonrandomized intervention study	See Figure 4–2.
Smith et al. (2008)	304	4 groups; means range from 63 to 73	Mild to moderate PTA (5, 1, 2, & 4k)	~50% Bilateral	"Whenever possible"	Nonrandomized intervention study	See Figure 4–2.
Smith et al. (2009)	131	74	Mild to severe sloping	Bilateral	Yes	Nonrandomized intervention study	See Figure 4–2.
Hickson et al. (2010)	1653	not reported, but based on distribution provided, likely in mid-70s	~1/3 mild to moderate sloping; ~1/3 mild to severe sloping	78% Bilateral	Not reported	Nonrandomized intervention study	See Figure 4–2.

List of Abbreviations and Acronyms: HFPTA = High-Frequency Pure-Tone Average (1, 2, & 4 kHz); IOI-HA = International Outcome Inventory for Hearing Aids; PP = Private Practice; PTA = Pure-Tone Average (0.5,1, & 2 kHz); VA = Veterans Affairs.

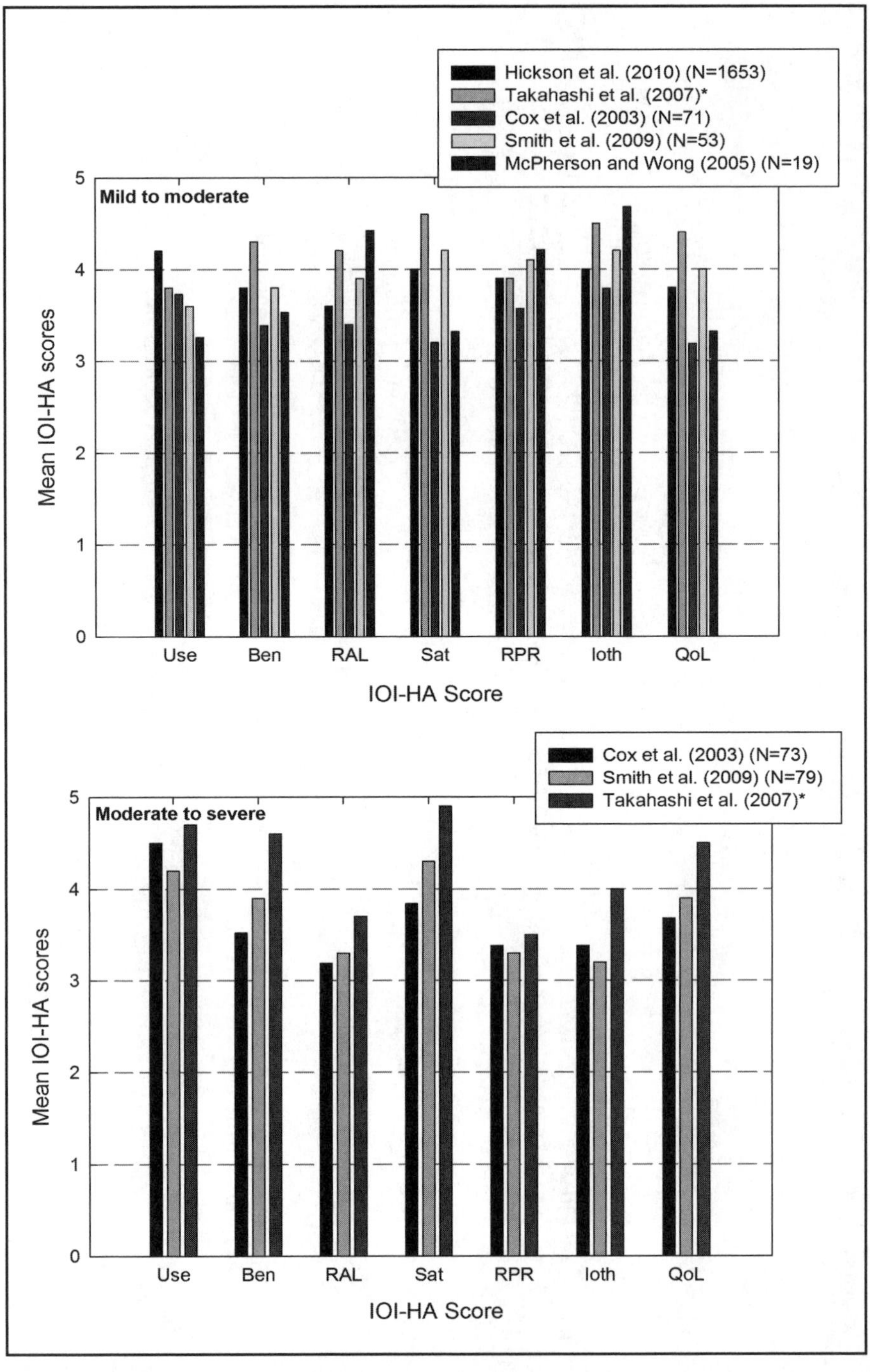

Figure 4–2. *Mean IOI-HA scores for several recent studies (see Table 4–3). Top panel pools several studies that assessed older adults with mild to moderate hearing loss and the bottom panel pools several studies for older adults with moderate to severe hearing loss. Use = hours of use per day; Ben = benefit; RAL = residual activity limitations; Sat = satisfaction; RPR = residual participation restrictions; Ioth = impact on others; QoL = quality of life. The sample size for Takahashi et al. (2007), replaced by an asterisk, was a total of 162 participants, but the authors did not indicate how the participants were distributed between the two hearing loss severity subgroups.*

Table 4–4. Summaries of Nine Studies of Aided Speech Understanding Pertaining to the Effectiveness of Hearing Aids

Author(s)	*N*	*Mean Age*	*Degree and Configuration of Hearing Loss*	*Unilateral/ Bilateral Fit*	*Real-Ear Verification*	*Research Design*	*Outcome Measures*	*Overall Results*
Humes et al. (1996)	20	72	Mild to severe sloping	Bilateral	Yes	Nonrandomized intervention study	NST, HINT (% correct)	Significant benefit for NST in quiet and HINT in noise and stable over 6 months.
Humes et al. (1997)	110	25–90; no additional details	Various: Mild to moderate gently sloping to moderate to severe gently sloping	Bilateral	Yes	Randomized double-blind study	NU-6 and CST	Both types of hearing aids demonstrated significant benefit for many listening conditions (quiet, noise, various levels) and for both words (NU-6) and sentences (CST); decrease in benefit at highest speech level (75 dB SPL) in noise.
Walden et al. (1998)	40	66	Mild to moderately severe sloping	Bilateral	Yes	Nonrandomized intervention study	CST in 4 different listening conditions	Aided scores significantly higher than unaided in all four conditions.
Humes et al. (1999)	55	>18; no additional details	Various: Mild to moderate gently sloping to moderate to severe gently sloping	Bilateral	Yes	Nonrandomized intervention study	NU-6 words and CST	Both types of hearing aids demonstrated significant benefit for many listening conditions (quiet, noise, various levels) and for both words (NU-6) and sentences (CST).

continues

Table 4–4. *continued*

Author(s)	*N*	*Mean Age*	*Degree and Configuration of Hearing Loss*	*Unilateral/ Bilateral Fit*	*Real-Ear Verification*	*Research Design*	*Outcome Measures*	*Overall Results*
Walden et al. (1999)	40	66	Mild to moderate sloping	Bilateral	Yes	Nonrandomized intervention study	CST in 4 different listening conditions	Aided scores significantly higher than unaided in all four conditions.
Larson et al. (2000)	360	67	Mild to severe sloping	Bilateral	Yes	Randomized double-blind study	NU-6 and CST	All 3 circuits improved speech recognition (both CST and NU6); decreased benefit (<5% improvement) at highest presentation level (74 dB SPL) in noise.
Humes et al. (2001)	173	73	Mild to severe sloping	Bilateral	Yes	Nonrandomized intervention study	NST, CST	Significant increases in NST and CST scores in quiet and noise from unaided to aided testing, except for CST at 80 dB SPL (0 dB SNR).
Humes et al. (2004)	53	74	Mild to severe sloping	Bilateral	Yes	Nonrandomized intervention study	NST and CST	Both devices provided significant benefit to wearers; no significant differences in benefits provided by either device at 1- or 6-month postfit intervals.
Saunders et al. (2006)	94	69	Mild to severe sloping	Bilateral	Not reported	Nonrandomized intervention study	SRT in noise using HINT	Aided SRT in noise (HINT) significantly better than unaided.

List of Abbreviations and Acronyms: CST = Connected Speech Test; HINT = Hearing in Noise Test; NST = City University of New York Nonsense Syllable Test; NU-6 = Northwestern University Auditory Test No. 6; SRT = Speech Reception Threshold.

SUMMARY

This chapter discussed some of the issues relevant to the study of the effectiveness of hearing aids in older adults and then completed a review of the evidence available. The following general findings emerged:

- Although a fair number of good-quality (Grade B) nonrandomized intervention studies (Level 3 evidence) have been completed in this area over the past two decades, only one randomized controlled trial (Level 2 evidence; Grade A) of hearing aid effectiveness (Yueh et al., 2001) is available. No studies have employed placebo groups as controls and the use of control groups has also been rare.
- The overwhelming majority of nonrandomized intervention studies have made use of similar study samples: older adults with mild to severe sloping sensorineural hearing loss fit bilaterally with hearing aids whose frequency-gain characteristics were verified via real-ear measurements. This facilitates pooling of the data and probably increases the likelihood for similar outcomes across studies, but does not aid generalization of findings to other groups of hearing-impaired adults or other protocols (i.e., unilateral amplification, failure to use real-ear measurements for verification, etc.).
- Keeping the two conclusions noted above in mind, the following general observations were drawn from the analyses of the existing nonrandomized intervention studies conducted:
    - Benefaction measures generally showed significant reductions in hearing handicap or the frequency of problems from unaided to aided conditions and generated typical responses of "helpful" and "satisfied";
    - Usage measures typically showed self-reported usage of 4 to 8 hours/day or "about three-quarters of the time"; and
    - Speech-understanding was significantly improved from unaided to aided test conditions, with the exception of high speech levels at low signal-to-noise ratios.

The general findings drawn from the outcomes of these nonrandomized intervention studies are consistent with the average data observed in recent comparisons of technologies for homogenous groups of older adults (Humes et al., 2009a, 2009b), suggesting that the influences of technology are minimal, at least over the range of technologies considered and when each has been well fit to prescriptive frequency-gain targets using real-ear verification.

In general, from the findings summarized above, it is clear that much more research needs to be conducted regarding the effectiveness of hearing aids in adults. Sufficient information is available from Level 3, Grade B nonrandomized interventional studies to design appropriate randomized controlled trials of hearing aid effectiveness in adults, including the use of placebos and controls. Data obtained to date are primarily from older adults with presbycusis and generalizations of the findings regarding hearing aid effectiveness from this review are necessarily restricted to this population. There is a need for additional research on hearing aid effectiveness in young and middle-aged adults.

REFERENCES

Alpiner, J. (1982). Evaluation of communication function. In J. Alpiner (Ed.), *Handbook of adult rehabilitative audiology*. Baltimore, MD: Williams & Wilkins.

Beecher, H. K. (1955). The powerful placebo. *Journal of the American Medical Association, 159*, 1602–1606.

Bentler, R. A., Niebuhr, D. P., Getta, J. P., & Anderson, C. V. (1993). Longitudinal study of hearing aid effectiveness. II: Subjective measures. *Journal of Speech and Hearing Research, 36*, 820–831.

Cox, R. M., & Alexander, G. C. (1995). The Abbreviated Profile of Hearing Aid Benefit (APHAB). *Ear and Hearing, 16*, 176–186.

Cox, R. M., & Alexander, G. C. (1999). Measuring satisfaction with amplification in daily life: The SADL Scale. *Ear and Hearing, 20*, 306–320.

Cox, R. M., & Alexander, G. C. (2001). Validation of the SADL questionnaire. *Ear and Hearing, 22*, 151–160.

Cox, R. M., & Alexander, G. C. (2002). The International Outcome Inventory for Hearing Aids (IOI-HA): Psychometric properties of the English version. *International Journal of Audiology, 41*, 30–35.

Cox, R. M., Alexander, G. C., & Beyer, C. M. (2003). Norms for the International Outcome Inventory for hearing aids. *Journal of the American Academy of Audiology, 14*(8), 403–413.

Cox, R. M., Alexander, G. C., & Gilmore, C. (1987). Development of the Connected Speech Test (CST). *Ear and Hearing, 8*(Suppl. 5), 119S–126S.

Cox, R. M., Alexander, G. C., & Gray, G. A. (2005). Hearing aid patients in private practice and public health (Veterans Affairs) clinics: Are they different? *Ear and Hearing, 26*, 513–528.

Cox, R. M., & Gilmore, C. (1990). Development of the profile of hearing aid performance (PHAP). *Journal of Speech and Hearing Research, 33*, 343–355.

Cox, R. M., Stephens, D., & Kramer, S. E. (2002). Translations of the International Outcome Inventory for Hearing Aids (IOI-HA). *International Journal of Audiology, 41*, 3–26.

Dillon, H. (1994). Shortened Hearing Aid Performance Inventory for the Elderly (SHAPIE): A statistical approach. *Australian Journal of Audiology, 16*, 37–48.

Dillon, H., Birtles, G., & Lovegrove, R. (1999). Measuring the outcomes of a national rehabilitation program: Normative data for the Client Oriented Scale of Improvement (COSI) and the Hearing Aid User's Questionnaire (HAUQ). *Journal of the American Academy of Audiology, 10*, 67–79.

Dillon, H., James, A., & Ginis, J. (1997). Client Oriented Scale of Improvement (COSI) and its relationship to several other measures of benefit and satisfaction provided by hearing aids. *Journal of the American Academy of Audiology, 8*, 27–43.

Formby, C., & Hawley-Kaczka, M. (2009). Intervention for reduced sound tolerance. *Tinnitus Research Institute (TRI) Newsletter, 9*, 62–65.

Forster, S., & Tomlin, A. (1988, May). *Hearing aid usage in Queensland.* Paper presented at the Audiological Society of Australia Conference, Perth.

Gatehouse, S. (1994). Components and determinants of hearing aid benefit. *Ear and Hearing, 15*(1), 30–49.

Gatehouse. S. (1999). Glasgow Hearing Aid Benefit Profile: Derivation and validation of a client-centered outcome measure for hearing aid services. *Journal of the American Academy of Audiology, 10*, 80–103.

Gatehouse, S., & Noble, W. (2004). The Speech, Spatial and Qualities of Hearing Scale (SSQ). *International Journal of Audiology, 43*, 85–99.

Giolas, T. G., Owens, E., Lamb, S. H., & Schubert, E. D. (1979). Hearing Performance Inventory. *Journal of Speech and Hearing Disorders, 44*, 169–195.

Gorsuch, R. L. (1983). *Factor analysis* (2nd ed.). Mahwah, NJ: Lawrence Erlbaum Associates.

Hickson, L., Clutterbuck, S., & Khan, A. (2010). Factors associated with hearing aid fitting outcomes on the IOI-HA. *International Journal of Audiology, 49*, 586–595.

Hosford-Dunn, H., & Halpern, J. (2000). Clinical application of the Satisfaction with Amplification in Daily Life scale in private practice I: Statistical, content, and factorial validity. *Journal of the American Academy of Audiology, 11*, 523–539.

Humes, L. E. (1999). Exploring dimensions of hearing aid outcome. *Journal of the American Academy of Audiology, 10*, 26–39.

Humes, L. E. (2001). Issues in evaluating the effectiveness of hearing aids in the elderly: What to measure and when. *Seminars in Hearing, 22*, 303–314.

Humes, L. E. (2003). Modeling and predicting hearing-aid outcome. *Trends in Amplification, 7*, 41–75.

Humes, L. E. (2007). Hearing-aid outcome measures in older adults. In C. A. Palmer & R. C. Seewald (Eds.), *Hearing care for adults 2006* (pp. 265–276) Stafa, Switzerland: Phonak AG.

Humes, L. E., Ahlstrom, J. B., Bratt, G. W., & Peek, B. F. (2009a). Studies of hearing aid outcome measures in older adults: A comparison of technologies and an examination of individual differences. *Seminars in Hearing, 30*, 112–128.

Humes, L. E., Christensen, L. A., Bess, F. H., & Hedley-Williams, A. (1997). A comparison of the benefit provided by well-fit linear hearing aids and instruments with automatic reductions of low-frequency gain. *Journal of Speech, Language, and Hearing Research, 40*, 666–685.

Humes, L. E., Christensen, L. A., Thomas, T., Bess, F. H., Hedley-Williams, A., & Bentler, R. (1999). A comparison of the aided performance and benefit provided by a linear and a two-channel wide dynamic range compression hearing aid. *Journal of Speech, Language, and Hearing Research, 42*, 65–79.

Humes, L. E., Garner, C. B., Wilson, D. L., & Barlow, N.N. (2001). Hearing-aid outcome measures following one month of hearing aid use by the elderly. *Journal of Speech, Language, and Hearing Research, 44*, 469–486.

Humes, L. E., Halling, D., & Coughlin, M. (1996). Reliability and stability of various hearing-aid outcome measures in a group of elderly hearing-aid wearers. *Journal of Speech and Hearing Research, 39*, 923–935.

Humes, L. E., Humes, L. E., & Wilson, D. L. (2004). A comparison of single-channel linear amplification and two-channel wide-dynamic-range-compression amplification by means of an independent-group design. *Journal of the American Academy of Audiology, 13*, 39–53.

Humes, L. E., & Wilson, D. L. (2003). An examination of the changes in hearing-aid performance and benefit in the elderly over a 3-year period of hearing-aid use. *Journal of Speech Language Hearing Research, 46*, 137–145.

Humes, L. E., Wilson, D. L., Barlow, N. N., & Garner, C. B. (2002a). Measures of hearing-aid benefit following 1 or 2 years of hearing-aid use by older adults. *Journal of Speech Language Hearing Research, 45*, 772–782.

Humes, L. E., Wilson, D. L., Barlow, N. N., Garner, C. B., & Amos, N. (2002b). Longitudinal changes in hearing aid satisfaction and usage in the elderly over a period of one or two years after hearing aid delivery. *Ear and Hearing, 23*, 428–438.

Humes, L. E., Wilson, D., & Thompson, E. (2009b). Hearing-aid outcome measures in older adults. In L. Hickson (Ed.), *Hearing care for adults 2009—The challenge of Aging* (pp. 131–138). Stafa, Switzerland: Phonak AG.

Jerram, J. C. K., & Purdy, S. C. (1997). Evaluation of hearing aid benefit using the Shortened Hearing Aid Performance Inventory. *Journal of the American Academy of Audiology, 8*, 18–26.

Johnson, J. A., Cox, R. M., & Alexander, G. C. (2010). Development of APHAB norms for WDRC hearing aids and comparisons with original norms. *Ear and Hearing, 31*(1), 47–55.

Joore, M. A., Potjewijd, J., Timmerman, A. A., & Anteunis, L. J. C. (2002). Response shift in the measurement of quality of life in hearing impaired adults after hearing aid fitting. *Quality of Life Research, 11*, 299–307.

Kochkin, S. (2000). MarkeTrak V: Consumer satisfaction revisited. *Hearing Journal, 53*(1), 38–55.

Kochkin, S. (2009). MarkeTrak VIII: 25-year trends in the hearing health market. *Hearing Review, 16*(11), 12–31.

Kramer, S. E., Goverts, S. T., Dreschler, W. A., Boymans, M., & Festen, J. M. (2002). International Outcome Inventory for Hearing Aids (IOI-HA): Results from The Netherlands. *International Journal of Audiology, 41*, 36–41.

Larson, V. D., Williams, D. W., Henderson, W. G., Luethke, L. E., Beck, L. B., Noffsinger, D., . . . Bratt, G.W. (2000). Efficacy of 3 commonly used hearing aid circuits. *Journal of the American Medical Association, 284*, 1806–1813.

McArdle, R., Chisolm, T.H., Abrams, H.B., Wilson, R.H., & Doyle, P.J. (2005). The WHO-DAS II: Measuring outcomes of hearing aid intervention for adults. *Trends in Amplification, 9,* 127–143.

McPherson, B., & Wong, E. T. L. (2005). Effectiveness of an affordable hearing aid with elderly persons. *Disability and Rehabilitation, 27,* 601–609.

Metselaar, M., Maat, B., Krijnen, P., Verschuure, H., Dreschler, W., & Feenstra, L. (2009). Self-reported disability and handicap after hearing-aid fitting and benefit of hearing aids: Comparison of fitting procedures, degree of hearing loss, experience with hearing aids and uni- and bilateral fittings. *European Archives of Otorhinolaryngology, 266,* 907–917.

Mulrow, C. D., Tuley, M. R., & Aguilar, C. (1992). Sustained benefits of hearing aids. *Journal of Speech and Hearing Research, 35,* 1402–1405.

Noble, W., & Gatehouse, S. (2006). Effects of bilateral versus unilateral hearing aid fitting on abilities measured by the Speech, Spatial, and Qualities of Hearing Scale (SSQ). *International Journal of Audiology, 45,* 172–181.

Olusanya, B. (2004). Self-reported outcomes of aural rehabilitation in a developing country. *International Journal of Audiology, 43,* 563–571.

Pfelffer, E. (1975). A short portable mental status questionnaire for the assessment of organic brain deficit in elderly patient. *Journal of the American Geriatric Society, 23,* 433–441.

Roberts, A. H., Kewman, D. G., Mercier, L. & Hovell, M. (1993). The power of nonspecific effects in healing: Implications for psychosocial and biological treatments. *Clinical Psychology Review, 13,* 375–391.

Saunders, G. H., & Cienkowski, K. M. (1997). Acclimatization to hearing aids. *Ear and Hearing, 18,* 129–139.

Saunders, G. H., & Forsline, A. (2006). The Performance-Perceptual Test (PPT) and its relationship to aided reported handicap and hearing aid satisfaction. *Ear and Hearing, 27*(3), 229–242.

Schum, D. J. (1992). Responses of elderly hearing aid users on the Hearing Aid Performance Inventory. *Journal of the American Academy of Audiology, 3,* 308–314.

Schwartz, C. E., & Sprangers, M. A. G. (1999). Methodological approaches for assessing response shift in longitudinal health-related quality-of-life research. *Social Science and Medicine, 48,* 1531–1548.

Smith, P., Mack, A., & Davis, A. (2008). A multicenter trial of an assess-and-fit hearing aid service using open canal fittings and comply ear tips. *Trends in Amplification, 12,* 121–136.

Smith, S. L., Noe, C. M., & Alexander, G. C. (2009). Evaluation of the International Outcome Inventory for Hearing Aids in a veteran sample. *Journal of the American Academy of Audiology, 20,* 374–380.

Stark, P., & Hickson, L. (2004). Outcomes of hearing aid fitting for older people with hearing impairment and their significant others. *International Journal of Audiology, 43,* 390–398.

Surr, R. K., Cord, M. T., & Walden, B. E. (1998). Long-term versus short-term hearing aid benefit. *Journal of the American Academy of Audiology, 9,* 165–171.

Strom, K. E. (2006). The HR 2006 dispenser survey. *Hearing Review, 15*(6), 16–39.

Takahashi, G., Martinez, C. D., Beamer, S., Bridges, J., Noffsinger, D., Sugiura, K., . . . Williams, D. W. (2007). Subjective measures of hearing aid benefit and satisfaction in the NIDCD/VA follow-up study. *Journal of the American Academy of Audiology, 18*(4), 323–349.

Tuley, M. R., Mulrow, C. D., Aguilar, C., & Velez, R. (1990). A critical reevaluation of the Quantified Denver Scale of Communication Function. *Ear and Hearing, 11,* 56–61.

Turner, C. W., Humes, L. E., Bentler, R., & Cox, R. M. (1996). A review of past research on changes in hearing-aid benefit over time. *Ear and Hearing, 17,* 14S–28S.

Uriarte, M., Denzin, L., Dunstan, A., Sellars, J., & Hickson, L. (2005). Measuring hearing aid outcomes using the Satisfaction with Amplification in Daily Life (SADL) questionnaire: Australian Data. *Journal of the American Academy of Audiology, 16,* 383–402.

Ventry, I. M., & Weinstein, B. E. (1982). The hearing handicap inventory for the elderly: A new tool. *Ear and Hearing, 3,* 128–134.

Walden, B. E. (1997). Toward a model clinical-trials protocol for substantiating hearing aid user-benefit claims. *American Journal of Audiology, 6,* 13–24.

Walden, B. E., Demorest, M. E., & Hepler, E. L. (1984). Self-report approach to assessing benefit derived from amplification. *Journal of Speech and Hearing Research, 27*, 49–56.

Walden, B. E., Surr, R. K., Cord, M. T., & Pavlovic, C. V. (1998). A clinical trial of the ReSound BT2 personal hearing system. *American Journal of Audiology, 7*, 85–100.

Walden, B. E., Surr, R. K., Cord, M. T., & Pavlovic, C. V. (1999). A clinical trial of the ReSound IC4 hearing device. *American Journal of Audiology, 8*, 65–78.

World Health Organization. (2001). *International Classification of Functioning, Disability and Health (ICF).* Geneva, Switzerland.

Yueh, B., Souza, P. E., McDowell, J. A., Collins, M. P., Loovis, C. F., Hedrick, S. C., . . . Deyo, R. A.(2001). Randomized trial of amplification strategies. *Archives of Otolaryngology—Head and Neck Surgery, 127*(10), 1197–1204.

Yesavage, J. A., Brink, T. L., & Rose, T. L. (1983). Development and validation of a geriatric depression screening scale: A preliminary report. *Journal of Psychiatric Review, 17*(1), 37–49.

CHAPTER 5

Hearing Aids for Children

Teresa Y. C. Ching

INTRODUCTION

The primary effects of hearing loss on children may be considered in terms of the International Classification of Functioning, Disability and Health (World Health Organization, 2007) classification b230 that relates to hearing function. A consequence of impairment in hearing function is the limitation it poses on children's activities and participation in real life. With the implementation of universal newborn hearing screening, it is now possible for congenital hearing loss to be detected shortly after birth. Early detection makes it possible for early intervention, a vital component of which is the provision of hearing aid amplification. This chapter reviews the evidence on hearing aid outcomes in terms of improving hearing functions as well as reducing restrictions on activity and participation for children. The primary goal is to provide an evidence-based guide to clinicians for maximizing hearing aid outcomes for children. In addition, the evidence can help inform families with hearing-impaired children and other professionals about what current research evidence reveals as best practices. Finally, it serves to identify gaps of knowledge to be addressed by further research.

In this chapter, the literature is reviewed under three broad areas: technology, prescription and fitting, and evaluation. The schemes for rating evidence listed in Table 1–5 and grading recommendation in Table 1–6 in Chapter 1 are adopted for classifying evidence in each area. The evidence is also categorized according to whether assessments were carried out under laboratory/ ideal conditions (Efficacious, EF) or in the real world (Effectiveness, EV).

TECHNOLOGY

A major goal of amplification is to provide an audible signal in as wide a frequency range as possible at comfortable listening levels. Audibility depends on a range of factors, including the dynamic range of sounds in the environment relative to the dynamic range of the listener, the amplification bandwidth and electroacoustic characteristics of hearing aids, the acoustics of the listening environment and the needs of the listener in different environments. Each of these aspects is outlined below together with technologies designed to address the listeners' needs, and research findings are examined with a view to guiding clinical choices.

Dynamic Range of Sounds: Compression

The huge dynamic range of sounds in the environment fits easily between the hearing threshold and discomfort levels of people with normal hearing. However, this becomes difficult for people with hearing loss because they lose sensitivity for low-intensity sounds yet perceive high-intensity sounds at close to normal loudness levels (Moore & Glasberg, 1986). To achieve audibility with amplification, the wide range of input levels needs to be compressed into the reduced dynamic range of people with hearing loss. Wide dynamic range compression (WDRC) in hearing aids does precisely this. For sounds that are sufficiently intense to exceed the compression threshold, gain is increased for low-level sounds (increased audibility) and decreased for high-level sounds (increased listening comfort and acoustic safety), without the need for manual adjustment of volume controls. This technology is particularly useful for infants and young children as they cannot manipulate volume controls.

Currently, the gains prescribed by major generic prescription rules such as the NAL (Dillon, 1999; Dillon, Keidser, Ching, Flax, & Brewer, 2011) and DSL (Scollie et al., 2005; Seewald, Cornelisse, & Ramji, 1997) procedures, and by all proprietary prescription rules, inherently contain compression. However, some clinicians are concerned about the likelihood for compression to reduce spectral contrasts of speech and to reduce signal-to-noise ratio by amplifying low-level background noise. Both may have detrimental effects on children who rely on the auditory input for acquiring speech and language. For this reason, research has been directed to comparing linear amplification with WDRC for children. The evidence, as summarized in Table 5–1, indicates that for children with mild to moderately severe hearing loss, the use of WDRC increases loudness of low-level speech and reduces loudness of high-level speech, and is associated with improved speech perception and horizontal localization at low-level inputs. There is also evidence to suggest that the use of WDRC is linked to improved functional performance in real-world environments.

Most of the current research findings relate to fast-acting, single or dual-channel WDRC with medium compression thresholds (around 40 to 50 dB) and moderate compression ratios (below 3:1). There is some evidence to suggest that children who were used to linear amplification required a familiarization period of up to 5 months after they were refitted with WDRC with very low compression thresholds (Guo, Valero, & Marcoux, 2002). When very low compression thresholds are used, the increased gain for low-level sounds can result in increased background noise and feedback oscillation in hearing aids. On the other hand, the use of very high compression thresholds reduces the potential advantage of WDRC for increasing audibility of low-level sounds. It seems reasonable to start with a compression threshold that allows all frequencies of speech to go into compression when the overall level of speech is around 52 dB SPL (Dillon, 1999). The best compression threshold for children is currently unknown.

There is also good quality evidence to suggest that low-level sounds need to be amplified to a higher sensation level for children than is best for adults while maintaining high-level sounds at a comfortable listening level (Ching, Scollie, Dillon, & Seewald, 2010). This implies that children need a higher compression ratio than adults. An increase in compression ratios necessarily reduces the amount of contrastive spectral information of speech (De Gennaro, Braida, & Durlach, 1986). Although direct evidence on the best compression ratio for children is currently

Table 5–1. Wide Dynamic Range Compression (WDRC) in Hearing Aids for Children

Evidence	*Source*	*Level*	*Grade*	*EFficacious/ EffectiVeness*
Moderately fast-acting single channel WDRC improved perception of nonsense words and sentences in quiet at low and high input levels for 10- to 27-year-olds with moderate to severe hearing loss. (n = 12)	Jenstad et al. (1999)	4	B	EF
Moderately fast-acting single channel WDRC increased loudness of low-level speech and reduced loudness of high-level speech, compared to linear amplification. (n = 10)	Jenstad et al. (2000)	4	B	EF
Moderately fast-acting single channel WDRC increased the dynamic range of audibility for 10- to 27-year-olds with moderate hearing loss.(n = 10)	Jenstad et al. (2000)	4	B	EF
Fast-acting single channel WDRC improved consonant discrimination for 4- to 14-year-olds with moderate to profound hearing loss, compared to linear amplification. (n = 14)	Marriage & Moore (2003)	4	C	EF
Low compression threshold nonlinear amplification improved sound discrimination and word perception at low input levels for 6- to 13-year-olds with moderate hearing loss. (n = 14)	Guo et al. (2002)	4	B	EF
Familiarization period of 5 months to optimize performance with low compression threshold nonlinear amplification for 6- to 13-year-old children with moderate hearing loss. (n = 14)	Guo et al. (2002)	4	B	EF
WDRC improves speech perception at low input levels for school-age children with mild to moderately severe hearing loss. (n = 20)	Ching et al. (2004)	2	A	EF
WDRC improves horizontal localization at low input levels for school-age children with mild to moderately severe hearing loss. (n = 20)	Ching et al. (2004)	2	A	EF
WDRC improves auditory functioning in real life for school-age children with mild to moderately severe hearing loss. (n = 20)	Ching et al. (2004)	2	A	EV

unavailable, the use of compression ratios below about 3:1 has not been associated with degradations in performance in any report.

It is also not known whether children should be prescribed fast or slow-acting compression. Research on adults (Gatehouse, Naylor, & Elberling, 2006) suggests that greater advantages for fast- than for slow-acting compression are obtained by people who are more alert and in more dynamic listening environments. On the other hand, fast-acting multichannel compression may destroy spectral information, even as it increases audibility. Although the compression speed (attack and release times) undoubtedly affects sound quality and amplification of background noise, and possibly speech intelligibility, current evidence from Cox and Xu (2010) suggests that fast-acting compression (attack time: <5 ms, release time: 30 ms) does not degrade speech intelligibility. There exists little scientific evidence to indicate whether short (<100 ms) or long (>500 ms) release times is more beneficial under any listening condition. Possibly, the major advantages of WDRC are obtained no matter whether fast or slow speeds are used.

Recommendation: Fit nonlinear hearing aids with wide dynamic range compression to infants and children with hearing loss.

High-Frequency Audibility: Amplification Bandwidth

Speech and environmental sounds contain energy over a very wide range of frequencies, with the high-frequency components often the most difficult to perceive by people with hearing loss. Research has shown that speech sounds, such as [f v θ ð s z ʃ ʒ tʃ dʒ] are among the most frequently misperceived and mispronounced phonemes, and are the latest to be acquired by children with hearing loss (Moeller et al., 2007). These deficits have been attributed to inadequate audibility and the limited bandwidth of hearing aids. Manufacturers of hearing aids generally report that the upper bandwidth of devices exceeds 6 kHz, with the upper frequency range defined as the 20-dB down point relative to the average gain at 1.0, 1.6, and 2.0 kHz (ANSI, 2009). Thus, a hearing aid with an average used gain of 40 dB would only have 20 dB of gain at the upper frequency limit. In many cases, this may be inadequate to ensure audibility of low-level high-frequency components of speech that contains important linguistic information (Boothroyd & Medwetsky, 1992). For instance, the peak energy of [s] spoken by female and child talkers occurs in the 6 to 9 kHz region, and so hearing aids may require an upper limit of 10 kHz to ensure audibility of [s]. The question is, is it beneficial or harmful to speech intelligibility in particular, and to the hearing aid fitting in general, to amplify to 10 kHz for children?

Research evidence (Table 5–2) reveals no significant benefit of bandwidth extension to 9 or 10 kHz on sentence perception, novel word learning in quiet or in noise, or listening effort of children with mild to moderate hearing loss. There is some evidence (Stelmachowicz, Lewis, Choi, & Hoover, 2007) to suggest that bandwidth extension increases children's perception of [s] and [z] spoken by female talkers but decreases perception of [f] and [v]. When the effect of bandwidth on rate of word learning was investigated (Pittman, 2008), it was found that children exposed to extended bandwidth learned new words with fewer repetitions than children exposed to limited bandwidth. This observed difference may be related not only to the bandwidth condition but also to the lesser degree of hearing loss in the former compared to the latter group. No research has investigated the usefulness of extended amplification bandwidth for children with severe or profound hearing loss.

Table 5–2. Amplification Bandwidth of Hearing Aids for Children

Evidence	*Source*	*Level*	*Grade*	*EFficacious/ EffectiVeness*
Extending bandwidth from 4 to 9 kHz increased the rate of learning new words (less repetitions) by 8- to 10-year-old children with mild to moderate hearing loss. (n = 14)	Pittman (2008)	4	C	EF
Extending amplification bandwidth from 4 to 9 kHz did not improve rapid word learning in quiet for 5- to 14-year-old children with mild to moderately severe sloping hearing loss. (n = 37)	Pittman et al. (2005)	4	C	EF
Extending amplification bandwidth from 5 to 10 kHz improved perception of /s/ and /z/ but decreased perception of /f/ and /z/ by 7- to 14-year-old children with mild to moderate hearing loss. (n = 24)	Stelmachowicz et al. (2007)	4	C	EF
Extending amplification bandwidth from 5 to 10 kHz did not affect perception of sentences by 7- to 14-year-old children with mild to moderate hearing loss. (n = 24)	Stelmachowicz et al. (2007)	4	C	EF
Extending amplification bandwidth from 5 to 10 kHz did not affect listening effort of 7- to 14-year-old children with mild to moderate hearing loss. (n = 24)	Stelmachowicz et al. (2007)	4	C	EF
Extending amplification bandwidth from 5 to 10 kHz did not affect learning of new words in noise for 7- to 14-year-old children with mild to moderate hearing loss. (n = 24)	Stelmachowicz et al. (2007)	4	C	EF

It must be remembered that gain increase in one frequency region is possible only at the expense of gains provided in other frequency regions, unless the amplified signal is also made louder overall. If too much gain is applied across all frequencies, the result can be discomfort, decreased intelligibility, or both. Even when audibility is provided across all frequencies, the amount of information that can be extracted from the audible signal diminishes as hearing loss increases (Ching, Dillon, Katsch, & Byrne, 2001), especially when listeners have "dead" regions in the cochlea with no functioning inner hair cells (Moore, 2001). The limitations to the benefit of high-frequency amplification include listener-related factors such as loudness discomfort, hearing sensitivity being too poor for amplified signals to be usable and presence of dead regions in the cochlea, as well as device-related factors such as practical limitations imposed by feedback oscillation and the limited maximum output of hearing aids. Overall, the evidence to date does not support linear extension of amplification bandwidth for children.

Recommendation: The evidence is insufficient to recommend for or against extension of amplification bandwidth to 10 kHz for infants and children.

High-Frequency Audibility: Frequency Transposition/ Frequency Compression

Alternative approaches to increasing audibility of high-frequency sounds use frequency lowering techniques (for a review, see Simpson, 2009), including frequency transposition and frequency compression. The rationale for these schemes is to enable high-frequency components of speech to be audible in lower frequencies where hearing loss is less severe. Two types of signal-processing schemes have been applied in commercial hearing aids widely fitted to children. One scheme implements linear frequency transposition (Kuk et al., 2006; Kuk, Keenan, Korhonen, & Lau, 2009). Signal components in a high-frequency source octave are transposed linearly by a fixed amount to a lower-frequency target octave. The size of shift is such that the dominant peak in the source octave is lowered in frequency by nominally one octave. The transposed signals are mixed with components that are already present in the target frequency region before amplification and other signal processing functions are applied. A second scheme uses frequency compression (Glista et al., 2009; Simpson, Hersbach, & McDermott, 2005). This approach does not involve mixing of frequency-shifted signals with other signals present in the lower frequency region. It reduces the signal bandwidth at the output relative to the range at the input of the hearing aid; and the amount of reduction depends on the cutoff frequency and the frequency compression ratio. For instance, a cut-off frequency of 2 kHz with a frequency compression ratio of 2:1 would result in each octave range of input frequencies above 2 kHz being compressed into a half-octave range, such that an input range of 2 to 4 kHz will have an output range of 2 to 2.8 kHz. Signals that are below the cutoff frequency are unchanged.

As shown in Table 5–3, recent investigations on the effect of frequency transposition on children with sloping high-frequency hearing loss revealed significant benefits for identification of consonants at low input levels and awareness of environmental sounds, compared to the children's personal hearing aids. These advantages may be due partly to the very low compression threshold used in fitting the test hearing aids (Guo et al., 2002) as well as other unknown differences in electroacoustic characteristics between the two sets of hearing instruments, rather than the use of transposition.

Current evidence on the effect of frequency compression for children (Table 5–4) indicates that perception of high-frequency sounds in quiet was improved for children with high-frequency hearing loss (Glista et al., 2009) and for children with moderate to moderately severe hearing loss (Wolfe et al., 2011). One study reported improvements in sentence perception in noise after children had used the hearing aids with frequency compression for 6 months. It is not clear whether the improvement was due to effects of practice or maturation or to familiarization with the device.

Indeed, previous studies suggested that auditory training with frequency transposition improved speech intelligibility over time (Auriemmo et al., 2009; Korhonen & Kuk, 2008), but recent evidence indicated that training did not increase the benefit from transposition per se, relative to the condition without transposition (Fullgrabe, Baer, & Moore, 2010).

The research to date suggests that children (and adults) who were fitted with new

Table 5–3. Frequency Transposition in Hearing Aids for Children

Evidence	*Source*	*Level*	*Grade*	*EFficacious/ EffectiVeness*
Frequency transposition improved recognition of phonemes presented at low input levels but not at medium input levels for 6- to 13-year-old children with sloping high-frequency loss (normal to moderate loss in the low frequencies and severe to profound loss in the high frequencies), after training over 6 weeks. (n = 10)	Auriemmo et al. (2009)	3	B	EF
Frequency transposition improved accuracy of /s/ and /z/ production in connected speech by children with sloping high-frequency loss, after training over 6 weeks. (n = 10)	Auriemmo et al. (2009)	3	B	EF
Weekly half-hour auditory training provided over a 6-week period improved children's perception of low-level consonants and production of high-frequency sounds. (n = 10)	Auriemmo et al. (2009)	3	B	EF
Frequency transposition increased awareness of environmental sounds for children with sloping hearing loss. (n = 10)	Auriemmo et al. (2009)	3	B	EF
Frequency transposition improved speech production in 9- to 14-year-old children with good low-frequency hearing but severe high-frequency hearing loss, after 24 weeks of familiarization. (n = 6)	Smith et al. (2009)	5	C	EF
Frequency lowering by slow playback improved aided thresholds and speech perception of some children with profound loss with up to 48 months of use. (n = 11)	MacArdle et al. (2001)	4	C	EF
Frequency lowering by slow playback improved aided thresholds and word recognition for 7 children with mild to moderate hearing loss and 12 children with severe to profound hearing loss after 4 weeks of usage. (n = 19)	Miller-Hansen et al. (2003)	4	C	EF

hearing aids that have either frequency transposition or frequency compression capabilities generally preferred the new hearing devices to their own devices that provided conventional amplification. The extent to which the preferences could be attributed to the new devices

Table 5–4. Frequency Compression in Hearing Aids for Children

Evidence	*Source*	*Level*	*Grade*	*EFficacious/ EffectiVeness*
Frequency compression improved perception of /s/ and /z/ for children aged between 6 and 17 years with sloping high-frequency hearing loss from moderately severe to profound, after familiarization of 16 weeks. (*n* = 11)	Glista et al. (2009)	3	B	EF
Frequency compression did not affect vowel perception for children. (*n* = 11)	Glista et al. (2009)	3	B	EF
Children with more severe high-frequency hearing loss obtained more benefit from frequency compression. (*n* = 11)	Glista et al. (2009)	3	B	EF
Children (aged between 6 and 15 years) with moderate to profound hearing loss perceived high-frequency words in quiet and in noise better after using hearing aids with frequency compression for 6 months, compared with their own hearing aids. No significant benefits specifically related to frequency compression were observed. (*n* = 13)	Bohnert (2009)	3	B	EF
Frequency compression improved production of high-frequency words for children with moderate to profound hearing loss after 6 months of use. (*n* = 13)	Bohnert (2009)	3	B	EF
Frequency compression improved audibility of high-frequency sounds in quiet for 6- to 12-year-old children with moderate to moderately severe hearing loss, after 6 weeks of familiarization. (*n* = 15)	Wolfe et al. (2011)	3	B	EF
Frequency compression improved sentence perception in noise for children with moderate to moderately severe hearing loss, after 6 months of familiarization. (*n* = 15)	Wolfe et al. (2011)	3	B	EF

or to the frequency transposition or compression in the devices remains to be investigated.

Although frequency lowering techniques were designed for people with minimal sensitivity in the high frequencies in mind, the application of these techniques is potentially beneficial for people who are not able to extract useful information from a signal in the high frequencies even when it is audible. In principle, frequency lowering enables high-frequency information to be more effectively extracted in regions where hearing sensitivity is better. However, transposition that superimposes a shifted signal to the signal already present leads to artefacts; and compression necessarily reduces spectral contrasts important for speech discrimination. These are important considerations for infants and young children because they rely on the auditory input to acquire speech and language, and they cannot provide feedback on the sound quality or efficacy of amplification.

In summary, there is insufficient evidence to recommend for or against frequency lowering in hearing aids for infants and children. It is not known what audiometric characteristics are associated with the greatest benefits from the processing schemes, and how best to adjust parameters to optimise benefits. Further research into candidacy and fitting procedures in the paediatric population is necessary. Nevertheless, if conventional amplification does not adequately provide an audible signal across speech frequencies to infants and children despite all efforts made to optimise the fitting for the individual, the use of amplification with frequency lowering should be evaluated before resorting to considerations for cochlear implantation.

Recommendations: (1) The evidence is insufficient to recommend for or against frequency transposition for infants and children. (2) The evidence is insufficient to recommend for or against frequency compression for infants and children.

Listening in Noise

Listening to speech in noisy situations is most challenging for people with hearing loss, and is even more so for children because they need a better signal-to-noise ratio (SNR) than adults to achieve equivalent levels of speech perceptual performance (Gravel, Fausel, Liskow, & Chobot, 1999; Jamieson, Kranjc, Yu, & Hodgetts, 2004). Improvement in SNR is therefore an important goal in the design of hearing devices.

The largest improvements in speech perception in noise have been shown to occur when wireless technology, such as frequency modulation (FM) systems, is used (Crandell & Smaldino, 2000; Hawkins, 1984; Lewis, Crandell, Valente, & Enrietto, 2004). Because an acoustic signal being picked up by a microphone in close proximity of the sound source can be transmitted as an electrical signal over long distances with high fidelity to a receiver, children are likely to benefit from the use of this technology whenever they have to listen to someone from a distance or in noisy environments. A necessary prerequisite for the advantage of wireless technology to occur, though, is that the user is able to pass the transmitter to different talkers as communication partners and listening venues change. For infants and young children, the use of this technology relies on the vigilant monitoring of an adult (Moeller, Donaghy, Beauchaine, Lewis, & Stelmachowicz, 1996).

Listening in Noise: Noise Reduction

Noise reduction systems in hearing aids also aim to improve SNR. Generally, one of two methods is used. The first uses a spectral subtraction method in which the noise spectrum is estimated from the gaps in the speech signal, and is then subtracted from the noisy speech spectrum in either the time or the frequency domain. The second method involves estimating the SNR within specific frequency bands before applying gain reduction in the frequency region that is poorer than other frequency regions. Theoretically, an algorithm that leads to a change in spectral balance of the amplified signal and noise, but which leaves unchanged the SNR at every frequency, can be expected only to improve quality and perhaps decrease listening fatigue, without affecting intelligibility. Many studies on adult listeners have indeed shown that noise reduction did not improve speech perception in noise when the spectrum of the noise was similar to that of the speech signal (Alcantara, Moore, Kuhnel, & Launer, 2003; Bentler, Wu, Kettel, & Hurtig, 2008a), but improved listening comfort (Boysman & Dreschler, 2000; Walden, Surr, Cord, Edwards, & Olson, 2000) and sound quality (Arehart, Hansen, & Gallant, 2003; Ricketts & Hornsby, 2005). There is no strong reason why the same benefits from noise reduction may not apply for children.

However, there are doubts about whether variations in the audible spectrum as a consequence of noise reduction may affect children's speech and language acquisition, because overhearing and incidental learning in real-world environments play an important role in early development (Akhtar, 2005). Even though speech is amplified with a frequency response that changes depending on the spectral characteristics of the noise present, such variations are small compared to the inherent variations in the acoustics of speech that may be attributed to different talker characteristics and physical environment. An evaluation of the effect of noise reduction on learning nonnative speech contrasts in noise by adults revealed no significant effect of the processing (Marcoux, Yathiraj, Cote, & Logan, 2006). A recent study on 16 children (ages 5 to 10 years) with mild to moderately severe hearing loss who had age-appropriate receptive language (Stelmachowicz et al., 2010) showed that single-channel spectral subtraction did not have a significant effect on perception of nonsense syllables, words, or sentences presented in speech-shaped noise at 0 to 10 dB SNR (Table 5–5). Whether similar results apply to other types of noise-reduction algorithms, other types of noise spectra, at poorer SNR, and most importantly, in real-world environments, remain to be investigated. In so far as noise reduction algorithms decrease the

Table 5–5. Noise Reduction in Hearing Aids for Children

Evidence	*Source*	*Level*	*Grade*	*EFficacious/ EffectiVeness*
Noise reduction did not degrade acquisition of novel, nonnative speech contrasts by adults (designed to simulate language acquisition by children). (n = 26)	Marcoux et al. (2006)	4	C	EF
Noise reduction (single-microphone, spectral subtraction algorithm) providing maximum attenuation of 6 dB did not degrade speech perception in noise at 0, +5, and +10 dB SNR for 5- to 10-year-old children with mild to moderately severe hearing loss who had age-appropriate vocabulary skills. (n = 16)	Stelmachowicz et al. (2010)	4	B	EF

saliency of background noise thereby improving listening comfort, the benefit applies to children as it applies to adults.

Recommendation: There is insufficient evidence to recommend for or against the use of noise reduction in hearing aids for infants and children.

Listening in Noise: Directional Microphones

When speech is embedded in noise and reverberation, directional microphones improve SNR of speech in front by attenuating sounds from nonfrontal sources. It is clear from physical principles that if a listener faces a talker, if the distance between the talker and the listener is not too much larger than the critical distance of a room, and if sufficient noise or reverberation is present, directional microphones will offer an improved SNR to the listener. Directional microphones have been shown to improve SNR by 7 to 8 dB in adults (Valente, Fabry, & Potts, 1995) and 3 to 4 dB in children (Gravel et al., 1999) in laboratory conditions. The effectiveness in real life is less certain.

Table 5–6 summarizes the research evidence on the effect of directional microphones for infants and children. When speech originated from the front and noise from the rear or the sides, directional microphones improved speech perception in noise by school-aged children. In real life, school-aged children did not rate omnidirectional and directional modes in their hearing aids differently. Research on infants and young children in real life indicated that they looked at the primary talker in everyday situations, and would be expected to obtain benefits of up to 3 dB improvement in signal-to-noise ratio in real life.

There are situations when directional microphones are not desirable, specifically when the hearing aid user is in a very quiet environment or when there is wind noise. A hearing aid with a directional response has a higher level of internal noise than if it had an omnidirectional response, because additional amplifier gain is applied in the directional response to the low frequencies to compensate for the reduction in sensitivity at these frequencies. The amplified noise may be audible and objectionable to the hearing aid user. When there is wind noise around a hearing aid, it is sensed by the hearing aid microphone with higher sensitivity than the target signal that is further away in the field, thereby resulting in reduced speech intelligibility. Consistent with these principles, research on adults has indicated a preference for omnidirectional mode in quiet environments (Kuk, 1996); a preference for switchable as opposed to fixed directionality in real life (Mueller, Grimes, & Erdman, 1983; Preves, Sammeth, & Wynne, 1999); and greater benefits of directionality in noisy situations with switchable rather than with fixed directionality (Ricketts, Henry, & Gnewikow, 2003). Preferences of adults for omnidirectional rather than directional processing in real-life situations appear to be dominated by perceived loudness of amplified speech and lower internal circuit noise levels (Wu & Bentler, 2010).

Despite the proven benefits of directionality for improving SNR for children, some clinicians express concerns about the potential detrimental effect of directionality in reducing audibility of sounds from the sides and the rear. These concerns are unnecessary, partly because current directional microphones are not that directional, and partly because even if sounds are attenuated by directional microphones, the compressor in a hearing aid with WDRC will increase gain for the sounds, typically by around half of the level decrease, as long as the sounds are sufficiently intense to exceed the compression threshold. Consequently, the net decrease in output level is

Table 5–6. Directional Microphone Technology in Hearing Aids for Children

Evidence	*Source*	*Level*	*Grade*	*EFficacious/ EffectiVeness*
Directional microphones improved speech perception in noise for children (aged 4 to 11 years) with mild to severe hearing loss when speech was presented from the front and noise from the rear. (*n* = 20)	Gravel et al. (1999)	4	C	EF
For school-age children with moderate hearing loss, directional microphones improved speech perception in simulated classroom environments when the primary talker was in front of the listener, but decreased speech perception when the primary talker was to the side or behind the listener. (*n* = 26)	Ricketts et al. (2007)	4	B	EF
Children aged 10 to 17 years did not rate directional vs. omnidirectional modes in their hearing aids differently in a range of real-life situations. (*n* = 26)	Ricketts et al. (2007)	4	B	EV
Reducing the frequency extent of directivity reduces both the SNR enhancement and decrement possible with directional microphones. (*n* = 26)	Ricketts et al. (2007)	4	B	EF
School-age children oriented toward a primary talker in multitalker situations in school settings. (*n* = 20 normal hearing and 20 mild to moderately hearing-impaired children)	Ricketts et al. (2008)	4	B	EF
For infants and children (ranging in age between 11 months old and 7 years), the overall effect of directional microphones in real life situations is effectively zero. Directionality is beneficial in some situations but detrimental in other situations. (*n* = 27)	Ching et al. (2009)	4	B	EV
Young children (11 months to 7 years of age) oriented to the talker of interest in different real-life scenarios. (*n* = 27)	Ching et al. (2009)	4	B	EV

only about half of that caused by a directional microphone acting alone.

The need for providing binaural directional amplification is even stronger for children who demonstrate a deficit in binaural processing, a deficit that has been found in many children with hearing loss from birth. They are not able to take advantage of the spatial separation between speech and noise to improve speech intelligibility, unlike children with normal binaural processing abilities (Ching, van Wanrooy, Dillon, & Carter, 2011; Litovsky, Johnstone, & Godar, 2006). Because young children are not able to operate manual switches, and it is not practical for a vigilant adult to always observe the changing listening environments and needs of a child to make intelligent decisions about program switching, an automatic switching arrangement in devices for young children is necessary. Benefits are possible as long as the switching chooses directional more often when speech is from the front and omnidirectional more often when speech is from the side or from the rear. The current evidence supports the use of automatically switchable directionality in hearing aids for infants and young children to enable them to monitor the environments around them as well as to enhance SNR in noisy situations when they look at the talker of interest.

Recommendation: Provide switchable directional microphone technology in hearing aids for infants and children.

PRESCRIPTION, FITTING, AND VERIFICATION

As the identification of infants with hearing loss is now possible with universal newborn hearing screening, it is important to provide them with timely amplification soon after diagnosis to support early development (Thompson et al., 2001). The process of amplification involves the determination of an audiogram, the selection of a prescription for deriving targets, and the use of verification methods to ensure that prescribed acoustic performance is achieved in hearing aids. Special considerations apply to providing amplification for infants. This is particularly the case before the infant is able to respond reliably to behavioral testing techniques, and before the small and growing ear canals of infants approximate average adult sizes.

There are now published protocols that describe systematic approaches to fitting hearing aids to infants and young children (Bagatto, Scollie, Hyde, & Seewald, 2010; King, 2010). Briefly, electrophysiologic testing techniques are used to evaluate auditory thresholds in response to frequency-specific stimuli for each ear. Evoked potential tests may include auditory brainstem responses (ABR), and/or auditory steady-state responses (ASSR) and/or transtympanic round window electrocochleography (ECochG). Air conduction thresholds measured using these electrophysiological methods are used to estimate behavioral hearing thresholds. The estimation procedure considers differences in stimuli and calibration methods used in testing (Stapells, 2000; Vander Werff, Prieve, & Georgantas, 2009) as well as differences in acoustic properties of ear canals between adults and children (Bagatto et al., 2005). Infants have smaller ear canals than young children who in turn have smaller ear canals than older children or adults. The size and volume of ear canals affect resonances in the ear, with smaller canals producing higher pressure levels at the eardrum for the same input (Voss & Herrmann, 2005). Fortunately, the application of appropriate corrections for estimating thresholds measured using different evoked potential tests is incorporated in the NAL and the DSL prescriptive procedures, both of which are widely used for fitting infants and children.

Consideration of ear canal acoustics is essential not only for defining hearing thresholds, but also for specifying the electroacoustic properties in hearing aids to achieve gain-frequency response targets of prescriptive procedures. The measurement of real-ear-to-coupler difference (RECD), that is, the difference between the level of a signal in the ear canal and the level of the same signal in an HA2-2cc coupler (Bagatto, Seewald, Scollie, & Tharpe, 2006; Moodie, Seewald, & Sinclair,

1994), can be used to quantify the effects of an infant's ear canal. For this reason, the RECD is an integral part of hearing aid fitting for infants and children. It can be used to derive coupler gain (CG) targets from real-ear-aided-gain prescriptions (REAG). The REAG is the increase in signal level when aided relative to the level of the signal in the sound field, and can be specified in terms of the sum of RECD and CG (REAG = RECD + CG). For the same REAG, higher coupler gains will be required as RECD decreases with age-related growth in ear canal size. If measurement of individual RECD is not possible, age-appropriate values may be used (Bagatto, Scollie, Seewald, Moodie, & Hoover, 2002; Feigin, Kopun, Stelmachowicz, & Gorga, 1989). Both the NAL and the DSL prescriptions provide REAG targets and CG targets for fitting, and both prescriptions incorporate age-appropriate RECDs in their fitting software. Hearing aids can be adjusted and verified in a coupler to ensure that targets are met.

Prescription

The NAL and DSL prescriptions differ in terms of gain-frequency responses for the same degree and configuration of hearing loss. A comparison of the prescriptions by Byrne and colleagues (Byrne, Dillon, Ching, Katsch, & Keidser, 2001) for 6 hypothetical audiograms indicated that the DSL prescribed higher low-frequency gain than NAL for flat hearing loss, higher high-frequency gain than NAL for sloping loss, and higher overall loudness for all losses. The DSL procedure also prescribed higher compression ratios than the NAL procedure.

Empirical evidence on the relative effectiveness of the two prescriptions for children is summarized in Table 5–7.

A cross-over controlled comparison for school-age children with mild to moderately severe hearing loss (Ching et al., 2010) indicated that the NAL and the DSL prescriptions were equally efficacious. In laboratory conditions, children rated speech amplified with either prescription to be similarly loud, after some familiarisation. They also perceived speech equally well with both prescriptions. In real-world environments, however, children preferred the DSL prescription when listening to softly spoken speech but the NAL prescription when listening to speech in noisy environments. Each prescription was effective in different listening conditions, but neither met the diverse needs of children in real life. The study also revealed that preferences of children were affected by previous auditory experience, despite prolonged periods of familiarization with each prescription.

To control for the effect of auditory experience, a recent randomized controlled comparison of hearing aid prescriptions was conducted. About 198 infants were randomly assigned to each prescription for first fitting, and the language development of both groups was assessed at 6 and 12 months after auditory intervention. The findings indicated that both prescriptions provided equally good support for language development over the first few years of life (Ching, Dillon, Day, & Crowe, 2007). On average, the choice of prescription was not associated with significant differences in auditory comprehension or expressive communication.

Recommendation: Fit hearing aids as early as possible, using either the NAL or the DSL prescription.

Verification

An integral part of the hearing aid fitting procedure is to verify in an HA2-2cc coupler that hearing aids have been adjusted to meet custom-derived targets as prescribed by

Table 5–7. Prescription and Verification of Hearing Aids for Children

Topic	*Evidence*	*Source*	*Level*	*Grade*	*EFficacious/ EffectiVeness*
Prescription	Speech perception in quiet and in noise by school-age children was similarly good with NAL and DSL prescriptions. (n = 48)	Scollie et al. (2010)	2	A	EF
	Loudness rating of speech amplified using either the NAL or the DSL prescription was similar. (n = 48)	Scollie et al. (2010)	2	A	EF
	NAL preferred for noisy real-life situations, and DSL for quiet situations. (n = 48)	Scollie et al. (2010)	2	A	EV
	The development of auditory comprehension was not significantly different between infants fitted with either the NAL or the DSL prescription. (n = 198)	Ching et al. (2007)	2	A	EV
	The development of expressive communication was not significantly different between infants fitted either with the NAL or the DSL prescription. (n = 198)	Ching et al. (2007)	2	A	EV
	Early fitting of infants with either the NAL or the DSL prescription facilitate language development over the first few years of life. (n = 198)	Ching et al. (2007)	2	A	EV
Verification	Speech Intelligibility Index overestimated speech perception of children with amplification. (n = 29)	Scollie et al. (2008)	3	B	EF
	Sound field–aided thresholds of children with moderately severe to profound hearing loss overestimated sensation levels of amplified speech. (n = 13)	Seewald et al. (1992)	3	B	EF

the chosen prescription (Bagatto et al., 2010; King, 2010; Seewald et al., 2005).

As the goal of amplification is to ensure that sounds are audible across a wide range of frequencies, aided audibility is sometimes used clinically to verify that the goal has been achieved. Aided speech audibility can be computed using information about a child's hearing threshold levels, the long-term average speech spectrum, and gains provided by a hearing aid (in terms of REAG or CG). Visual displays of audibility can be generated within the fitting software of the NAL and the DSL prescriptions, and also by some commercial real-ear gain analyzers. These displays are useful for viewing how much of an assumed speech spectrum is audible to the child when hearing aids are worn.

The amount of audible signal can also be quantified by using the Speech Intelligibility Index (SII, ANSI, 1997), and clinical applications have been developed to quantify audibility of different types of speech spectra with amplification for children (e.g., the Situational Hearing Aid Response Profile or SHARP, Stelmachowicz, Lewis, & Creutz, 1997). These representations of audibility, however, do not indicate how well a child can extract information from the audible signal for understanding speech. Greater audibility can be achieved by simply turning up the volume control of hearing aids, which will no doubt increase in loudness but not necessarily increase in intelligibility. Indeed, there is research evidence to indicate that an increase in the hearing loss of a listener is associated with a decrease in the amount of speech information that can be extracted from an audible signal (Ching, Dillion, & Byrne, 1998; Ching et al., 1998; Ching et al., 2001; Sherbecoe & Studebaker, 2003). There is evidence (see Table 5–7) to suggest that SII (or the amount of audible signal) overestimates the speech performance of adults (Ching et al., 1998; Ching et al., 2001) and school-age children (Scollie, 2008).

Measures of aided thresholds in the sound field have also been used commonly to verify the fit in infants and young children. These measures have poor reliability, are susceptible to circuit and amplified room noise, and are very time consuming to measure even for children who are able to provide reliable behavioural responses (Hawkins, 2004). The value of aided threshold measurements for quantifying audibility diminishes with the use of nonlinear signal processing in hearing aids. Because aided thresholds are often measured in response to audiometric test signals that are low in level relative to the sound pressure levels of conversational speech, they tend to overestimate the available gain and therefore the levels at which amplified speech will be received by the infant in the aided condition. Measures of aided thresholds in the sound field are nonetheless very useful for quantifying audibility for children who use bone-conduction hearing aids because verification using real-ear measures in these cases is not applicable.

It is important to remember that audibility represents the sensation level of a signal with amplification. It does not provide information about listening comfort or about the effectiveness of amplification for the child (Byrne & Ching, 1997; Jordt et al., 1997).

Recommendation: Adjust and verify that hearing aids meet prescriptive targets in a coupler. Estimates of audibility should not be used as the primary method of hearing aid verification.

EVALUATION OF OUTCOMES

Evaluation of amplification outcomes is the basis of evidence-based clinical practice. Whereas verification serves to ascertain that prescriptive targets are achieved, evaluation checks that amplification needs of individual children are met or indicate how the hearing aids need to be optimized according to user requirements. Table 5–8 summarizes evidence on the need to evaluate and the methods for evaluating infants and children.

Why Evaluate?

The need to evaluate individual fitting that was based on a prescription is clearly indicated in research showing an association between differences in hearing aid characteristics and auditory performance of children. A difference in gain-frequency response of >3 dB/octave has a significant effect on functional performance of young children in real life, as observed by parents and teachers (Ching, Hill, & Dillon, 2008). Of the samples of children whose amplification was evaluated in previous studies, about one-third to one-quarter of children preferred or functioned more effectively in real-world environments when they used hearing aids that provided more or less low- or high-frequency emphasis than prescribed targets used for fitting (Ching et al., 2008; Ching et al., 2010). With developments in technology, features provided by signal-processing in hearing aids also need to be evaluated for applicability to infants and children.

How to Evaluate?

Common methods for evaluating amplification include subjective testing of speech perception (Bess et al., 1996; Bess & Paradise, 1994; Boothroyd, 1991) and paired-comparison judgments of quality or intelligibility (Ching, Hill, Birtles, & Beecham, 1999; Ching, Newall, & Wigney, 1994; Ching et al., 1994; Ching et al., 1998; Eisenberg & Levitt, 1991) for older children. Speech tests are less sensitive and more time-consuming than paired-comparison judgments for evaluating alternative gain-frequency responses in hearing aids (Studebaker, 1982). For infants and young children who are not able to provide verbal feedback about the appropriateness of the fit or participate in behavioral tests, evaluations may be based on direct observations of auditory behaviors by parents, or on objective measurement of auditory evoked potentials using electrophysiological techniques.

Parental questionnaires have been widely used to document children's behaviour and development in health-related domains, including the monitoring of auditory responses (Stelmachowicz, 1999; for a review, see Ching & Hill, 2007). Several questionnaires exist for parents of older children, including the Meaningful Auditory Integration Scale (MAIS, Robbins, Renshaw, & Berry, 1991) and the infant-toddler version (Zimmerman-Phillipps, Osberger, & Robbins, 1998), a parental questionnaire to evaluate children's Auditory Behavior in Everyday Life or ABEL (Purdy, Rarringon, Moran, Chard, & Hodgson, 2002) and the Children's Abbreviated Profile of Hearing Aid Performance (C-APHAP), Kopun & Stelmachowicz, 1998). There are very few published outcome assessment tools for infants. The Family Expectation Worksheet is one such tool which involves families rating the degree of success achieved for each agreed amplification goal (Palmer & Mormer, 1998, 1999). If goals are not met, then appropriateness of the fit and functionality of hearing aids are reviewed. Another questionnaire is the Parents' Evaluation of Aural/oral performance of Children (PEACH, Ching & Hill, 2007). Normative data and critical differences are published, thereby allowing direct comparisons of auditory behaviors of hearing-impaired children with their normal-hearing peers. The reliability and validity of the PEACH are supported by research (Ching et al., 2008).

Table 5–8. Evaluation of Hearing Aids for Children

Topic	*Evidence*	*Source*	*Level*	*Grade*	*EFficacious/ EffectiVeness*
Need to evaluate	Difference in hearing aid gain of more than 3 dB results in a difference in loudness comfort, intelligibility judgment and everyday functioning. (*n* = 48)	Ching et al. (2010); Scollie et al. (2010)	2	A	EF & EV
	Difference in hearing aid frequency response of more than 3 dB/octave results in a difference in everyday functioning for school-age children (*n* = 22, Ching et al., 1999) and young children with severe to profound hearing loss. (*n* = 30, Ching et al., 2008)	Ching et al. (1999); Ching et al. (2008)	2	A	EV
How to evaluate	Parental reports are sensitive to differences in frequency response in hearing aids for infants and young children with severe and profound hearing loss. (*n* = 30)	Ching et al. (2008)	2	A	EV
	Self-reports are sensitive to differences in hearing aid gains for school-age children with severe to profound hearing loss (*n* = 22, Ching et al., 1999) and children with mild to moderately severe hearing loss. (*n* = 48, Ching et al., 2010)	Ching et al. (1999); Ching et al. (2010)	2	A	EV
	Speech tests are limited in sensitivity to differences in hearing aid gain-frequency responses for school-age children with mild to moderately severe hearing loss. (*n* = 48)	Scollie et al. (2010)	2	A	EF
	Paired-comparison judgments can be used reliably to evaluate differences in gain-frequency response in hearing aids for school-age children (*n* = 15, Ching et al., 2008; *n* = 48, Ching et al., 2010).	Ching et al. (2008); Ching et al. (2010)	2	A	EF & EV

Table 5–8. *continued*

Topic	*Evidence*	*Source*	*Level*	*Grade*	*EFficacious/ EffectiVeness*
How to evaluate *continued*	Paired-comparison judgments of clarity by mild to moderately hearing-impaired children between 7 and 12 years of age do not reveal a difference in perceived quality for speech amplified using different hearing aid output compression characteristics. (n = 20)	Stelmachowicz et al. (1999)	2	A	EF & EV
	Presence of aided cortical auditory evoked potentials to speech stimuli is associated with better functional performance in real life in infants. (n = 31)	Golding et al. (2007)	4	B	EF
	Detection of cortical auditory evoked potentials to speech stimuli is indicative of audibility in normal-hearing infants. (n = 14)	Carter et al. (2010)	4	C	EF
	Detection of cortical auditory evoked potentials is associated with development of receptive language skills and speech perception in children with auditory neuropathy. (n = 15)	Rance et al. (2002)	4	B	EF

Objective recording of cortical auditory evoked potentials (CAEP) offers a unique opportunity to assess audibility of speech sounds presented in the sound field (Purdy & Kelly, 2008). Cortically generated responses can be reliably evoked by speech stimuli at supra-threshold levels in infants and children, even though intersubject variability of the response shape is high (Carter, Golding, Dillon, & Seymour, 2010; Cone-Wesson & Wunderlich, 2003). Because signals have to pass through the entire auditory system before a response is generated in the cortical region, the presence of CAEP suggests that the listener gets sufficient information from the amplified speech to learn to make use of it.

The research evidence on using CAEP for evaluating amplification is shown in Table 5–8. The presence of CAEPs has been found to correlate with auditory perception and normal receptive language at 1 year of age (Kurtzberg, 1989). In children with auditory neuropathy spectrum disorders, the presence of aided cortical responses was related to speech perception with amplification (Rance, Cone-Wesson, Wunderlich, & Dowell, 2002).

In infants and children below 3 years of age, the number of detected CAEPs to speech stimuli was positively correlated with age-corrected PEACH scores (Golding et al., 2007). These results suggest that detection of CAEPs to speech stimuli is a valid measure of aided functional performance in infants and children.

Notwithstanding the efficiency of evaluations carried out in controlled clinical settings, the effectiveness of amplification must be evaluated in real-life situations. There is evidence to indicate that children's performance in structured settings do not correlate well with performance in natural environments in which amplification is used (Vidas, Hassan, & Parnes, 1992). This is clearly demonstrated in the evaluation of the relative effectiveness of the NAL or the DSL prescription for school-age children (Ching et al., 2010). Even though children demonstrated speech perceptual performance as well as their normal-hearing peers, both in quiet and noisy situations in laboratory settings, they reported much difficulty in speech communication in real life (Scollie, Ching, Seewald, Dillon, Britton, Steinberg, & Corcoran, 2010; Scollie, Ching, Seewald, Dillon, Britton, Steinberg, & King, 2010). In a similar vein, evaluations of hearing aid technologies revealed significant benefits in laboratory conditions that were not commensurate with actual effects in real-world environments (e.g. Bentler, Wu, Kettel, & Hurtig, 2008b). On the other hand, preferences in real life were not always linked to benefits in controlled conditions (Ching et al., 2010; Cox & Xu, 2010). It is for this reason that evidence summarised in the Tables in this chapter have distinguished between those that relate to assessments conducted in laboratory/ideal conditions (Efficacious), and those that relate to effects in real-world environments (Effectiveness). This distinction must be considered in the interpretation of findings for clinical applications and counseling purposes.

Recommendation: Evaluate the effectiveness of amplification for infants and young children using parental reports and/or objective electrophysiologic measures.

SUMMARY

This chapter addresses the technical aspects of hearing aid selection, fitting, verification, and evaluation, within the context of a comprehensive management scheme for children who need hearing aids. Specific recommendations and statements are made after reviewing the existing scientific evidence.

There is good quality evidence to support the use of wide-dynamic-range compression and automatically switchable directional-microphone technology for infants and children. The current evidence on extended amplification bandwidth, frequency transposition, frequency compression, and noise reduction for children is insufficient to assess the balance of benefits and harms of the technology. Selection of hearing aids using either the NAL or the DSL prescription is efficacious, and evaluations using subjective and objective means are recommended to ensure that amplification meets the needs of the individual child.

REFERENCES

Akhtar, N. (2005). The robustness of learning through overhearing. *Developmental Science*, *8*(2), 199–209.

Alcantara, J. L., Moore, B. C., Kuhnel, V., & Launer, S. (2003). Evaluation of the noise reduction system in a commercial digital hearing aid. *International Journal of Audiology*, *42*, 34–42.

American National Standards Institute. (1997). *ANSI S3.5, Methods for calculations of the speech intelligibility index*. New York, NY: Author.

American National Standards Institute. (2009). *ANSI S3.22, Specification of hearing aid characteristics.* (ANSI S3.22-2009). New York, NY: Author.

Arehart, K. H., Hansen, J. H., & Gallant, S. (2003). Evaluation of an auditory masked threshold suppression algorithm in normal-hearing and hearing-impaired listeners. *Speech Communication, 40,* 575–592.

Auriemmo, J., Kuk, F., Lau, C., Marshall, S., Thiele, N., Pikora, M., . . . Stenger, P. (2009). Effect of linear frequency transposition in speech recognition and production of school-aged children. *Journal of the American Academy of Audiology, 20,* 289–305.

Bagatto, M., Moodie, S., Scollie, S., Seewald, R., Moodie, S., Pumford, J., & Liu, R. (2005). Clinical protocols for hearing instrument fitting in the Desired Sensation Level method. *Trends in Amplification, 9*(4), 199–226.

Bagatto, M., Scollie, S. D., Hyde, M., & Seewald, R. (2010). Protocol for the provision of amplification within the Ontario Infant hearing program. *International Journal of Audiology, 49*(S1), S70–S79.

Bagatto, M., Scollie, S. D., Seewald, R. C., Moodie, K. S., & Hoover, B. M. (2002). Real-ear-to-coupler difference predictions as a function of age for two coupling procedures. *Journal of the American Academy of Audiology, 13*(8), 407–415.

Bagatto, M., Seewald, R. C., Scollie, S. D., & Tharpe, A. M. (2006). Evaluation of a probe-tube insertion technique for measuring the real-ear-to-coupler difference (RECD) in young infants. *Journal of the American Academy of Audiology, 17*(8), 573–581.

Bentler, R., Wu, Y. H., Kettel, J., & Hurtig, R. (2008a). Digital noise reduction: Outcomes from laboratory and field studies. *International Journal of Audiology, 47*(8), 447–460. doi: 901531759 [pii]

Bentler, R., Wu, Y. H., Kettel, J., & Hurtig, R. (2008b). Digital noise reduction: Outcomes from laboratory and field studies. *International Journal of Audiology, 47,* 447–460.

Bess, F. H., Chase, P. A., Gravel, J. S., Seewald, R. C., Stelmachowicz, P. G., Tharpe, A. M., & Hedley-Williams, A. (1996). Amplification for infants and children with hearing loss. *American Journal of Audiology, 5*(1), 53–68.

Bess, F. H., & Paradise, J. L. (1994). Universal screening for infant hearing impairment: Not simple, not risk-free, not necessarily benificial and not presently justified. *Pediatrics, 93*(2), 330–334.

Bohnert, A. (2009). *Hearing aids with multichannel non-linear frequency compression: A study with adults and children.* Paper presented at the British Academy of Audiology, Liverpool, UK.

Boothroyd, A. (1991). *Speech perception measures and their role in the evaluation of hearing aid performance.* Paper presented at the 1991 National Conference of Pediatric Amplification., Boys Town National Research Hospital, Omaha, NE.

Boothroyd, A., & Medwetsky, L. (1992). Spectral distribution of /s/ and the frequency response of hearing aids. *Ear and Hearing, 13,* 150–157.

Boysman, M., & Dreschler, W. A. (2000). Field trials using a digital hearing aid with active noise reduction and dual-microphone directionality. *Audiology, 39,* 260–268.

Byrne, D., & Ching, T. Y. C. (1997). Optimising amplification for hearing-impaired children: I. Issues and Procedures. *Australian Journal of Education of the Deaf, 3*(1), 21–28.

Byrne, D., Dillon, H., Ching, T. Y. C., Katsch, R., & Keidser, G. (2001). NAL-NL1 procedure for fitting nonlinear hearing aids: Characteristics and comparisons with other procedures. *Journal of the American Academy of Audiology, 12,* 37–51.

Carter, L., Golding, M., Dillon, H., & Seymour, J. (2010). The detection of infant cortical auditory evoked potentials (CAEPs) using statistical and visual detection techniques. *Journal of the American Academy of Audiology, 21,* 347–356.

Ching, T., Hill, M., Van Wanrooy, E., & Agung, K. (2004). The advantages of wide-dynamic-range compression over linear amplification for children. *NAL Annual Report, 2003/2004,* 45–49.

Ching, T. Y. C., Brien, A. O., Dillon, H., Chalupper, J., Hartley, L., Hartley, D., . . . Hain, J. (2008). Directional effects on infants and young children in real life: Implications for amplification. *Journal of Speech, Language, and Hearing Research, 52,* 1241–1254.

Ching, T. Y. C., Dillon, H., & Byrne, D. (1998). Speech recognition of hearing-impaired listeners: predictions from audibility and the limited role of high-frequency amplification. *Journal of the Acoustical Society of America, 103*(2), 1128–1140.

Ching, T. Y. C., Dillon, H., Day, J., & Crowe, K. (2007). The NAL study on longitudinal outcomes of hearing-impaired children: Interum findings on language of early and later-identified children at 6 months after hearing aid fitting. *Proceedings of the Fourth International Conference: A Sound Foundation Through Early Amplification* (pp.185–199), Stafa, Switzerland.

Ching, T. Y. C., Dillon, H., Katsch, R., & Byrne, D. (2001). Maximizing effective audibility in hearing aid fitting. *Ear and Hearing, 22*(3), 212–224.

Ching, T. Y. C., & Hill, M. (2007). The Parent's Evaluation of Aural/Oral Performance of Children (PEACH) Scale: Normative data. *Journal of the American Academy of Audiology, 18*(3), 220–235.

Ching, T. Y. C., Hill, M., Birtles, G., & Beecham, L. (1999). Clinical use of paired comparisons to evaluate hearing aid fitting of severely/profoundly hearing-impaired children. *Australian and New Zealand Journal of Audiology, 21*(2), 51–63.

Ching, T. Y. C., Hill, M., & Dillon, H. (2008). Effects of variations in hearing aid frequency response on real-life functional performance of children with severe or profound hearing loss. *International Journal of Audiology, 47*, 461–475.

Ching, T. Y. C., Newall, P., & Wigney, D. (1994). Audio-visual and auditory paired comparison judgments by severely and profoundly hearing-impaired children: Reliability and frequency response preferences. *Australian Journal of Audiology, 16*(2), 99–106.

Ching, T. Y. C., Scollie, S. D., Dillon, H., & Seewald, R. C. (2010). A cross-over, double-blind comparison of the NAL-NL1 and the DSLv.4.1 prescriptions for children with mild to moderately severe hearing loss. *International Journal of Audiology, 49*, S4–S15.

Ching, T. Y. C., van Wanrooy, E., Dillon, H., & Carter, L. (2011). Spatial release from masking in normal-hearing children and children who use hearing aids. *Journal of the Acoustical Society of America, 129*(1), 368–375.

Cone-Wesson, B., & Wunderlich, J. (2003). Auditory evoked potentials from the cortex: Audiology applications. *Current Opinions in Otolaryngology, Head and Neck Surgery, 11*, 372–377.

Cox, R. M., & Xu, J. (2010). Short and long compression release times: speech understanding, real-world preferences, and association with cognitive ability. *Journal of the American Academy of Audiology, 21*(2), 121–138.

Crandell, C. C., & Smaldino, J. (2000). Classroom acoustics for children with normal hearing and with hearing impairment. *Language, Speech, and Hearing Services in Schools, 31*, 362–370.

De Gennaro, S., Braida, L., & Durlach, N. (1986). Multichannel syllabic compression for severely impaired listeners. *Journal of Rehabilitation Research and Development, 23*(1), 17–24.

Dillon, H. (1999). NAL-NL1: A new procedure for fitting non-linear hearing aids. *Hearing Journal, 52*(4), 10–16.

Dillon, H., Keidser, G., Ching, T. Y. C., Flax, M., & Brewer, S. (2011). The NAL-NL2 prescription procedure. *Phonak Focus, 40*, 1–10.

Eisenberg, L. S., & Levitt, H. (1991). Paired comparison judgments for hearing aid selection in children. *Ear and Hearing, 12*, 417–430.

Feigin, J. A., Kopun, J. G., Stelmachowicz, P., & Gorga, M. P. (1989). Probe-tube microphone measures of ear canal sound pressure levels in infants and children. *Ear and Hearing, 10*(4), 254–258.

Fullgrabe, C., Baer, T., & Moore, B. C. (2010). Effect of linear and warped spectral transposition on consonant identification by normal-hearing listeners with a simulated dead region. *International Journal of Audiology, 49*(6), 420–433. doi: 10.3109/14992020903505521

Gatehouse, S., Naylor, N., & Elberling, C. (2006). Linear and nonlinear hearing aid fittings—2. Patterns of candidature. *International Journal of Audiology, 45*, 153–171.

Glista, D., Scollie, S., Bagatto, M., Seewald, R., Parsa, V., & Johnson, A. (2009). Evaluation of nonlinear frequency compression: Clinical outcomes. *International Journal of Audiology, 48*(9), 632–644. doi: 10.1080/14992020902971349

Golding, M., Pearce, W., Seymour, J., Cooper, A., Ching, T., & Dillon, H. (2007). The relationship between obligatory cortical auditory evoked potentials (CAEPs) and functional measures in young infants. *Journal of American Academy of Audiology, 18*, 117–125.

Gravel, J. S., Fausel, N., Liskow, C., & Chobot, J. (1999). Children's speech recognition in noise using omni-directional and dual-microphone hearing aid technology. *Ear and Hearing, 20*(1), 1–11.

Guo, J., Valero, J., & Marcoux, A. (2002). The effect of non-linear amplification and low compression threshold on receptive and expressive speech ability in children with severe to profound hearing loss. *Journal of Educational Audiology, 10*, 1–14.

Hawkins, D. B. (1984). Comparison of speech recognition in noise by mildly-to-moderately hearing-impaired children using hearing aids and FM systems. *Journal of Speech and Hearing Disorders, 49*, 409–418.

Hawkins, D. B. (2004). Limitations and uses of the aided audiogram. *Seminars in Hearing, 25*(1), 51–62.

Jamieson, D. G., Kranjc, G., Yu, K. C., & Hodgetts, W. E. (2004). Speech intelligibility of young school-aged children in the presence of real-life classroom noise. *Journal of American Academy of Audiology, 15*, 508–517.

Jenstad, L. M., Seewald, R., Cornelisse, L. E., & Shantz, J. (1999). Comparison of linear gain and wide dynamic range compression hearing aid circuits: aided speech perception measures. *Ear and Hearing, 19*, 117–126.

Jenstad, L. M., Seewald, R., Cornelisse, L. E., & Shantz, J. (2000). Comparison of linear gain and wide dynamic range compression hearing aid circuits: Aided loudness measures. *Ear and Hearing, 21*(1), 32–44.

Joint Committee on Infant Hearing. (2007). Year 2007 Position statement: Principles and guidelines for early hearing detection and intervention programs. *Pediatrics, 120*(4), 898–921. doi: 10.1542/peds.2007-2333

Jordt, J., Ching, T. Y. C., Byrne, D., Dillon, H., Della Flora, R., Hill, M., . . . Kirievsky, L. (1997). Optimising amplification for hearing-impaired children: II. Aided speech audiogram. *Australian Journal of Education of the Deaf, 3*(1), 21–28.

King, A. M. (2010). The national protocol for paediatric amplification in Australia. [Research article]. *International Journal of Audiology, 49*(S1), S64–S69. doi: 10.3109/1499202090 3329422

Kopun, J. G., & Stelmachowicz, P. (1998). Perceived communication difficulties of children with hearing loss. *American Journal of Audiology, 7*(1), 30–38.

Korhonen, P., & Kuk, F. (2008). Use of linear frequency transposition in simulated hearing loss. *Journal of American Academy of Audiology, 19*(8), 639–650.

Kuk, F. (1996). Subjective preference for microphone types in daily listening environments. *Hearing Instruments, 49*(4), 29.

Kuk, F., Keenan, D., Korhonen, P., & Lau, C. C. (2009). Efficacy of linear frequency transposition on consonant identification in quiet and in noise. *Journal of the American Academy of Audiology, 20*(8), 465–479.

Kuk, F., Korhonen, P., Peeters, H., Keenan, D., Jessen, A., & Anderson, H. (2006). Linear frequency transposition: Extending the audibility of high-frequency information. *Hearing Review, 13*(10), 42–48.

Kurtzberg, D. (1989). Cortical event-related potential assessment of auditory system function. *Seminars in Hearing, 10*, 252–262.

Lewis, M. S., Crandell, C. C., Valente, M., & Enrietto, H. J. (2004). Speech perception in noise: Directional microphones versus frequency modulation (FM) systems. *Journal of American Academy of Audiology, 6*, 426–439.

Litovsky, R. Y., Johnstone, P. M., & Godar, S. P. (2006). Benefits of bilateral cochlear implants and/or hearing aids in children. *International Journal of Audiology, 45*(S1), S78–S91.

MacArdle, B. M., West, C., Bradley, J., Worth, S., Mackenzie, J., & Bellman, S. C. (2001). A study of the application of a frequency transposition hearing system in children. *British Journal of Audiology, 35*(1), 17–29.

Marcoux, A. M., Yathiraj, A., Cote, I., & Logan, J. (2006). The effect of a hearing aid noise reduction algorithm on the acquisition of novel speech contrasts. *International Journal of Audi-*

ology, 45(12), 707–714. doi: 10.1080/14992020600944416

Marriage, J. E., & Moore, B. C. J. (2003). New speech tests reveal benefit of wide-dynamic-range, fast-acting compression for consonant discrimination in children with moderate-to-profound hearing loss. *International Journal of Audiology, 42*(7),418–425.

Miller-Hansen, D. R., Nelson, P. G., Widen, J. E., & Simon, S. D. (2003). Evaluating the benefit of speech recoding hearing aids in children. *American Journal of Audiology, 12,* 106–113.

Moeller, M. P., Donaghy, K. F., Beauchaine, K. L., Lewis, D. E., & Stelmachowicz, P. G. (1996). Longitudinal study of FM system use in non-academic settings: effects on language development. *Ear and Hearing, 17,* 28–41.

Moeller, M. P., Hoover, B., Putman, C., Arbataitis, K., Bohnenkamp, G., Peterson, B., . . . Stelmachowicz, P. (2007). Vocalizations of infants with hearing loss compared with infants with normal hearing: Part I—phonetic development. *Ear and Hearing, 28*(5), 605–627. doi: 10.1097/AUD.0b013e31812564ab00003446-200709000-00002 [pii]

Moodie, K. S., Seewald, R., & Sinclair, S. T. (1994). Procedure for predicting real ear hearing aid performance in young children. *American Journal of Audiology, 3,* 23–31.

Moore, B. C. (2001). Dead regions in the cochlea: diagnosis, perceptual consequences, and implications for the fitting of hearing aids. *Trends in Amplification, 5*(1), 1–34.

Moore, B. C., & Glasberg, B. (1986). A comparison of two-channel and single-channel compression hearing aids. *Audiology, 25,* 210–226.

Mueller, H. G., Grimes, A., & Erdman, S. (1983). Subjective ratings of directional amplification. *Hearing Instruments, 34*(2), 14–16.

Palmer, C., & Mormer, E. (1998). Defining the children's and parents' expectations of the hearing aid fitting. *Hearing Journal, 51*(9), 80.

Palmer, C., & Mormer, E. (1999). Goals and expectations of the hearing aid fitting. *Trends in Amplification, 4*(2), 61–71.

Pittman, A. (2008). Short-term word-learing rate in children with normal hearing and children with hearing loss in limited and extended high-frequency bandwidths. *Journal of Speech, Language, and Hearing Research, 51,* 785–797.

Pittman, A. L., Lewis, D. E., Hoover, B. M., & Stelmachowicz, P. G. (2005). Rapid word-learning in normal-hearing and hearing-impaired children: Effects of age, receptive vocabulary, and high-frequency amplification. *Ear and Hearing, 26*(6), 619–629.

Preves, D. A., Sammeth, C. A., & Wynne, M. K. (1999). Field trial evaluations of a switched directional/omnidirectional in-the-ear hearing instrument. *Journal of the American Academy of Audiology, 10,* 273–284.

Purdy, S., Rarringon, D. R., Moran, C. A., Chard, L. L., & Hodgson, S. A. (2002). A parental questionnaire to evaluate children's auditory behaviour in everyday life (ABEL). *American Journal of Audiology, 11,* 72–82.

Purdy, S. C., & Kelly, A. S. (2008). Auditory evoked response testing in infants and children. In J. R. Madell & C. Flexer (Eds.), *Pediatric audiology: Diagnosis, technology and management* (pp. 132–144). New York. NY: Thieme Medical.

Rance, G., Cone-Wesson, B., Wunderlich, J., & Dowell, R. C. (2002). Speech perception and cortical event related potentials in children with auditory neuropathy. *Ear and Hearing, 23,* 239–253.

Ricketts, T. A., & Galster, J. (2008). Head angle and elevation in classroom environments: Implications for amplification. *Journal of Speech, Language, and Hearing Research, 51,* 516–525.

Ricketts, T. A., Galster, J., & Tharpe, A. M. (2007). Directional benefit in simulated classroom environments. *American Journal of Audiology, 16,* 130–144.

Ricketts, T. A., Henry, P., & Gnewikow, D. (2003). Full time directional versus user selectable microphone modes in hearing aids. *Ear and Hearing, 24,* 424–439.

Ricketts, T. A., & Hornsby, W. Y. (2005). Sound quality measures for speech in noise through a commercial hearing aid implementing digital noise reduction. *Journal of the American Academy of Audiology, 16,* 270–277.

Robbins, A. M., Renshaw, J. J., & Berry, S. W. (1991). Evaluating meaningful auditory integration in profoundly hearing-impaired children. *American Journal of Otolaryngology, 12,* 144–150.

Schwartz, D. M., & Larson, V. D. (1977). A comparison of three hearing aid evaluation procedures for young children. *Archives of Otolaryngology, 103,* 401–406.

Scollie, S., Seewald, R., Cornelisse, L. E., Moodie, S., Bagatto, M., Laurnagaray, D., . . . Pumford, J. (2005). The Desired Sensation Level Multistage Input/Output Algorithm. *Trends in Amplification, 9,* 159–197.

Scollie, S. D. (2008). Children's speech recognition scores: The Speech Intelligibility Index and proficiency factors for age and hearing level. *Ear and Hearing, 29*(4), 543–556.

Scollie, S. D., Ching, T. Y. C., Seewald, R., Dillon, H., Britton, L., Steinberg, J., & Corcoran, J. (2010). Evaluation of the NAL-NL1 and DSLv.4.1 prescriptions for children: preference in real world use. *International Journal of Audiology, 49*(S1), S49–S63.

Scollie, S. D., Ching, T. Y. C., Seewald, R., Dillon, H., Britton, L., Steinberg, J. A., & King, K. A. (2010). Children's speech perception and loudness rating when fitted with hearing aids using the DSL v.4.1 and the NAL-NL1 prescriptions. *International Journal of Audiology, 49*(S1), S26–S34.

Seewald, R., Cornelisse, L. E., & Ramji, K. V. (1997). DSL v4.1 for Windows: A software implementation of the Desired Sensation Level (DSL[i/o]) method for fitting linear gain and wide-dynamic-range compression hearing instruments. Users' manual. London; Ontario: University of Western Ontario Hearing Health Care Research Unit.

Seewald, R., Hudson, S. P., Gagne, J.-P., & Zelisko, D. L. (1992). Comparison of two procedures for estimating the sensation level of amplified speech. *Ear and Hearing, 13*(3), 142–149.

Seewald, R., Moodie, S., Scollie, S., & Bagatto, M. (2005) The DSL Method for pediatric hearing instrument fitting: Historical perspective and current issues. *Trends in Amplification, 9*(4), 145–157.

Sherbecoe, R. L., & Studebaker, G. A. (2003). Audibility index prediction of normal-hearing and hearing-impaired listeners' performance on the Connected Speech Test. *Ear and Hearing, 24,* 71–88.

Simpson, A. (2009). Frequency-lowering devices for managing high-frequency hearing loss: A review. *Trends in Amplification, 13*(2), 87–106.

Simpson, A., Hersbach, A. A., & McDermott, H. J. (2005). Improvements in speech perception with an experimental nonlinear frequency compression hearing device. *International Journal of Audiology, 44*(5), 281–292. doi: 10.1080/14992020500060636

Smith, J., Dann, M., & Brown, P. M. (2009). An evaluation of frequency transposition for hearing impaired school-age children. *Deafness and Education International, 11*(2), 62–82.

Stapells, D. R. (2000). Frequency-specific evoked potential audiometry in infants. In R. C. Seewald (Ed.), *A sound foundation through early amplification: Proceeedings of an international conference* (pp. 13–32). Stafa, Switzerland: Phonak AG.

Stelmachowicz, P. (1999). Hearing aid outcome measures for children. *Journal of the American Academy of Audiology, 10*(1), 14–25.

Stelmachowicz, P., Lewis, D., & Creutz, T. (1997). *The Situational Hearing Aid Response Profile (SHARP).* Omaha, NE: Boys Town National Research Hospital.

Stelmachowicz, P., Lewis, D., Hoover, B., & Keefe, D.H. (1999). Subjective effects of peak clipping and compression limiting in normal and hearing-impaired children and adults. *Journal of the Acoustical Society of America, 105*(1), 412–422.

Stelmachowicz, P., Lewis, D., Hoover, B., Nishi, K., McCreery, R., & Woods, W. (2010). Effects of digital noise reduction on speech perception for children with hearing loss. *Ear and Hearing, 31*(3), 345–355. doi: 10.1097/AUD.0b013e3181cda9ce

Stelmachowicz, P. G., Lewis, D. E., Choi, S., & Hoover, B. (2007). Effect of stimulus bandwidth on auditory skills in normal-hearing and hearing-impaired children. *Ear and Hearing, 28*(4), 483–494.

Studebaker, G.A. (1982) Hearing aid selection: An overview. In G. A. Studebaker and F. H. Bess (Eds.), *The Vanderbilt hearing aid report: State of the art—Research needs* (pp. 147–155). Upper Darby, PA: Instrumentation Associates.

Thompson, D. C., McPhillips, H., Davis, R. L., Lieu, T. A., Homer, C. J., & Helfand, M.

(2001). Universal newborn hearing screening: Summary of evidence. *Journal of the American Medical Association, 286*(16), 2000–2010. doi: 10.1001/jama.286.16.2000

Valente, M., Fabry, D. A., & Potts, L. G. (1995). Recognition of speech in noise with hearing aids using dual microphones. *Journal of the American Academy of Audiology, 6*, 440–449.

Vander Werff, K. R., Prieve, B. A., & Georgantas, L. M. (2009). Infant air and bone conduction tone burst auditory brain stem responses for classification of hearing loss and the relationship to behavioral thresholds. *Ear and Hearing, 30*(3), 350–368.

Vidas, S., Hassan, R., & Parnes, L. S. (1992). Real-life performance considerations of four pediatric multi-channel cochlear implant recipients. *Journal of Otolaryngology, 21*, 387–393.

Voss, S. E., & Herrmann, B. S. (2005). How does the sound pressure generated by circumaural, supra-aural, and insert earphones differ for adult and infant ears? *Ear and Hearing, 26*(6), 636–650.

Walden, B. E., Surr, R. K., Cord, M. T., Edwards, B. M., & Olson, L. (2000). Comparison of benefits provided by different hearing aid technologies. *Journal of the American Academy of Audiology, 11*, 540–560.

Wolfe, J., John, A., Schafer, E., Nyffeler, M., Boretzki, M., Caraway, T., & Hudson, M. (2011). Long-term effects of non-linear frequency compression for children with moderate hearing loss. *International Journal of Audiology, 50*(6), 396–404. doi:10.3109/14992027.2010.551788

World Health Organization. (2007). *International Classification of Functioning, Disability and Health (ICF)* (1st ed.). Geneva, Switzerland: Author.

Wu, Y.-H., & Bentler, R. A. (2010). Impact of visual cues on directional benefit and preference: Part II—Field tests. *Ear and Hearing, 31*(1), 35–46. doi: 10.1097/AUD.1090b1013e3181bc1769b.

Zimmerman-Phillipps, S., Osberger, M. J., & Robbins, J. M. (1998). Infant-Toddler: Meaningful Auditory Integration Scale (IT-MAIS). In W. Eastabrooks (Ed.), *Cochlear implants for kids*. Washington, DC: AG Bell Association for the Deaf.

CHAPTER 6

Evidence-Based Practice and Emerging New Technologies

Gitte Keidser

INTRODUCTION

A challenge for engineers working in the hearing aid industry has always been to work within the constraints of size and power. When hearing aids were analogue, it would take considerable time to bring an idea from concept to commercial product, as a completely new design of the electronic layout was usually required. In the digital era, however, the journey from concept to commercial product may require no more than a change to the code in the central processing unit (CPU) of the instrument. As a result, new hearing aid processing strategies and features are often introduced every 6 months, typically launched at the large annual meetings organized by the American Academy of Audiology (AAA) in the United States of America in April, and the Union of Hearing Aid Acousticians (EUHA) in Germany in October. The new features are, however, not always directly aimed at improving the hearing performance of hearing-impaired people, but sometimes have the goal of making the instruments more convenient to wear (e.g., synchronization of volume control and program changes across ears, Powers & Burton, 2005), or easing the clinician's job (e.g., data logging; Fabry, 2005).

The issue for Evidence-Based Practice (EBP), however, is that the introduction of digital technology has not proportionally reduced the time it takes to evaluate a new product in a well-designed study, and to have the findings reach the public domain through a peer-reviewed process. It may come as a surprise that it easily can take up to 30 months for study outcomes to appear in a peer-reviewed journal. The steps involved in designing and executing a comprehensive study that meets the criteria for a high-level and statistically well powered study are listed in Table 6–1. In my experience, the preparations for a project (steps 1 to 4) can take 6 months or more to complete. Depending on the scope of the study and the number of participants, data collection can take up to 9 months, especially when the study is based on a field test conducted in a crossover design with about 30 participants. It can take 3 months to complete the study and produce a manuscript (steps 6 to 7), and may take longer depending on the complexity of the data set. The review process in step 8 can be expected to take up to 6 months, allowing for one revision, but can take much longer if substantial changes to the manuscript are requested, resulting in several iterations of the review process. Finally, a 6-month wait from the time a manuscript is

Table 6–1. An Overview of the Steps Involved in Designing, Conducting, and Publishing a Study That Will Produce High-Level, Evidence-Based Data

Steps
1. Identify research questions, including a search for information to obtain a good understanding of the aim and function of the technology in question (e.g., literature review or objective tests)
2. Devise test protocol, including ensuring all test parameters are justified and determining the sample size required to obtain sufficient statistical power
3. Implement test protocol, including obtaining ethics approval, collecting all hardware and software required for testing, and making sure that all test equipment is functional and calibrated
4. Recruit test participants
5. Collect data
6. Enter and analyze data
7. Write up and submit paper
8. Paper review process
9. Publication

accepted until it appears in the journal is not uncommon. Unfortunately, such time frames mean that, in the highly competitive environment in which hearing aid manufacturers operate, it is not viable to wait for evidence based data supporting a new technology to be available in peer-reviewed publications before introducing it on the market. This means that some technologies are commercially available long before the evidence for their effectiveness is published. What should clinicians do in such situations when they want to apply EBP to their clinical work? This chapter provides some ideas for where to obtain relevant information about new hearing aid technology in the intervening time, and how to process it. Examples of emerging technologies for which peer-reviewed data are currently very limited, or nonexistent, are introduced. The available data related to these new inventions are discussed, and recommendations are made for which further evidence is needed.

WHEN PEER-REVIEWED EVIDENCE IS NOT AVAILABLE

This section briefly introduces three procedures the clinician can follow when peer-reviewed evidence is not readily available. Each procedure is presented and discussed in more details in the following sections.

New features in hearing aids are rarely introduced without some supporting data, or at least a description of the motivation for the implementation and the processing strategy. Sporadic data collected either in-house or by an independent institution using a prototype of the final product, or a computer simulation of the invention, may be available at the time a new technology is launched, or shortly thereafter. Such data are often based on simple analytical studies conducted in controlled laboratory environments or short field tests based on a small sample size, and are presented through non-peer-reviewed channels such as white papers produced by the manufacturer or trade journals. The fact that these publications have not been refereed should not exclude them from the review of research evidence (e.g., Cox, 2005), because the decision to bypass the peer review process could be one based on time. Nevertheless, non-peer-reviewed presentations should be appraised with extra care and with special attention to the design and statistical power. These days, online presentations are quickly becoming a popular means of early distribution of information by manufacturers.

As long as mainly non-peer-reviewed publications are available, it is recommended to also look at the rationale and theory behind the new feature and to review the literature on the basic research that has led to the particular signal processing strategy. Although this information does not directly prove that the new strategy is effective for hearing aid wearers, the evidence can be used to obtain a better understanding of what, specifically, the new strategy is expected to achieve, and in which situations it may be beneficial. This knowledge can be used to develop an informed opinion about how likely it is that the new strategy will have a significant impact on a hearing aid user's performance in specific listening environments. An example is outlined in the detailed section below.

A further, and not unreasonable, approach would be for the clinician to obtain some personal experience with the effectiveness of the feature in question from test box measurements and from listening to the hearing aid processing in targeted listening situations. This is evidence, although at a low level (Level 6) in terms of the EBP hierarchy in Table 1–5 in Chapter 1, but it may well be the only evidence available.

White Papers and Trade Journal Articles

White papers and trade journal articles would not turn up using the database search engines referred to in Chapter 1. The best place to look for the manufacturers' white papers, or any information about a recent release, is on the manufacturer's global Web site, typically addressed www.companyname.com. Most sites will have a section for professionals that is accessed from the main home page. In this section you may find access to a "library," "publications," or "presentations" where available information is found. "Downloads" may be found under the specific products. Note that not all manufacturers engage in publication of white papers, but if they do, these are also most likely available directly from the local supplier. Searching for information on the manufacturers' Web sites provides the best result if the proprietary name of the technology and/or the product in which it is available is known.

The two most common trade journals used to disseminate audiology and hearing aid-related research are *The Hearing Journal* (http://journals.lww.com/thehearingjournal/pages/default.aspx) and *The Hearing Review* (http://www.hearingreview.com). Both provide a search engine and access to their most recent and archived articles free of charge. *Audiology Online* (www.audiologyonline.com) is another Web site that is increasingly used by manufacturers to distribute information about new products and features in a timely manner, especially through the live and recorded courses hosted by the Web site. These courses can be accessed through registration free of charge. Fees only apply if you wish to accrue continuing education points for a membership in one of the American or Canadian audiological societies.

Statistical strength and the type of evidence are still the foremost characteristics to examine when scrutinising non-peer-reviewed publications and presentations (referred to as internal validity in Chapter 1), but it is unusual to find sufficient information about these characteristics in such publications. The recommendation here is to disregard data sets based on fewer than ten participants (unless the data concern a special population from which recruitment of larger numbers is clearly very difficult), and data presented without any statistical analyses to support the interpretation of the results. Otherwise, the larger the sample size and the lower the significance level is below 0.05, the more confidence one can have in the findings. This is because increasing the number of observations will reduce the variation (i.e., standard deviation) in data and hence a greater effect size is expected. Furthermore, the lower the significance level is, the greater is the chance that the same significant result will be obtained in a repeated study. Consider two studies, A and B, which both show a statistically significant benefit from a directional microphone of 3.5 dB, and a similar spread in data. Because the result of study A is obtained on 25 participants and reaching a significance level of 0.00006 whereas in study B the result is based on 12 listeners and a significance level of 0.02, study A will on its own present a more conclusive outcome. Of course, reviewed together, the two studies would provide stronger evidence for the benefit of directional microphones. Chapters 1, 2, and the Appendix also provide details of study characteristics to examine when evaluating evidence.

Another factor to look for is how closely the evaluation of the technology under investigation mimics real-life usage. The early studies found in non-peer-reviewed publications are often limited to laboratory experiments. Laboratory tests offer the controllability and repeatability that are essential to quantitative scientific research, and although such data can be informative, the limitations introduced by evaluating the feature in an environment without the dynamic changes, additional cues, and distracters present in most real-world listening conditions should not be ignored. Furthermore, early studies published in either peer-reviewed or non-peer-reviewed journals may be conducted using a computer simulation (offline or real-time processing) of the new signal processing strategy. For example, to investigate the effect of extending the hearing aid bandwidth on speech intelligibility, Moore, Füllgrabe, and Stone (2010) used stimuli that had been processed off-line through a computer-simulated hearing aid. At the test appointment the pre-processed stimuli were presented to study participants through headphones. To evaluate the effect of a new transient noise reduction algorithm, Keidser, O'Brien, Latzel, and Convery (2007) presented stimuli that were picked up by the microphones on a pair of hearing aids on the participant's ear, and directed to a computer for real-time processing before being sent back to the earphone receivers in the hearing instruments. Apart from the microphones and receivers, the hearing instruments were empty shells. In the case of such simulations, it is important to consider whether the invention has been evaluated in isolation or in interaction with common hearing aid signal processing strategies such as wide dynamic range compression (WDRC), feedback cancellation, and noise reduction (NR). If the simulation was presented through headphones or a loudspeaker, the results may be different from those if the same strategy was presented through a hearing instrument due to the possible effect of the microphone placement on the hearing aid and the coupling to the ear.

Scrutinizing Basic Research

A prerequisite for following this path is that sufficient information about the feature of interest and its implementation is disclosed by the manufacturer. This information may be found in product brochures or in any publication presenting evaluation data. These publications may also provide preliminary references for the basic research that forms the rationale behind the new strategy. The steps for scrutinizing basic research follow the first three steps described in Chapter 1 for evaluating the evidence directly related to the technology or intervention in question. That is, a specific question is defined, the evidence to answer the question is searched, and the available evidence is evaluated. However, instead of relating the evidence directly to the client, in this case the evidence is related to the claims of the new strategy. The knowledge is used to make an informed decision about how likely the strategy is to be effective for its stated purpose.

For example, recently, a new signal processing strategy that limits directionality to the high frequencies was introduced with the claim that it would help hearing aid users localize sounds better. The strategy is explained in detail and reviewed in a later section of this chapter. To support the claim manufacturers described how spectral cues used to localize sounds get distorted when the ear is occluded with a hearing aid, and presented the results of objective measurements that demonstrated how the new strategy, relative to conventional signal processing, produced a directivity pattern that better resembled that available to the open ear. However, the objective measurements do not guarantee the efficiency of the signal processing strategy. If no evaluation data on hearing-impaired listeners were available to review, the clinician could ask to what extent distortion of spectral cues caused by occluding the ear affect localization performance and how. Such data may provide an insight into how important the new strategy may be to hearing aid users. A literature search would reveal that localization performance by normal-hearing listeners is dramatically reduced when the external ear is occluded in some form to distort spectral cues produced by the pinna (e.g., Gardner & Gardner, 1973; Hofman, Van Riswick, & Van Opstal, 1998; Musicant & Butler, 1984). It also has been found that hearing aid users with milder sensorineural hearing loss generally localize sound better unaided than aided with conventional devices (Byrne & Noble, 1998; Van den Bogaert, Klasen, Moonen, Van Deun, & Wouters, 2006). This would suggest that the new signal processing has potential to be beneficial to hearing aid users. However, it is worth noting that Hofman et al. (1998) found that while there was a dramatic reduction in localization performance immediately after normal-hearing listeners had their ears occluded with a mould, over time while wearing the mould, their ability to localize sounds improved. The finding that the brain can recalibrate to different cues, which is supported by Zahorik, Bangayan, Sundareswaran, Wang, and Tam (2006), could suggest that long-term hearing aid users may not benefit from the new strategy immediately after fitting, or may require some time to show the optimum benefit. Such knowledge is valuable in guiding the expectations of clients.

Gather Personal Experience

To explore modern hearing aid features, a hearing aid analyser offering a variety of noise and speech, or speechlike, stimuli and a chamber that allows the hearing aid to be positioned such that the microphone can be reliably aligned with the loudspeaker in any azimuth is required for test box measurements. A hearing aid listening tube or instant fit tips and a field setup with at least two loudspeakers are needed for obtaining a personal listening experience. Test box measurements are best used to verify the effect of a feature and to quantify the resulting response change. For example, with noise presented from 180 degrees, is gain reduced when switching from omnidirectional to directional microphone mode? Or, how much is gain reduced when the instrument is exposed to various noise stimuli and the noise reduction strength is set to minimum, medium, or maximum relative to the off position?

Listening experiences provide a better idea of the real-life effectiveness of the feature. Ideally, the function of the technology is trialed in the real-world listening situations it is designed to target, but valuable experiences can also be gathered from listening to different simulated environments in the clinic. For this purpose, it is desirable to be able to present speech and noise through different loudspeakers that surround you and allow you to position yourself in different directions relative to the speech and noise. CDs containing different speech and noise stimuli are widely available. It should be noted that test box measurements and unilateral listening tests (e.g. through a listening tube) are sufficient to evaluate most current technologies. However, proper evaluation of newer signal processing strategies, which utilize information about the sound arriving at the microphone on each of two instruments, require a listening test in which the paired devices are worn bilaterally.

EMERGING NEW TECHNOLOGIES

New strategies in hearing aids seem to be focused on three areas in particular: (1) improvement of the signal-to-noise ratio (SNR), (2) restoration of binaural hearing, and (3) personalization of the hearing aid processing. It is well established that hearing-impaired people require a better SNR than normal-hearing people for understanding speech in noise (e.g., Plomp, 1978), and that hearing aids distort the binaural cues that are used for localization of sounds and to ease conversation when with a group of people or in competing noise (e.g., Byrne & Noble, 1998). The former problem has been a research focus for a long time and has resulted in the introduction of increasingly sophisticated directional microphone modes and noise reduction algorithms (e.g,. Chung, 2004), whereas attention to the latter problem is more recent and has been sparked by the possibility of binaurally linking the signal processing in bilaterally fitted hearing aids. There is no doubt that rapid advancement in the area of wireless sound transmission, enabling increased data transmission and faster communication between two hearing aids, opens up new possibilities to both improving the SNR and restoring binaural cues. The motivation to personalize the hearing aid processing arises from the general acceptance of the fact that hearing aid wearers have different needs and different preferences, and that younger hearing aid candidates especially are likely to enjoy taking some control of their instruments. In a world where technology and experimentation are such an integral part of our life, it seems natural to start handing over some of the decision-making processes and controls to the hearing aid wearer.

Table 6–2 lists some of the more recently established hearing aid features that address one of the three areas outlined above and for which there currently is no strong evidence to support the feature as implemented in the final product. By "established," I mean that the feature is included in hearing instruments by several manufacturers and is thus considered widely available, although the specific implementation of the feature can vary greatly among manufacturers. The following sections provide more background about each of these features, discuss the limited information currently available about the effectiveness of the features, and identify the research needed to support recommendation of these features in hearing rehabilitation. Suggestions for test box measurements or personal listening tests are not made as these would depend on the equipment and real-life opportunities available.

NEW STRATEGIES FOR IMPROVING THE SNR AND THE EVIDENCE

One of the most recent contributions to this area is the introduction of a feature that enables the hearing aid wearer to direct the

Table 6–2. An Overview of Established Features in Hearing Instruments That Have Not Been Thoroughly Evaluated in the Final Products

Area of Interest	*New Feature*	*Specific Aim*
Improve SNR	Selective directional focus	To direct the focus of the directional beam to a target talker situated either to the front, right, left, or rear side of the hearing aid wearer
Restore binaural cues	High-frequency directionality	To provide spectral cues similar to those produced by the pinna
	Binaural gain control	To provide ILD cues similar to those experienced in the unaided ear
	Extended high-frequency bandwidth	To make available high-frequency sounds that are important for directional hearing audible
Personalize the processing	Trainability	To enable the hearing aid wearer to fine-tune and optimize the amplification characteristics in their everyday listening environments

Note: SNR = Signal-to-Noise Ratio; ILD = Interaural Level Difference.

sensitivity of the directional microphones to the front, to either side of the head, or to the rear. This means hearing aid wearers do not need to turn their heads to face a speaker situated next to or behind them to obtain an optimum SNR. This may be an advantage in situations where the hearing aid wearer needs to keep looking to the front while conversing with someone situated next to them (e.g., when driving a vehicle). Currently, there are no peer-reviewed studies published that have evaluated this feature as implemented in a hearing instrument.

A search in the public domain revealed three evaluation studies of the final product described in publications produced by the manufacturers.[1] One of these has been further published in a trade journal (Nyffeler & Dechant, 2009). In terms of the speech reception threshold (SRT) required for 50% speech recognition in noise, all three studies used a crossover design and at least 20 participants to demonstrate a significant directional benefit with the selective directional focus feature relative to omnidirectional and conventional fixed directional microphones when speech was presented from 180 degrees and noise was presented from other directions (Fig. 6–1). None of these publications would be regarded as achieving a high level of evidence (see Chapter 1), mainly due to insufficient statistical interpretation of data; that is, the papers lack clear information about such parameters as the statistical analysis used, variation in data, degrees of freedom, or significance level. However, it should be noted that the average directional benefit measured when speech is presented at 180 degrees azimuth in all three

[1]References to manufacturers' own publications are not given in this chapter, because these quickly become outdated and later disappear from the public domain.

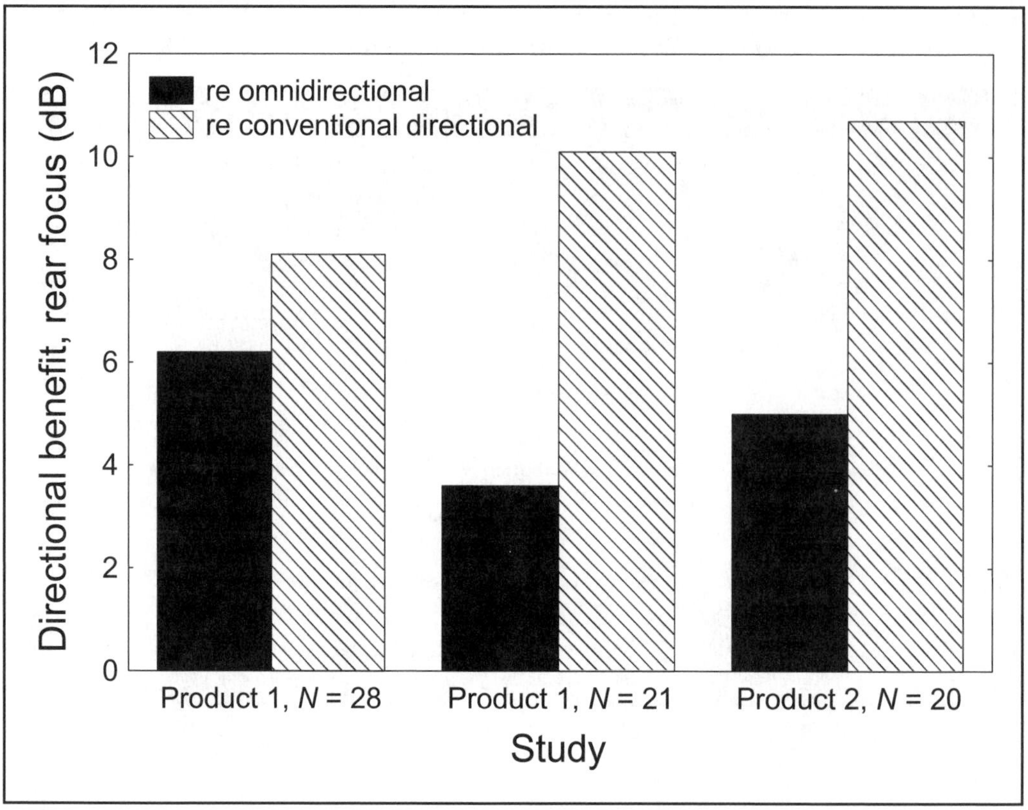

Figure 6–1. *The average directional benefit measured when the directional beam was pointing at the rear of the listener relative to an omnidirectional and a fixed, forward-pointing directional mode. Data that stem from three different studies using two different products, different populations, and sample sizes (N) were obtained from the manufacturers' white papers.*

studies is comparative to the directional benefit measured with conventional fixed directional microphones over omnidirectional microphones when speech is presented at 0 degrees azimuth (e.g., Chung, 2004). In the condition where the sensitivity of the microphone is directed to the front, the real-world effectiveness of directional microphones is supported by evidence based research (e.g., Bentler, 2005), and therefore, it seems justifiable to expect this new feature to be effective in achieving better speech understanding when the speaker is not situated directly in front of the hearing aid wearer.

In one of the products evaluated above (Product 1 in Fig. 6–1), the directional focus to either side of the head is achieved by transferring the microphone signal from the chosen focus ear (e.g. right) to the opposite instrument (e.g., left), where the original microphone signal is attenuated by 20 dB (Biggins, 2009). This approach, which significantly increases the SNR presented to the hearing aid wearer, is supported by the findings by Richards, Moore, and Launer (2006). In that study, speech performance of normal-hearing and hearing-impaired listeners was measured when a simulated conversation in a car was presented in various binaural listening configurations under headphones using linear amplification. The study demonstrated that both groups performed best when speech and noise arriving at the ear closer to the talker were presented to both ears. The low number of study participants (<10 in each group) and the simplified representation of the real situation are factors that reduce the impact of this study. In fact, according to Moore (2007), subsequent work has revealed that due to reflections from the windshield, speech in a car is not received mainly in the ear closer to the talker, but also in the ear away from the talker. Some more fundamental questions that have not been answered through the speech testing presented in these publications are: to what extent does the hearing aid wearer find it acceptable to have the audio input intensely focused away from a real-world visual scene? What proportion of hearing aid wearers find the feature useful? Of those who do find it useful, what characteristics do they have, and how often do they use the feature? These questions are important to consider when a clinician discusses amplification options with individual clients—the fourth step in the EBP process, as described in Chapter 3.

NEW STRATEGIES FOR RESTORING BINAURAL CUES AND THE EVIDENCE

The cues important for binaural hearing, which is necessary for localising sounds and for being able to focus on a target sound among a myriad of sound sources, are well established in normal-hearing listeners. They include the interaural time (ITD) and level (ILD) differences resulting from the head shadowing effect, and monaural high-frequency spectral differences created by the pinna (e.g., Blauert, 1999). That is, sounds that are not presented directly in front of or behind the listener will arrive sooner and louder to the ear closer to the sound source than the ear further away. Similarly, a sound will have a slightly different spectral shape when arriving at the eardrum depending on the direction from which it enters the ear canal. ITD and ILD cues are used primarily for left/right discrimination and require access to information arriving at each side of the head. In contrast, the monaural spectral cue, which in particular is used for front/back and up/down discrimination, requires access to high-frequency information and an unobstructed ear. Originating directly from the theory, different features currently address different aspects of these requirements and three of these (high frequency directionality, binaural gain and extended high frequency bandwidth) are discussed in this section.

High-Frequency Directionality

Natural pinna cues are often not available to hearing instrument wearers, either because of the microphone location on the instruments, which means that sounds are picked up for amplification before they are filtered by the pinna, or because the external ear is occluded with an earmould or the instrument itself. Limiting the microphone directionality to the high frequencies, however, alters the spectral shape of sound as a function of arrival azimuth in a way similar to the unobstructed pinna (Fig. 6–2). This signal processing strategy may therefore enhance front/back and up/down localization. To date, only one study evaluating the effect of high-frequency directionality has been published in a peer reviewed journal (Keidser, O'Brien, Hain, McLelland, & Yeend, 2009). In this study, localization performance with high-frequency directionality was compared to the performance with omnidirectional and full-band directional microphones in both the laboratory and the

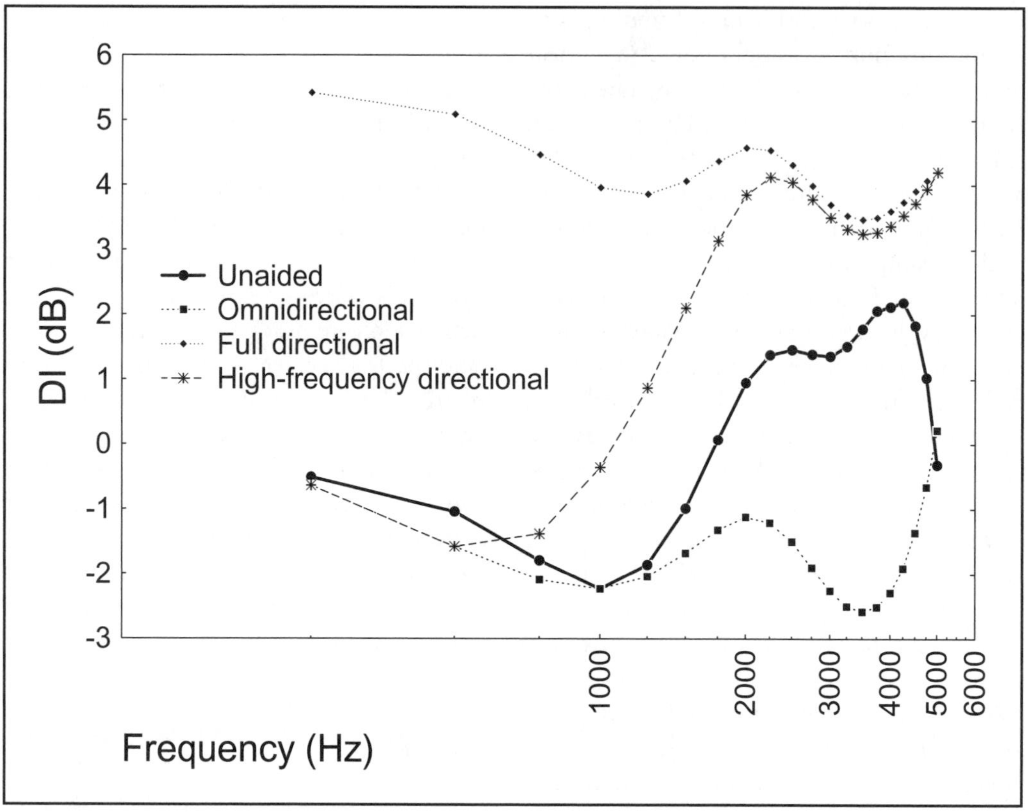

Figure 6–2. *The directional index (DI) measured as a function of frequency on the Knowles Electronics Manikin for Acoustic Research (KEMAR) when unaided, and when fitted with an omnidirectional, a full directional, and a high-frequency (from 1 kHz) directional microphone. The raw data for these measurements were kindly provided by Siemens Hearing Instruments.*

field. Data were collected from a relatively small sample (21 participants) in a randomized crossover design. Although objective data collected in the laboratory showed a small but significant ($p = 0.004$) improvement in front/back localization with high-frequency directionality compared to the other conditions, subjective reports from the field test revealed no effect from this feature. The difference in outcomes again shows the importance of considering both intervention efficacy (i.e., laboratory results obtained in ideal conditions with a specified population) and effectiveness (i.e., real-world results obtained in average conditions with an average population), as discussed in Chapter 1.

Moving to non-peer-reviewed publications, one study published in a trade journal, which evaluated a different implementation of the feature, confirms the findings above (O'Brien, Yeend, Hartley, Keidser, & Nyffeler, 2010). A more recent trade journal article (Groth & Laureyns, 2011) and a publication from one manufacturer both report studies in which front/back discrimination measured in the laboratory was significantly improved with different implementations of high-frequency directionality. A cross-over design was used in all studies with participation of 23, 20, and 14 hearing-impaired listeners, respectively. In O'Brien et al. (2010) all results are interpreted using appropriate statistics with all input and output parameters, including degree of freedom and significant levels, clearly presented. Consequently, the current trend is that limiting directionality to the high frequencies can improve front/back discrimination in a controlled environment, but the effect does not seem to be significant enough to have an impact on hearing aid wearers in real life. As individual variations in performance were noted by Keidser et al. (2009), it would be interesting to conduct research into why this feature is more helpful to some than others and why the feature seems to be less effective in real life than in the laboratory. The effect of high-frequency directionality on localization in the vertical plane also needs to be investigated.

Binaural Gain Control

Unsynchronized operation of such common features as WDRC, NR, and adaptive directional microphones in bilaterally fitted hearing instruments can cause distortions to the ILD cue used to resolve left/right localization (Fig. 6–3). This is because any one of these features will, in each instrument, change gain adaptively in response to the overall level and

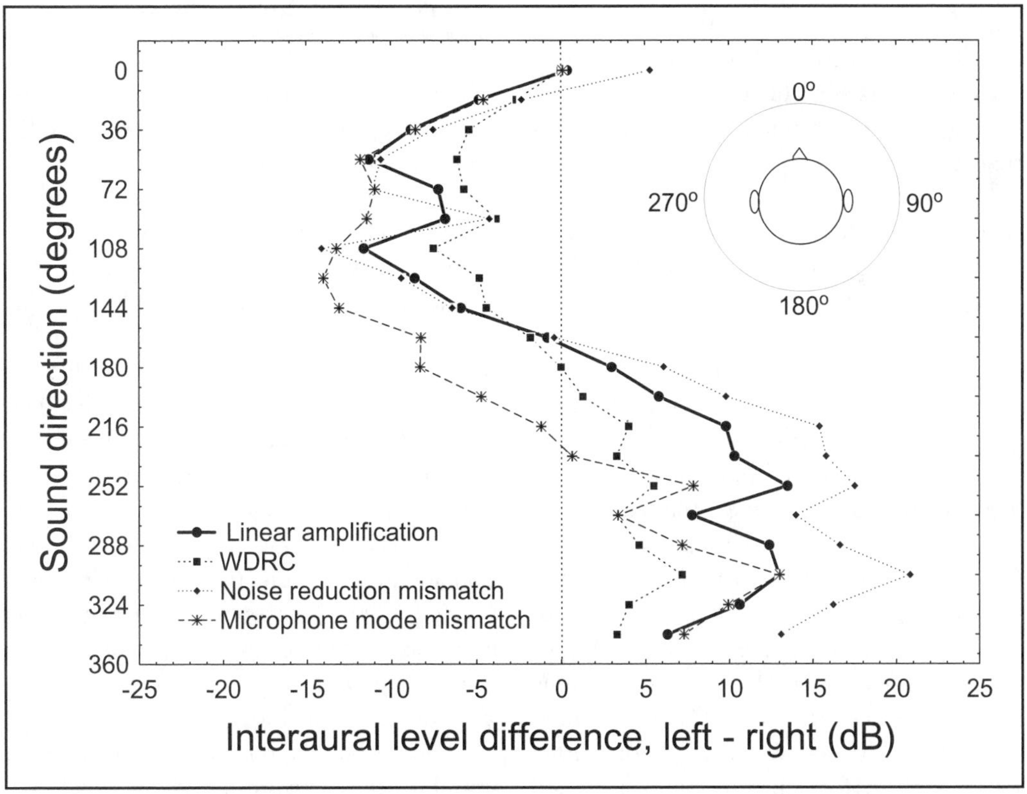

Figure 6–3. *The interaural level difference (left minus right ear) measured as a function of azimuth on KEMAR when fitted with two instruments providing linear amplification (no distortion to ILD), WDRC, NR mismatch across ears, and directional microphone mode mismatch across ears. Data are extracted from the Keidser et al. (2006) study.*

SNR arriving only at the microphone of that instrument. For example, in the case of WDRC, less gain is applied to the ear closer to the sound source where the sound is louder, whereas more gain is applied to the ear farther away from the sound source where the sound is softer, a response that will reduce the natural ILD. The greater the compression ratio in the instruments, the greater the resulting reduction of ILD. Synchronization of noise reduction and directional microphone mode has been possible for some time and is commercially available in several products. More recently, manufacturers have utilized wireless communication between two instruments to coordinate gain changes applied by WDRC in the two instruments to ensure that the typical ILD caused by the head shadow effect is maintained (e.g., Wilson, Lindley, & Schum, 2007).

There are currently no peer-reviewed studies that have evaluated the effect of this strategy on horizontal localization performance. One non-peer-reviewed paper shows a small but significant ($p < 0.05$) improvement in the left/right discrimination of 30 bilaterally fitted hearing aid wearers when binaural communication between the two instruments was enabled (Sockalingam, Holmberg, Eneroth, & Shulte, 2009). One potential caveat in this study is that the stimulus used for localization testing was a bird chirp, which is likely to have been a high-frequency weighted sound. It is well established that the ITD cue is dominant as long as the signal has audible components at frequencies below 1.5 kHz, whereas the ILD cue is more pronounced at higher frequencies (e.g., Wightman & Kistler, 1992). This means that as long as there is no distortion to ITD and the sound contains audible low-frequency information, localization performance by the hearing aid wearers should not be severely affected. This is partly supported by Keidser, Rohrseitz, Dillon, Hamacher, Carter, and Convery (2006), who demonstrated that although the ILD cues were distorted by WDRC and NR, this did not have a significant effect on left/right localization performance measured on 12 hearing aid wearers using a broadband test stimulus. Consequently, it is possible that the benefit of binaural gain control is limited to high-frequency weighted sounds, which are experienced less often in everyday life. Further research in this area needs to systematically investigate the effect of the feature on everyday sounds with different frequency contents while also taking the effect of the ITD cue into consideration. The real-life benefit of binaural gain control also needs to be verified.

EXTENDED HIGH-FREQUENCY BAND

Extending the bandwidth of the hearing aid response has been a goal in hearing aid design for a long time and gradual progress has been made over the years as technology made it possible. The parameters driving this development include the responses of the microphone and the receiver and signal processing power. Recent technological advancement has allowed the hearing aid bandwidth to be extended to 10 kHz. One possible advantage of this feature is access to high-frequency speech components and hence improved speech understanding (e.g., Moore et al., 2010). Because pinna cues used for localization are most prominent at frequencies above 5 kHz (Fig. 6–4), access to higher frequencies may also improve localization performance in hearing aid wearers, provided pinna cues are available, or somehow restored.

Byrne and Noble (1998) report some unpublished data from a study in which participants were asked to localize sounds that were amplified linearly up to 10 kHz, using an experimental hearing aid, and delivered through a completely-in-the-canal style mould

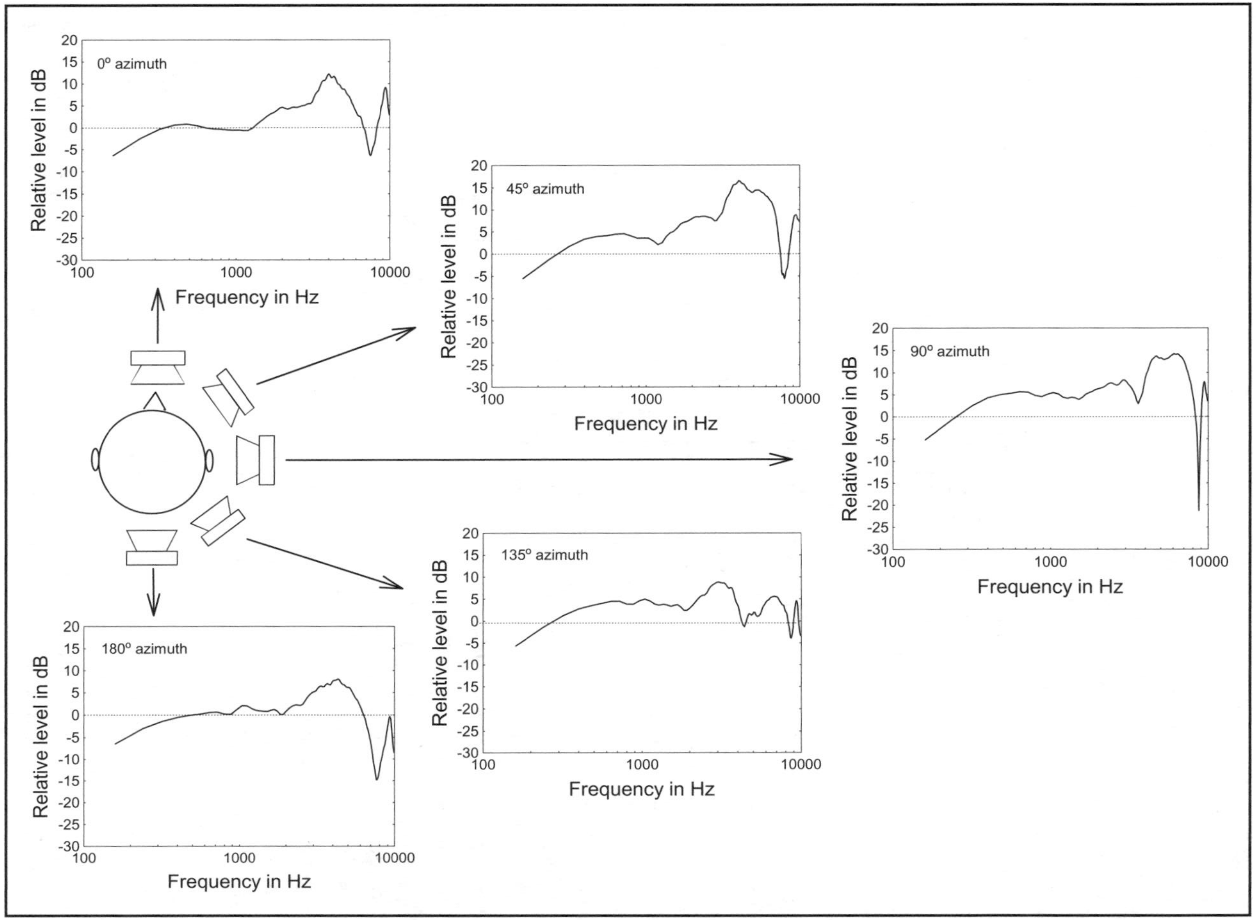

Figure 6–4. *The changes in spectral shape caused by the pinna shadowing effect as the sound (white noise) moves from the median plane in front of KEMAR (0 degrees azimuth), to the side (90 degrees azimuth), and to the back of KEMAR (180 degrees azimuth). The raw data for these measurements were kindly provided by Dr. Jorge Mejia from the National Acoustic Laboratories.*

that left the pinna function intact. They found that a few hearing-impaired listeners with good high-frequency hearing and good unaided vertical localization performance produced their optimum and near-perfect result when the bandwidth was 8 kHz. Beck and Sockalingam (2010) refer to two recent field tests with participation of 58 and 39 participants in which a device with extended bandwidth was evaluated against a conventional instrument. Both studies reported that the participants found the spatial perception in everyday life significantly improved with the new instrument ($p < 0.05$). These studies do not, however, suggest in which dimension localization was improved. Additionally, the instruments used in both studies had other features activated that aim at improving the spatial perception, such as those outlined above. Therefore, there is currently very limited information available to lend direct support to extending high-frequency gain for hearing-impaired listeners in order to improve their spatial perception. In fact, Keidser et al. (2009) has speculated that due to long-term deprivation from high-frequency information, hearing-impaired listeners have learned to utilize spectral differences at mid frequencies (1 to 2 kHz) to determine whether sounds are coming from the front or the back. It is also possible that extending the frequency band is most effective when combined with other processing strategies aimed at improving spatial perception.

A current complication in evaluating instruments with extended high-frequency bands is the lack of knowledge regarding how much gain should be prescribed and the difficulty in verifying the hearing aid output across the higher frequencies (e.g., Kuk & Baekgaard, 2009). Further research in this area needs to first address the more fundamental question of how to prescribe and verify the extended amplification characteristics, and second, to demonstrate that gain at higher frequencies, either alone or combined with other processing strategies aimed at enhancing spatial perception, can improve localization in hearing aid wearers. In addressing the latter question, acclimatization should be considered. The issue of acclimatization is also discussed in Chapter 4.

NEW STRATEGIES FOR PERSONALIZING THE PROCESSING AND THE EVIDENCE

It is highly recommended that hearing aids are fitted using a prescriptive formula for setting the hearing aid parameters. It is also widely acknowledged that the prescribed setting is based on average data and that fine-tuning of the hearing aid parameters based on real-life experiences with the instruments is a crucial part of the fitting process (e.g., Dillon, 2001, pp. 302–320). Fine-tuning in a clinical setting can be complicated and cumbersome. This is partly due to difficulties in determining the particular needs of a client, and partly because the fine-tuned response cannot be immediately verified. Trainable instruments, which give the hearing aid wearer access to a set of controls that enable them to self-adjust selected hearing aid parameters to reach their preferred amplification settings, attempt to address this problem. These devices include a learning algorithm, which collects and stores information about the hearing aid parameter settings chosen by the hearing aid wearer in different listening environments and the acoustic characteristics of the environment at the time a new setting is selected. Over time, based on the acoustic input, the instruments will use this information to automatically apply the wearer's preferred settings (Dillon, Zakis,

McDermott, Keidser, Dreschler, & Convery 2007). Several commercial products are trainable, of which most offer training of environment-specific overall gain. This is achieved by applying the average volume control setting selected by the wearer over time for each class of sound recognized by the instrument's environmental classifier (e.g., Groth, Nelson, Jespersen, & Christensen, 2008). For example, a wearer may choose to increase the volume relative to the baseline setting when listening to speech in quiet, but to reduce the volume when in noisy environments. If this is a consistent pattern, then over time the hearing aid will automatically set overall gain higher when the instruments' environmental classifier decides that the wearer is listening to speech in quiet, and set gain lower when it decides the environment consists only of noise. Thereafter, further training of the instrument would not be required.

The implementation described above is a very simple representation of trainability that utilizes only a very crude classification of sounds based on their acoustic characteristics. If one considers that the acoustics of background noises, for example, vary across multiple dimensions, including intensity, spectral, and temporal characteristics (e.g., Keidser, 2009), it would seem reasonable to expect better outcomes from training algorithms that analyse a continuum of acoustic parameters. At least one manufacturer has recently introduced a training algorithm that enables independent training of input-dependent gain in four channels, which means that the static compression characteristics can be varied in each of four channels and hence the gain-frequency response shape can be changed at various input levels (Chalupper, Junius, & Powers 2009).

A literature search on trainable, or self-learning, hearing instruments, including non-peer-reviewed publications, revealed no studies that had aimed to evaluate the potential real-life benefit of training the device to adjust overall gain in specific environments. The search, however, produced four peer-reviewed articles on the trainable concept. One of these papers (Zakis, McDermott, & Dillon, 2007) describes the evaluation of a sophisticated training algorithm implemented in a programmable research device. This device provided slow-acting WDRC and modulation depth-based NR in three channels. Using one control, the hearing aid wearer could alternate between three different gain adjustments: overall gain, response slope, and mid-frequency gain. The static compression parameters and the noise suppression strength in each hearing aid channel were trained using information about the intensity level and estimated SNR overall and in each of the three channels, and the preferred gain settings in each channel. After a training period of up to 4 weeks, 13 hearing-impaired people compared their trained response with the baseline response in a double-blind field trial. At the end of the trial, nine participants showed a significant preference for the trained response. Only one preferred the baseline response. The double-blind evaluation was achieved by having the two responses randomly assigned to each of two programs every time the device was switched on, thus totally excluding a biased effect on the preference. This well-designed study therefore suggests that hearing-impaired people can manage a complex control to train the device to produce amplification characteristics that, overall, provided a better listening experience across everyday listening environments compared to a prescribed response. The weaknesses of this study include the low number of test participants, and the fact that participants were not randomly selected from a typical clinical population, but were recruited from a group of volunteers who could manage a nonstandard device and who were willing to wear the body-worn style device in real life.

That hearing-impaired people can handle different and complex control configurations to reliably select their preferred responses in a variety of listening situations was confirmed by Dreschler, Keidser, Convery, and Dillon (2008), whereas three independent studies have shown that the baseline response from which training begins significantly affects the preferred gain setting (Dreschler et al., 2008; Keidser, Dillon, & Convery, 2008; Mueller, Hornsby, & Weber, 2008). All three studies used a randomized crossover design with participation of 21 to 24 hearing-impaired people. In two of the studies (Dreschler et al., 2008; Keidser et al., 2008), gain manipulations were collected in the laboratory using a numerical keypad as the controller and real-time linear processing of sounds that were presented in the free field to the listeners' unaided ears. Consequently, these studies used an overly simplistic representation of trainability. In Mueller et al. (2008), participants were fitted with a commercial product that enabled training of overall gain through the usage pattern of the volume control. Adjustments were made in the field starting from two different baseline conditions that shared the same gain-frequency response shape but differed in overall gain by 12 dB. Although this study suffers from a problem with floor and ceiling effects in the adjustment range from the two starting points, rendering some data invalid, the finding is in agreement with the two laboratory studies. All three studies demonstrated that lower gain levels generally were selected when starting from the baseline setting that provided less gain relative to a baseline setting that provided more gain (Fig. 6–5). Keidser et al. (2008) further showed that while some individuals were able to consistently select the same preferred response from two different baseline responses, most participants had no real preference when selecting from among a wide range of responses.

Taken together, current publications on trainability would suggest that at least some hearing-impaired people can manage and benefit from trainability, but that the starting point must be appropriately prescribed to reduce the likelihood of wearers who are likely to make few changes to the amplification choosing a potentially harmful setting. It is probable that more complex training algorithms will be introduced in hearing instruments in the future. To build up better evidence-based knowledge about this feature, future studies need to investigate the benefit of trainable instruments in a large clinical population, and to determine the degree of algorithm complexity the average client can handle. From our current knowledge, it seems that some hearing-impaired people are more likely than others to benefit from trainability, in which case determining the profile of candidates for trainability would be a desirable goal. The importance of assessing the individual needs and abilities of people with hearing impairment who seek rehabilitation is discussed in Chapter 3.

SUMMARY

In the field of audiology, new technology is often available years before peer-reviewed evidence. In the meantime, clinicians should critically scrutinize the findings of available non-peer-reviewed publications for consistency, with a specific focus on sample size, statistical analyses, and the realism of the test paradigm used (implementation and listening situation). For further information, the literature on basic research supporting the new technology could be reviewed to obtain a better understanding of what the technology is likely to achieve. Finally, with the right

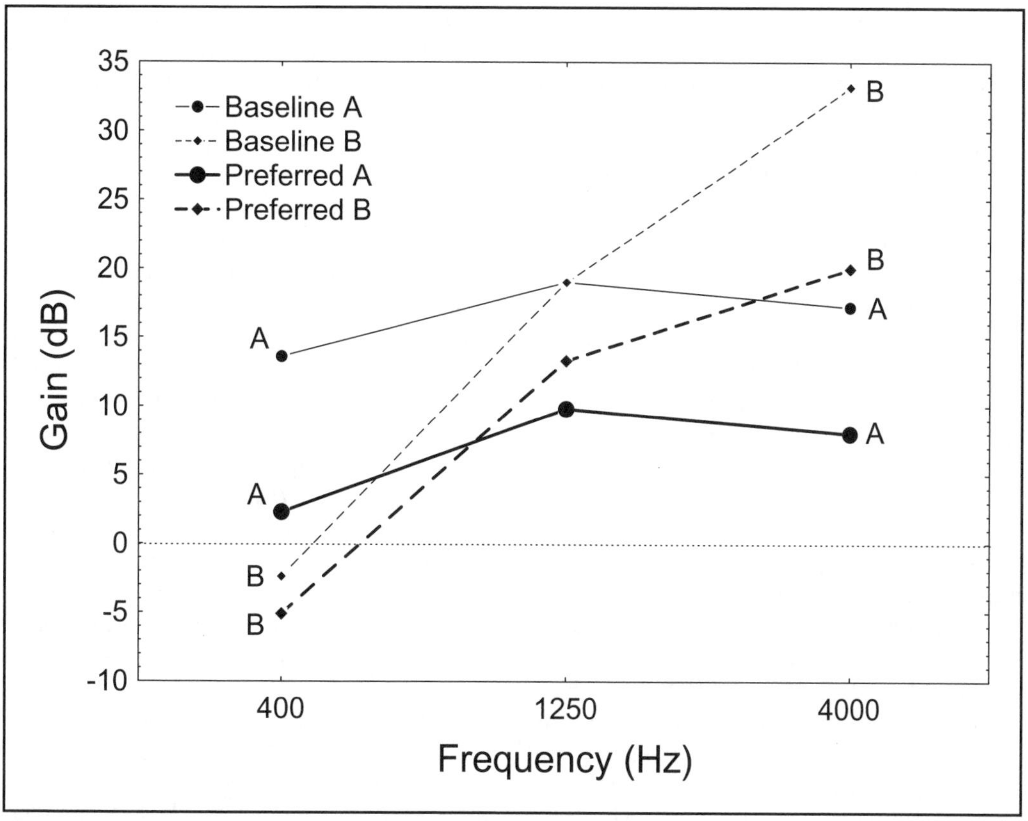

Figure 6–5. *The baseline responses* (A and B, thin lines) *and the average preferred responses across 12 different listening environments and 24 participants when starting from each baseline response* (A and B, thick lines). *Data are from the study by Keidser et al. (2008).*

equipment, experience with the operation and effectiveness of the technology can be obtained through test box measurements and personal listening sessions.

REFERENCES

Beck, D. L. & Sockalingam, R. (2010). Facilitating spatial hearing through advanced hearing aid technology. *Hearing Review, 17*(4), 44–47.

Bentler, R. A. (2005). Effectiveness of directional microphones and noise reduction schemes in hearing aids: A systematic review of the evidence. *Journal of the American Academy of Audiology, 16*(7), 473–484.

Biggins, A. (2009). Benefits of wireless technology. *Hearing Review, 16*(11), 40–43.

Blauert, J. (1999). *Spatial hearing. The psychophysics of human sound localization.* Cambridge, MA: MIT Press.

Byrne, D., & Noble, W. (1998). Optimizing sound localization with hearing aids. *Trends in Amplification, 3*, 551–573.

Chalupper, J., Junius, D., & Powers, T. (2009). Algorithm lets users train aid to optimize compression, frequency shape, and gain. *Hearing Journal, 62*(8), 26–33.

Chung, K. (2004). Challenges and recent developments in hearing aids. Part I. Speech understanding in noise, microphone technologies and noise reduction algorithms. *Trends in Amplification, 8*(3), 83–124.

Cox, R. M. (2005). Evidence-based practice in provision of amplification. *Journal of the American Academy of Audiology, 16*(7), 419–438.

Dillon, H. (2001). *Hearing aids*. Sydney, Australia: Boomerang Press.

Dillon, H., Zakis, J., McDermott, H., Keidser, G., Dreschler, W., & Convery, E. (2007). The trainable hearing aid: What will it do for clients and clinicians? *Hearing Journal, 59*(4), 30–36.

Dreschler, W. A., Keidser, G., Convery, E., & Dillon, H. (2008). Clientbased adjustments of hearing-aid gain: The effect of different control configurations. *Ear and Hearing, 29*, 214–227.

Fabry, D. A. (2005). DataLogging: A clinical tool for meeting individual patient needs. *Hearing Review, 12*(1), 32–36.

Gardner, M. B., & Gardner, R. S. (1973). Problem of localization in the median plane: Effect of pinnae cavity occlusion. *Journal of the Acoustical Society of America, 53*(2), 400–408.

Groth, J., & Laureyns, M. (2011). Preserving localization in hearing instrument fittings. *Hearing Journal, 64*(2), 34–38.

Groth, J., Nelson, J., Jespersen, C. T., & Christensen, L. (2008). Automatic hearing instrument adjustments based on environmental listening situations. *Hearing Review, 15(4*), 40–48.

Hofman, P. M., Van Riswick, J. G. A., & Van Opstal, A. J. (1998). Relearning sound localization with new ears. *Nature Neuroscience, 1*, 417–421.

Keidser, G. (2009). Many factors are involved in optimizing environmentally adaptive hearing aids. *Hearing Journal, 62*(1), 26–32.

Keidser, G., Dillon, H., & Convery, E. (2008). The effect of the base line response on self-adjustments of hearing aid gain. *Journal of the Acoustical Society of America, 124(*3), 1668–1681.

Keidser, G., O'Brien, A., Hain, J-U., McLelland, M., & Yeend, I. (2009). The effect of frequency-dependent microphone directionality on horizontal localization performance in hearing-aid users. *International Journal of Audiology, 48*(11), 789–803.

Keidser, G., O'Brien, A., Latzel, M., Convery, E. (2007). Evaluation of a noise-reduction algorithm that targets non-speech transient sounds. *Hearing Journal, 60*(2), 29–39.

Keidser, G., Rohrseitz, K., Dillon, H., Hamacher, V., Carter, L., & Convery, E. (2006). The effect of multichannel wide dynamic range compression, noise reduction, and the directional microphone on horizontal localization. *International Journal of Audiology, 45*, 563–579.

Kuk, F., & Baekgaard, L. (2009). Considerations in fitting hearing aids with extended bandwidths. *Hearing Review, 16*(11), 32–38.

Moore, B. C. J. (2007). Binaural sharing of audio signals: Prospective benefits and limitations. *Hearing Journal, 60*(11), 46–48.

Moore, B. C. J., Füllgrabe, C., & Stone, M. A. (2010). Effect of spatial separation, extended bandwidth, and compression speed on intelligibility in a competing-speech task. *Journal of the Acoustical Society of America, 128*(1), 360–371.

Mueller, G. H., Hornsby, B. W. Y., & Weber, J. E. (2008). Using trainable hearing aids to examine real-world preferred gain. *Journal of the American Academy of Audiology, 19*, 758–773.

Musicant, A. D., & Butler, R. A. (1984). The influence of pinnae-based spectral cues on sound localization. *Journal of the Acoustical Society of America, 75*(4), 1195–1200.

Nyffeler, M., & Dechant, S.(2009). Field study on user control of directional focus: Benefits of hearing the facets of a full life. *Hearing Review, 16*(1), 24–28.

O'Brien, A., Yeend, I., Hartley, L., Keidser, G., & Nyffeler, M. (2010). Evaluation of frequency compression and high-frequency directionality. *Hearing Journal, 63*(8), 32–37.

Plomp, R. (1978). Auditory handicap of hearing impairment and the limited benefit of hearing aids. *Journal of the Acoustical Society of America, 63*(2), 533–549.

Powers, T. A., & Burton, P. (2005). Wireless technology designed to provide true binaural amplification. *Hearing Journal, 58*(1), 25–34.

Richards, V., Moore, B. C. J., & Launer, S. (2006). Potential benefits of across-aid communication for bilaterally aided people: Listening in a car. *International Journal of Audiology, 45*(3), 182–189.

Sockalingam, R., Holmberg, M., Eneroth, K., & Shulte, M. (2009). Binaural hearing aid communication shown to improve sound quality and localization. *Hearing Journal, 62*(10), 46–47.

Van den Bogaert, T., Klasen, T. J., Moonen, M., Van Deun, L., & Wouters, J. (2006). Horizontal localization with bilateral hearing aids: Without is better than with. *Journal of the Acoustical Society of America, 119*(1), 515–526.

Wightman, F. L., & Kistler, D. J. (1992). The dominant role of low-frequency interaural time differences in sound localization. *Journal of the Acoustical Society of America, 9*, 1648–1660.

Wilson, G., Lindley, G., & Schum, D. (2007). A new Epoch in hearing history. *Hearing Review Products Report, July/August*, 32–35.

Zahorik, P., Bangayan, P., Sundareswaran, V., Wang, K., & Tam, C. (2006). Perceptual recalibration in human sound localization: Learning to remediate front-back reversals. *Journal of the Acoustical Society of America, 120*(1), 343–359.

Zakis, J. A., McDermott, H. J., & Dillon, H. (2007). The design and evaluation of a hearing aid with trainable amplification parameters. *Ear and Hearing, 28*, 812–830.

PART III

Cochlear Implants

CHAPTER 7

Evidence About the Effectiveness of Cochlear Implants for Adults

Richard C. Dowell

THE DEVELOPMENT OF COCHLEAR IMPLANTATION AND THE NEED FOR AN EVIDENCE-BASED APPROACH

Cochlear implantation has developed over a period of 30 years to be a significant part of clinical audiology practice across the world. For adults with acquired severe or profound hearing loss, this procedure has been demonstrated to be one of the most effective surgical procedures in modern medicine (Fig. 7–1). The success rate in terms of demonstrable benefit for auditory skills exceeds 90% of the treated population and the effect size (Cumming & Finch, 2001), in terms of improvements to speech perception can be estimated at between 1.3 and 1.8 (Cohen's *d*). This indicates that in the key measure of speech perception, the application of cochlear implants improves the mean result for the population of interest (severely and profoundly deaf adults) by more than one standard deviation. In terms of the size of improvement, a recent study of a group of 310 postlingually deafened adults (Dowell, Fellows, & Hollow, 2007) showed that sentence perception improved from a median preoperative score of 14% to a postoperative median of 90%, and with competing noise at 10dB SNR, from 0% to 43%. The quality of life improvements for many recipients are also reported as highly significant and well-correlated with measurements of speech perception (Hawthorne et al., 2004).

Cochlear implant systems represent the first successful replacement of a sensory system using a human-machine interface (Clark, 2003). A cochlear implant bypasses the defective peripheral auditory apparatus by eliciting sound percepts through electrical stimulation of the auditory nerve. Rehabilitation of severe hearing loss through cochlear implantation is a truly multidisciplinary activity where audiologists play the key role in evaluation, recommendation, counseling, and postsurgical management for individual patients (Dowell, 2005). The ideal cochlear implant audiologist needs solid scientific knowledge in areas of auditory physiology, acoustic phonetics, amplification and hearing devices, electrophysiological assessment, and auditory rehabilitation, plus excellent communication skills and working knowledge of relevant otological and general medical issues.

Despite the overwhelming evidence that now supports cochlear implantation, the initial research that led to modern implant sys-

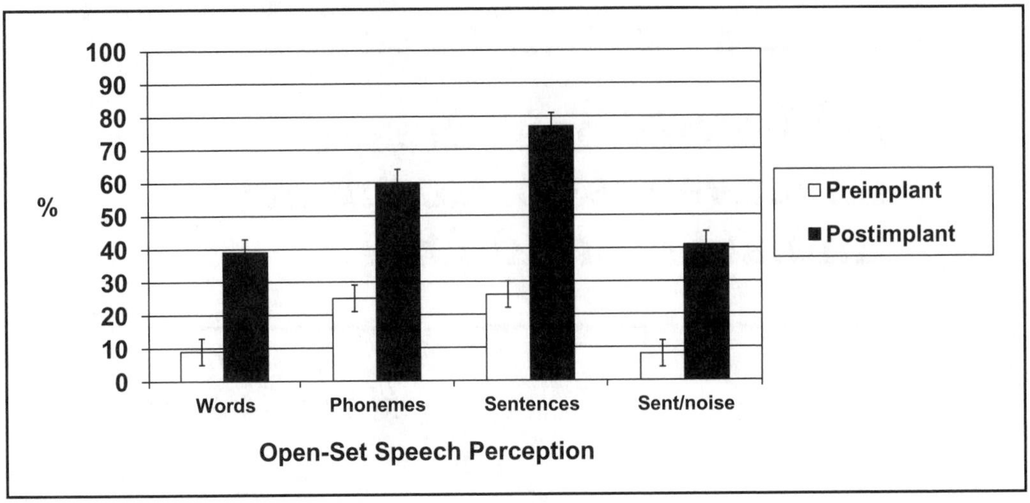

Figure 7–1. *Pre- and postoperative mean speech perception scores for 310 consecutive adult patients with acquired hearing loss who received cochlear implants in Melbourne Australia between 1994 and 2006. Preoperative results are obtained using optimized hearing aids and postoperative results are at approximately 3 months after surgery using the cochlear implant alone. Recorded speech materials are presented at 60 dBA (65 dB SPL). Scores are shown for open set monosyllabic words (phoneme and word scores), CUNY sentences in quiet, and at a signal to noise ratio of +10 dB.*

tems and their clinical application was not well supported in its early years, and viewed with skepticism by the hearing research, otological, and audiological communities. The level of suspicion about the effectiveness of cochlear implants in their early incarnation was understandable to some degree. Opinions from respected auditory researchers, based on animal experiments, suggested that the concept of electrical stimulation in the auditory system could not work effectively for assisting human communication (Lawrence, 1964). Audiologists shied away from the idea of surgical intervention and the risks that could be involved, and tended to focus on demonstrating the benefits of noninvasive rehabilitation techniques using amplification and tactile devices. Even otologists viewed the opening of the cochlea (to place a stimulating electrode) as something that probably could only lead to further damage of the auditory system. There also were objections to the concept based on the knowledge obtained from postmortem temporal bone studies that suggested that profoundly deaf patients may have only limited numbers of cochlea nerve cells surviving (Kerr & Shuknecht, 1968).

This climate of skepticism meant that the science and clinical application of cochlear implants had to proceed cautiously and use rigorous evaluation to demonstrate safety and efficacy. Looking back, it is fitting to write the story of the development of cochlear implantation from the perspective of evidence-based practice, a story that provides ample support for the benefits of this approach in clinical audiology and other health care fields.

This chapter outlines some of the important questions that have been addressed in order to develop cochlear implantation to its current level and brings the reader up to date with current evidence on outcomes and factors affecting performance in adult recipients.

Attempts are made to bring this evidence together within an information transmission model of the cochlear implant system which may help the reader to understand how these multiple technical and patient factors contribute to overall success. The conclusion provides a few practical guidelines, based on evidence from clinical studies, that may assist in discussing options with patients who are considering cochlear implantation. In addition, some of the current and future challenges are discussed where good clinical evidence will be needed to provide the best advice to hearing-impaired people.

BASIC SCIENCE QUESTIONS IN COCHLEAR IMPLANTATION

Early Attempts at Electrical Stimulation of the Auditory Nerve

To have a full understanding of the issues in the clinical application of cochlear implants it is necessary to have a basic knowledge of the scientific foundations of electrical stimulation of the auditory nerve. The idea that electrical stimulation of the auditory system may provide assistance to those with hearing loss has probably been around since the discovery of electrophonic hearing in the 1930s (Wever & Bray, 1930), but it is a French team (Djourno & Eyries, 1957) that is widely attributed with first demonstrating the feasibility of electrical stimulation of the auditory nerve in humans. Sporadic research efforts from that time up until the late 1970s repeatedly showed that deaf patients perceived auditory sensations when the VIIIth nerve was electrically stimulated, but the technical problems of providing reliability and signal processing sophistication for a clinical implant device were insurmountable at the time (Atlas, Herndon, Simmon, Dent, & White, 1983; Clark, 1969; Eddington, Dobelle, & Brackmann, 1978; Fourcin, Rosen, & Moore, 1979; Hochmair, Hochmair-Desoyer, & Burian, 1979; House & Urban, 1973; Michelson, 1971; Pialoux, Chouard, & Meyer, 1979; Simmons, 1966).

Partly because of these issues, only simple single electrode devices were used clinically in significant numbers during the 1970s (House, Berliner, & Eisenberg, 1981). Although the generation of an auditory percept in a deaf person must have seemed like a breakthrough at the time, the real problem for developing a useful cochlear implant system was to provide effective transfer of useful acoustic information. Without patients having access to useful information in real time, particularly for speech sounds, there was no possibility of providing benefit for communication. There are three stages in this information transfer process in an effective cochlear implant system. The first involves the detection and analysis of acoustic signals, the next involves determining how the acoustic information should be presented to the auditory nerve (the so-called sound or speech processing strategy) and the last is the mechanism for delivering the electrical signals to the VIIIth nerve. The basic and applied sciences involved in these stages include acoustics and electrical engineering in stage one, speech science and psychophysics in stage two and auditory physiology, surgery, and electrode design for stage three. The safety of the implant system also requires careful consideration of the electrical parameters and implanted materials for biocompatibility. Therefore, researchers had to find a solution to a significant research question. If we put this research question into the PICO format described in Chapter 1, we could be asking, "For those with profound sensorineural hearing loss (P), does electrical stimulation of the cochlear (I) provide, safe, reliable and real-time information (C) to facilitate speech understanding (O)?"

Safety and Biocompatibility in Cochlear Implants

Safety and biocompatibility (the "I" component of the research question) in the implanted part of a cochlear implant (known as the receiver/stimulator) were key issues in the development of the systems we have today. The generation of action potentials in neural tissue can be achieved with any type of electrical stimulus but most of these are highly toxic to the surrounding body tissues. This is due to the biochemical reactions that occur at the interface between metal electrodes and body fluid which can be highly damaging to local cells. This is particularly true when direct current stimulation is used and the interface reactions occur in only one direction. For this reason, modern cochlear implants tend to use biphasic charge-balanced current pulses for stimulation within the cochlea. Under these conditions, equal amounts of charge flow in each direction over a short time interval (<100 µs) and the products of interface reactions do not have a chance to build up to toxic levels. Careful studies in the late 1970s and early 80s established that such stimulation was safe and effective in animal models (Shepherd, Franz, & Clark, 1990) and also established a safe limit in terms of charge density for electrical stimulation within the cochlea. These results guided the engineering design of cochlear implant stimulators (Clark, Black, Forster, Patrick, & Tong, 1978), and 30 years of experience with implanted human subjects suggests that the design standards are appropriate given that no systematic change in electrical thresholds has been evident.

The safety of the electrical stimulus was obviously crucial to any long term treatment of hearing loss using cochlear implants, but other key design problems involved the materials for an implanted device, the isolation of electronic components from corrosive body fluids and the provision of a power source for the internal components. In particular, the stimulating electrodes required an inert metal that could provide consistent electrical stimulation for up to 24 hours a day for a lifetime with no significant deterioration or change in properties. Most metals under these conditions corrode rapidly and some, such as copper, are toxic in relatively small concentrations. These significant engineering challenges all required considerable investigation and some ventures down cul-de-sacs before cochlear implant systems arrived at their current state of development. Platinum is used for intracochlear electrodes, titanium and ceramic materials for containing the implanted electronic components, sophisticated hermetic sealing techniques are used to ensure that fluid cannot penetrate to the electronics in the long term, and power is provided to the receiver/stimulator via a radio frequency link rather than implanted batteries. The reliability of modern systems has improved markedly over the last 20 years to where failure rates for the current Cochlear Ltd system are less than 0.2% per year. For more details on the technical and engineering aspects of cochlear implants, the reader is referred to Graeme Clark's comprehensive volume *Cochlear Implants: Fundamentals and Applications* (Clark, 2003). Therefore, although safety concerns were addressed in the early stage of implant development, outcomes from long-term use have provided further evidence about this.

Speech Science and the Psychophysical Basis of Cochlear Implants

Evidence for the use of cochlear implants to deliver speech information evolved over time and speech coding strategies were refined based on the evidence. The groundwork for our understanding of how humans decipher the acoustic code of speech was set in the 1950s and 1960s through classic studies at the Haskins laboratories, among others, in the United States (see for instance, Liberman, Delattre, Gerstman, & Cooper, 1954). This work formed the basis of our understanding of acoustic phonetics, developed the concept of the phoneme as the fundamental unit of speech, and identified some aspects of the rapid, sophisticated auditory analysis that takes place when humans communicate. A complete review of this area is not needed here but a few major results are of relevance to the understanding of cochlear implant systems. Simplifying and summarizing a great deal of work in acoustic phonetics, it is reasonable to identify two major sources of acoustic information in speech that are highly significant for comprehension. These are the changes in the instantaneous spectrum and, independently, in the amplitude envelope of the speech signal. In particular, rapid changes within the spectral shape or the amplitude envelope of connected speech provide many of the important cues for recognizing consonants, which carry much of the information content. For instance, rapid changes in spectral peaks (in particular the second formant) cue the place of articulation for some consonant groups, and a silent period followed by a short noise burst provides a strong cue for differentiating stop consonants. It is clear that a cochlear implant system would need to be able to transfer dynamic information about the spectral shape and amplitude envelope of the acoustic signal in real time if it was to provide useful speech perception.

So, forgetting for a moment about the engineering challenges of extracting these parameters from the environment, how can this information be delivered using electrical stimulation of the auditory nerve? The first attempts at providing information via a cochlear implant were necessarily simple and involved presenting the raw speech signal in electrical form to a single electrode inside, or adjacent to, the cochlea. It would have been fortuitous if this approach resulted in speech understanding, but evidence quickly accumulated that a more sophisticated approach was required. Studies of the perceptual characteristics elicited by electrical stimulation of the auditory nerve in deaf subjects were carried out by a number of researchers during the 1960s (Simmons, 1966) and 1970s (Eddington et al., 1978) but it was only after systematic work, notably by Tong and others in Melbourne (Tong, Clark, Blamey, Busby, & Dowell, 1982; Tong, Dowell, Blamey, & Clark, 1983) and Robert Shannon in the United States (Shannon, 1983), that a clear picture emerged of the fundamental psychophysics of cochlear implantation.

In summary, it has been demonstrated that the discrimination of the frequency of stimulation delivered at a single site within the cochlea is very poor compared with normal hearing. Frequency difference limens (DLs) for postlingually deaf adults were between 10 and 20% for low frequencies from 50 to 200 Hz, and little or no discrimination of frequencies was possible above 300 Hz (Tong et al., 1982). This is in stark contrast to normal hearing listeners where frequency DLs are less than 0.5% over a wide range of frequencies (Sek & Moore, 1995). Just why this frequency (or rate) discrimination is so poor remains one of the major mysteries of cochlear implant science to this day. It is surprising because animal studies have demonstrated that the phase-locking of action potentials to electrical stimulation is strong, at least up to approximately 1000 Hz (Rose, Brugge, Anderson, & Hind, 1971). Thus, the temporal information related to frequency is available in the timing of action potentials within the auditory nerve, and we know that central mechanisms exist in the normal auditory system that can analyze fine timing cues to a high level of precision. It seems, however, that the central mechanisms are not geared to deal with timing information in the form it is presented by a cochlear implant electrode. The possibility of presenting mid and high frequency spectral information via a single electrode in the cochlea was therefore limited and researchers had to consider other ways of providing the essential spectral information for speech.

The situation for amplitude discrimination was more encouraging as many studies demonstrated that the loudness percept for an electrical signal could be controlled reasonably precisely by varying the amount of current delivered at an electrode (Shannon, 1983; Tong et al., 1982; Tong et al., 1983). For the pulsatile signals used most commonly in cochlear implant systems, loudness depended on the amount of electrical charge delivered in each pulse that could be controlled by varying the current (the height of the pulse) or the duration (the width of the pulse). A number of issues emerged relating to the provision of amplitude information in a practical cochlear implant system. The useful dynamic range for electrical stimulation was very narrow (10–15 dB) compared to the range of sound pressure levels in the acoustic environment (80–100 dB). This range could also be significantly different for different subjects and electrode sites. In addition, when electrical signals were presented at more than one site in the cochlea, loudness varied in an uncontrolled fashion due to physical interactions of the electrical signals. The compression of the wide range of acoustic amplitudes onto the narrow range available for electrical stimulation has been one of the major engineering challenges in developing sound processors for cochlear implants. Work on refining the control of amplitude continues today and it has been demonstrated that subtle changes can alter speech perception performance in particular acoustic environments. These issues overlap with many issues in modern hearing devices such as maximum output limiting, wide dynamic range compression, and noise reduction algorithms.

The variation of dynamic range across individuals and electrodes has resulted in the development of the procedure known as "mapping" which occupies a significant proportion of time in the postoperative management of cochlear implant users. In this procedure, controlled electrical stimulation pulse trains are presented to individual electrodes and the threshold (T-levels) and maximum comfortable level (C-levels or M-levels) are measured in terms of the current being delivered. Once these are established the information which defines the useful dynamic range for each electrode site is stored within the user's cochlear implant system (usually in the external sound processor). This "map" is then unique for the individual user at a particular time and allows the cochlear implant system to function within a comfortable loudness range for that individual.

The problem of uncontrolled interaction of electrical signals presented simultaneously at different sites in the cochlea has been overcome by using so-called sequential stimulation. This shifts all the pulses slightly in time so that stimulation at multiple sites is not in fact truly simultaneous. The short delays involved, however, mean that the stimulation is effectively simultaneous from the perspective of the neural elements. Due to the need to use sequential stimulation, there is a benefit in using narrow pulse widths for stimulation as this allows more electrode sites to be activated in a quasisimultaneous manner within a fixed time period. Default pulse widths for the Cochlear Ltd. cochlear implant system for instance, are 25 μs /phase allowing pulse rates of more than 15,000 Hz.

Perhaps the most important psychophysical finding relevant to cochlear implant systems is that the pitch percepts generated at different sites in the cochlea follow the tonotopic arrangement of the auditory system with more basal electrodes generating higher pitch (sharper) auditory percepts progressing to lower pitch (duller) percepts toward the apical end of the cochlea (Tong et al., 1982; Shannon, 1983). This perceptual arrangement is highly reliable in postlingually deaf adult cochlear implant recipients although the ability to discriminate these percepts (and therefore different electrode sites in the cochlea) varies across subjects. This "place-pitch" discrimination ability has provided the means for transferring spectral information from the acoustic environment to multichannel cochlear implant users, at first with fairly crude systems that provided only major spectral peak information, progressing to today's sound coding strategies such as SPEAK (McDermott, McKay, & Vandali, 1992), ACE (Skinner, Holden, Whitford, Plant, Psarros, & Holden, 2002), and CIS (Wilson, 2000) that provide a relatively sophisticated representation of the instantaneous spectrum in real time. Henry and others showed that the speech perception ability of cochlear implant recipients was highly correlated with their ability to discriminate different electrode sites (Henry, McKay, McDermott, & Clark, 2000). The road to providing finer representation of speech signals represents an effort to continuously search, evaluate and audit the evidence to answer the research question stated above. These efforts address EBP Steps 2 (searching for evidence to answer the question), 3 (evaluating the available evidence) and 5 (evaluating the outcomes of the EBP process), as described in Chapter 1.

CLINICAL APPLICATION OF SINGLE CHANNEL COCHLEAR IMPLANTS AND THE SINGLE/MULTICHANNEL CONTROVERSY

The first clinical application of a cochlear implant system on a significant scale was the use of the House single-channel device developed by William House in Los Angeles (House & Urban, 1973; House et al., 1981). William House is considered one of the pioneering clinicians who helped to drive the cochlear implant field forward in spite of skepticism from the scientific and clinical communities. It is hard to be sure how important this work was to later developments but it is clear that his drive to alleviate the considerable problems faced by his profoundly deaf patients stimulated the scientific community to take notice of the issues. A proliferation of anecdotal evidence that the House implant could provide significant benefit eventually led to the first systematic assessment of auditory outcomes in the cochlear implant field by Bilger, Black, and Hopkinson (1977). This study made it clear that patients using the House device could not understand speech without visual cues, but did gain some awareness of environmental sounds and could discriminate some aspects of speech sounds that assisted lipreading. This was perhaps disappointing to the proponents of single channel devices, but silenced some of the more hard-nosed skeptics who felt that the concept of cochlear implantation was seriously flawed and would never provide benefit to patients. This effort was clearly an example of the application of a clinician's expert knowledge to customize a hearing device to meet clients' needs and a motivation to initiate an EBP process. The outcomes with these devices then motivated a redefinition of the "I" (intervention) in the PICO format question and a repeat of the EBP process.

Research in Vienna led by Hochmair and Hochmair-Desoyer in the late 1970s provided a more sophisticated approach to a single channel cochlear implant system and some open-set speech discrimination was reported for two patients (Hochmair-Desoyer, Hochmair, Fischer, & Burian, 1980). Both the House and Hochmair technology were taken up by the 3M company and later marketed as the 3M-House and 3M-Hochmair cochlear implant systems. Many researchers continued to work on the more challenging problems related to producing a useful multiple channel cochlear implant system but the limited technology of the day and the lack of sophistication in manufacture meant that patient trials were often affected by implant and electrode failures. Expectations of what may be possible with a cochlear implant system were so low among scientists and audiologists that the modest benefits of single channel devices seemed like the way to proceed. A number of tactile devices for the hearing impaired were under development at this time and some rehabilitative audiologists felt that these devices held greater promise with less risk compared with cochlear implants. It was the group at the University of Melbourne under Graeme Clark working with the Nucleus company (later to become Cochlear Ltd.) who were able to produce the first reliable multichannel cochlear implant system for clinical use in 1982. A careful clinical trial of this device, initially in Australia (Dowell, Martin, Clark, & Brown, 1985) and later across a number of centers in the United States showed that substantial benefits were possible for auditory visual communication in postlingually deaf adults and that a proportion of patients showed some ability to understand speech in an open-set context without visual cues. Skepticism remained, however, until outcomes were published by Gantz and colleagues from the University of Iowa for four different cochlear implant designs showing that only the multichannel systems had the potential for patients to understand speech without lipreading (Gantz, McCabe, Tyler, & Preece, 1987). The clinical trial of the Australian cochlear implant system which culminated in market approval by the US Food and Drug Administration (FDA) in 1985 introduced the need for a strong evidence-based approach in cochlear implant work. Outcomes were assessed for each patient individually both pre- and postoperatively using a battery of assessments that covered a wide range of auditory abilities. There were rigorous procedures to ensure that preoperative performance had been optimized through the use of appropriate hearing devices (or in some cases, tactile devices) and each patient's results were assessed statistically for evidence of significant improvement rather than relying only on group data. The comparatively modest gains (compared to today's outcomes) for speech perception in a majority of cases plus the relatively low incidence of complications from surgery or technical failures, was sufficient for the FDA to agree that the device was safe and effective. From that point on, the modern era of cochlear implantation began with a rapid increase in patient numbers around the world and continuing research and development to improve implant technology. Multichannel systems using an array of intracochlear electrodes with radio frequency transmission of coded information and power supply have since become the standard in the industry.

THE DEVELOPMENT OF IMPROVED SOUND CODING FOR COCHLEAR IMPLANTS

As described above, one of the keys to providing useful speech information to profoundly deaf subjects was in the transmission of spectral information in real time. This was very limited in single channel systems as mid and high frequency information was poorly discriminated when applied at one electrode site, but with the advent of reliable multichannel systems, important spectral information could be transferred reliably and open set speech perception became a reality. A simple approach was needed in the early 1980s due to the limitations of the technology of the time. Work by Tong and colleagues (Tong et al., 1983) led to the implementation of the F0F2 coding strategy in the Nucleus (Cochlear Ltd.) system. In terms of spectral information, this processor attempted to estimate the main mid-frequency spectral peak in an acoustic signal and this estimate controlled the position of the electrical stimulation in the cochlea. For a speech signal, this usually captured the second formant (F2) of the phonemes, providing a substantial amount of acoustic phonetic information for both consonants and vowels. It was demonstrated that postlingually deaf adults could learn to recognize this information and use it to improve auditory visual communication, recognize vowels and consonants, and understand a limited amount of speech without visual cues (Dowell, Martin, Tong, Clark, Seligman, & Patrick, 1982; Dowell et al., 1985). Although this represented a significant step forward for cochlear implants, the speech perception obtained was not generally sufficient for the device to be used in the auditory alone mode (e.g., for telephone use), but importantly, the outcomes were consistent with the perception of second formant information combined with amplitude and voicing cues.

This F0F2 coding scheme was highly susceptible to competing noise as the estimate of the second formant in a speech signal was easily scrambled by additional acoustic inputs. The first step forward from this simple "one-electrode-at-a-time" approach was the introduction of the F0F1F2 scheme which provided estimates of both the second and first formant of a speech signal which independently controlled electrical stimulation at two sites in the cochlea (using the sequential stimulation described above). In initial evaluations of the F0F1F2 coding scheme (Dowell, Seligman, Blamey, & Clark, 1987), speech perception results for vowels, consonants, open-set words, open-set sentences, and in competing noise were all improved significantly in subjects using the F0F1F2 strategy compared with F0F2. Furthermore, the results, particularly for vowels and consonants, were consistent with the addition of first formant information. Thus, an evidence-based approach using analysis of speech based on established knowledge from acoustic phonetics, and the psychophysical results for electrical stimulation of the auditory nerve, had provided a way to give additional information in a form that could be discriminated in real time by deaf patients.

This process continued in work undertaken in Melbourne in the late 1980s and early 1990s resulting in two further improvements to speech coding, the Multipeak strategy introduced in 1989 (Skinner et al., 1991) and the SPEAK strategy (McDermott et al., 1992), resulting in further improvements to speech perception for adult patients. These two schemes again involved refinement of the presentation of spectral information within the cochlea with the MULTIPEAK system providing formant and high frequency information at four electrode sites, and the SPEAK scheme providing stimulation at up to 10 independent sites. The SPEAK scheme in particular brought the speech perception for most adult cochlear implant users into the range where auditory alone communication was possible, with mean speech perception scores for sentence material exceeding 80% across the clinical population (Skinner, Fourakis, Holden, Holden, & Demorest, 1996). Another sound coding scheme used extensively in cochlear implant systems was the CIS (continuous interleaved sampling) scheme developed and refined by Blake Wilson and colleagues (Wilson, 2000). Historically, this system was developed for cochlear implant devices that included a relatively small number of intracochlear electrodes (4 to 8, compared with 22 in the Nucleus device). Partly for this reason, this coding used all available electrodes, pairing specific acoustic filters with each electrode to provide spectral information in a tonotopic fashion. In essence, despite many engineering differences and further refinements, the CIS and SPEAK schemes still form the basis of sound coding in virtually all cochlear implant systems available today.

These coding schemes and variations that have been developed from them follow the same principles in terms of information transmission, namely that the instantaneous spectrum of a sound is represented in terms of the pattern of electrical stimulation along the accessible part of the cochlea, and amplitude information is represented by variations in the current level of signals presented at individual electrodes. Advances in technology over the last 20 years have allowed the sound analysis to become more sophisticated, occur more rapidly, and be implemented in smaller devices, but there has been little overall improvement in average speech perception outcomes for adult patients since the mid-1990s (see below). Figure 7–2 summarizes the relationship between sound coding developments and open set speech perception abilities in postlingually deaf adult cochlear implant users derived from a number of published studies (Dowell et al., 1985; Dowell et al., 1987; Hollow et al., 1997; Skinner et al., 1991; Skinner et al., 1996).

EXPANSION OF CLINICAL APPLICATION AND FACTORS AFFECTING PERFORMANCE

By the mid-1990s, the skepticism surrounding cochlear implantation had diminished and audiologists and otologists around the world became involved in the wider application of these devices. The generally good speech perception results for adults fueled optimism about providing help to a wider group of patients with hearing impairment. Older patients, those with a congenital component to their hearing loss and those with useful residual hearing, began to be considered for cochlear implantation. It had been clear that sound coding technology had been responsible for the major improvements in patients' auditory skills to that point, but it was equally obvious that results varied over a wide range and that other factors affected outcomes for these patients. Clinicians became interested in being able to predict outcomes for individual patients based on measureable preimplant characteristics. This was clinically important in terms of

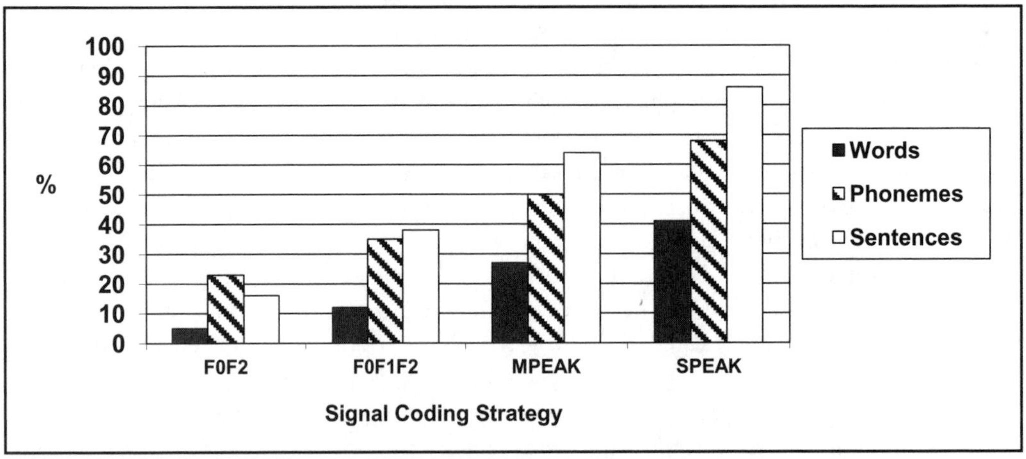

Figure 7–2. *Summary of mean speech perception scores for groups of adult cochlear implant patients with acquired hearing loss obtained approximately 3 months after implant surgery using four different speech coding strategies. The results indicate the rapid improvement in auditory skills for adult cochlear implant users between 1982 and 1994. Scores are shown for open-set auditory alone perception of words, phonemes, and sentences.*

providing realistic advice to patients, particularly in view of the cost of cochlear implantation. It was also important to collect evidence in a careful and unbiased way across large numbers of subjects to avoid clinical practice being driven by "expert hunches" often based on very limited experience and, in some cases, on no actual measurement.

Many studies investigated a range of factors that may conceivably affect cochlear implant outcomes and the reader is directed to Blamey et al. (1996) for a summary of the literature in this area. Blamey's review and subsequent analysis of data for 808 adults from a number of locations around the world indicated that cochlear implant outcomes were affected significantly by the duration of profound deafness, age at implantation, and experience in using the cochlear implant. There was only a negligible effect shown for etiology of deafness and a large amount of variance remained unexplained (at least 65%). These results were consistent with a number of other studies that indicated that duration of deafness was related to speech perception outcomes, and others that had shown a small effect for age at implant. There had been discussion in the literature for some time that the differing effects of pathology on the cochlea and factors such as auditory deprivation would influence cochlear implant results due to damage to the spiral ganglion cells, the neural elements that are stimulated by a cochlear implant. Blamey, however, concluded that the results he and others had observed were not well explained by variations in ganglion cell numbers and that central effects including learning, neural plasticity and the degeneration associated with aging, must play a role in determining outcomes.

Blamey did not address factors such as the number of electrodes available for stimulation and the individual dynamic range of stimulation but subsequent studies have found significant effects for these electrical stimulation parameters. A reduced number of electrodes for stimulation obviously reduces the spectral resolution of the signal applied to the cochlea and therefore has the potential to affect speech perception. With the current sound coding schemes, these effects appear to be minimal until the number of electrodes is reduced by 50% (in the Cochlear system, from 22 electrodes to 11) but this may well depend on the type of speech assessment, the coding scheme and the level of competing noise. It has been difficult to readily assess the effect of electrode number as a large majority of patients have straightforward surgeries and are able to have all implanted electrodes "mapped" into their sound processor. Only a small proportion of cases have incomplete electrode insertion or some other factor that limits the use of all electrodes, and it has therefore been difficult to isolate the precise effect of electrode number.

Studies from this time did not tend to address the effect of residual hearing on outcomes as the "traditional" cochlear implant patient between 1985 and 1995 had no useful residual hearing and in most cases, nothing to lose from undergoing the procedure. Over the last 15 years, this situation has changed dramatically with over 60% of prospective adult patients having useful auditory skills (open-set speech perception) prior to cochlear implant surgery. In many cases they do have something to lose: the remaining hearing in the implanted ear, any binaural advantage they may have from bilateral hearing aids, and the potential problems of integrating the different auditory signals from the two ears.

RESIDUAL HEARING AND EVIDENCE-BASED RECOMMENDATIONS

Clinical practice in cochlear implantation has become relatively straightforward as more experience has been gained. The improvement of sound coding, and the miniaturization of internal and external components of cochlear implant systems, plus the streamlining of the "mapping" procedures has enabled audiologists to focus on the rehabilitative and counseling side of patient care. The fitting of a cochlear implant has become increasingly similar to the fitting of hearing aids and vice versa with the programming technology and options for compression, directional microphones and noise reduction coalescing as researchers strive toward the same goals. One major change in cochlear implant application stems from the improvement in outcomes such that many hearing-impaired adults are considering a cochlear implant not as a replacement for lost auditory skills, but as an alternative to amplification. Over 60% of adult patients who have received cochlear implants in Melbourne, Australia, over the last 10 years have had useful auditory skills in one or both ears (as measured by aided open-set speech perception performance). The question for these people and their audiologists is not whether a cochlear implant will work for them but whether it will provide better auditory skills than their current hearing aids. Although a number of factors have been identified that can help to predict outcomes for adults ("duration of profound deafness" stands out among studies from 1985 to 2000), all research into predictive factors have found that over 50% of variance in outcomes remains unexplained by measureable, individual patient factors. In addition, all cochlear implant patients risk the loss of residual hearing in the ear to be implanted, and an individual's ability to integrate auditory information from a cochlear implant on one side and an amplification device on the other is unpredictable.

An approach that may be helpful for decision making in these cases is to use existing data on cochlear implant outcomes to provide statistical information about the likelihood of improvement with a cochlear implant for patients with residual auditory skills. To this end, a study was undertaken in Melbourne to assess the efficacy of such an approach (Dowell, Hollow, & Winton, 2004). Outcome data for an unselected group of 262 adult cochlear implant users were analyzed, in particular to define the distribution of speech perception scores obtained. Multivariate analysis demonstrated that the onset of hearing loss (pre- or postlingual), duration of severe hearing loss, age at implantation, and presurgical aided speech perception were significant predictors of cochlear implant outcomes at the three month post surgical evaluation. The distribution of speech perception outcomes was then reviewed in particular for the adults with postlingual hearing loss and useful auditory skills prior to their cochlear implant. For open-set sentence testing, the median for the distribution of scores was 91% with the first quartile at 70%. This implies that 50% of these adults exceeded a score of 91% with their cochlear implant and 75% exceeded a score of 70%.

Based on these findings, new evidence-based criteria were proposed for providing recommendations to adult patients with residual hearing. As always in clinical practice, individual factors for patients such as their age, additional health problems, communication needs, and so forth, are important in making any recommendation, but the primary goal of cochlear implant programs is to improve auditory skills, particularly for speech perception, so recommendations must consider the likelihood of achieving this goal. Prospective cochlear implant patients were included within an experimental cohort if their best aided speech perception for sentences was between 40% and 70% and if their score in the ear to be implanted was less than 40%. These guidelines were outside those that had been used (e.g., by the FDA in the US) up until that time. Based on the distribution of scores for cochlear implant adults, patients fitting these guidelines would have a 75%

chance of improving their best-aided speech perception and a 95% chance of improving speech perception in the ear to be implanted. These likelihoods were considered to be adequate for a recommendation of cochlear implantation and had the advantage of being straightforward enough for the average patient to understand.

Forty-five adults fitting these revised criteria were implanted between 2000 and 2003, and underwent the standard postoperative program and evaluations at the Melbourne cochlear implant clinic. Comparisons of their pre- and postsurgical speech perception results for open set sentences are shown in Figures 7–3 and 7–4. These results indicated that 36 out of 45 patients (80%) improved their best aided speech perception following cochlear implants, and 44 out of 45 (98%) improved their speech perception for the implanted ear. These outcomes are very close to the predictions based on the distribution of scores for previous cochlear implant users, and provide clear verification of the usefulness of this evidence-based approach. A similar approach has been followed in more recent years to refine these guidelines for adults and children considering cochlear implant (Leigh, Dettman, Dowell, & Sarant, 2011) at Melbourne.

CHANGING POPULATIONS AND PREDICTION OF OUTCOMES

The last decade has seen a rapid expansion in the clinical application of cochlear implants with the number of adults using these devices

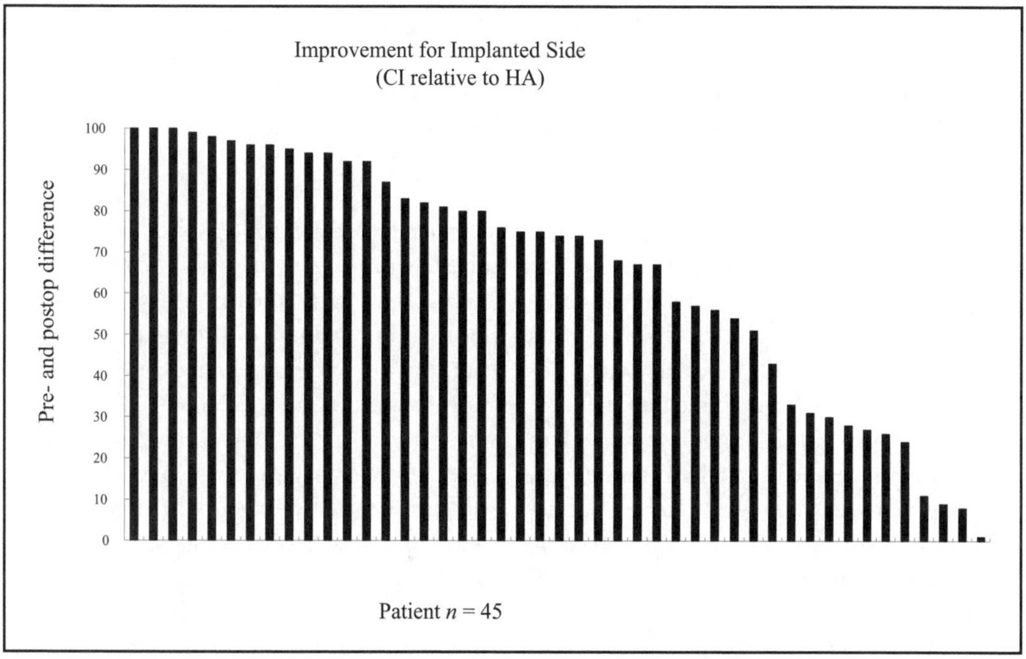

Figure 7–3. *Improvement in speech perception for the implanted ear for 45 adult cochlear implant recipients with significant residual auditory skills prior to surgery. Each bar represents the difference between preoperative open set sentence scores with an optimized hearing aid in the ear to be implanted, and scores with the cochlear implant alone approximately 3 months postoperative. Forty-four of 45 patients (98%) showed improvement for the implanted ear after the procedure (Dowell, Hollow, & Winton, 2004).*

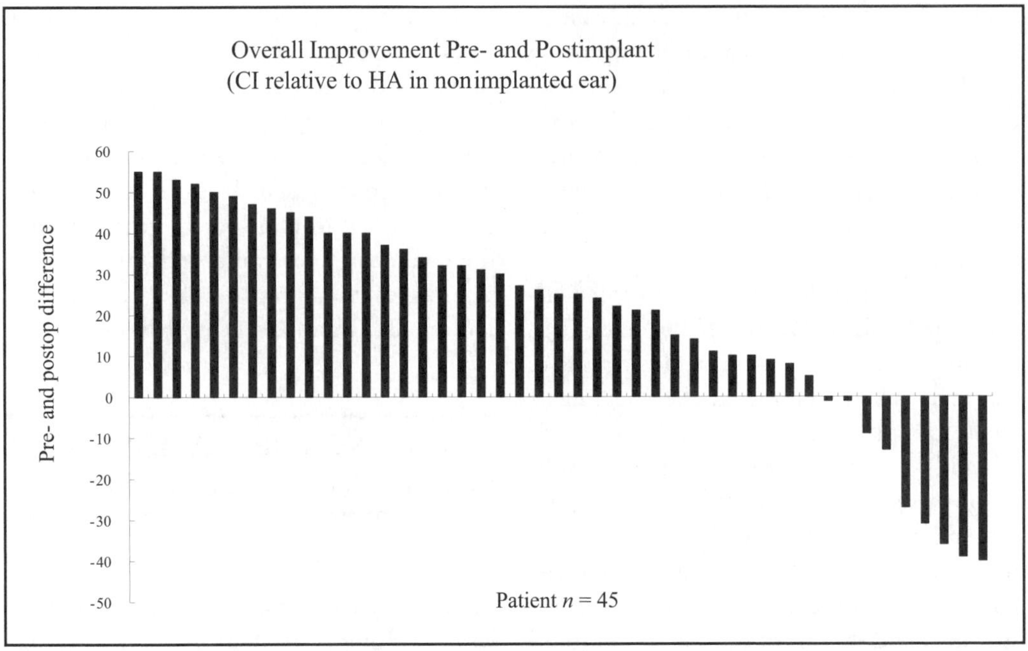

Figure 7–4. *Improvement in overall speech perception for 45 adult cochlear implant recipients with significant auditory skills prior to surgery. Each bar represents the difference between the preoperative open set sentence scores in the best aided condition, and scores with the cochlear implant alone approximately 3 months postoperative. Thirty-six out of 45 patients (80%) showed improvement over the best-aided preoperative condition in the postoperative assessment (Dowell Hollow, & Winton, 2004).*

around the world now exceeding 150,000. The indications have broadened to include adults with a congenital or prelingual component to their hearing loss, older patients in their 80s or even 90s, patients with useful residual hearing (as discussed above) and patients with psychiatric or neurological issues that may not have been considered in the past. The case manager audiologist faces a daunting task in assisting patients and their families in making an informed decision about a cochlear implant. Humans cannot help being biased by their own direct experience. For an individual, this may be advice given to them by a neighbor or a friend who knows someone with a cochlear implant. The particular cochlear implant user may be doing very well or very poorly and their hearing history and other characteristics may be similar or entirely different to the patient who is considering a cochlear implant, but this will not stop the information having a disproportionate effect. Audiologists and surgeons are not immune from the effects of the "N = 1 experiment" when it is part of their recent direct experience. For instance, a surgeon who has just seen a recently implanted patient with a long duration of deafness with a good outcome (or at least reporting so), may be more inclined to recommend a cochlear implant for another patient with similar characteristics, despite the well-described finding that outcomes can be adversely affected by long-term auditory deprivation. This is where adherence to an evidence-based approach combined with good communication across a multidisciplinary team is important for avoiding disappointing or unexpected outcomes.

In order to bring the reader up to date on factors affecting cochlear implant outcomes in adults, the results of a recent study will be presented in this final section (Dowell, Fellows, & Hollow, 2007). This study analyzed outcomes for a consecutive series of 465 adults who received cochlear implants in Melbourne, Australia between 1994 and 2006. This represents one of the largest clinical studies of speech perception outcomes in an unselected adult population. This type of study does not represent the highest level of evidence in clinical research as it is impossible to have either the subjects or experimenters blinded to the treatment condition (with and without the cochlear implant). The sampling is also not entirely random but opportunistic, in that the clients who have been treated represent a subgroup of hearing-impaired adults who take the steps to investigate cochlear implantation and indeed have gone through with the procedure. This subgroup may differ in a number of important ways from the larger population of all hearing-impaired adults who could benefit from a cochlear implant. But importantly, the number of subjects is relatively large and all subjects are included. The strength of evidence in this study is also enhanced due to the fact that all subjects underwent cochlear implantation in the same clinic with the same audiological and surgical personnel, the data have been collected prospectively following a fixed protocol, and each subject acts as his or her own control in the pre- and postoperative comparisons. All subjects underwent audiological evaluation, surgery, postoperative care, programming, and assessment within the same clinical centre at the Royal Victorian Eye and Ear Hospital in Melbourne. Prior to surgery, and approximately 3 months after the first programming session, each patient was evaluated with a battery of speech perception tests: CNC monosyllabic words (scored for both words and phonemes correct), CUNY open set sentences presented in quiet, and with multitalker competing noise at a signal to noise ratio (SNR) of +10 dB. Speech materials were presented using recorded material at a peak signal level of 60 dBA (65 dB SPL). In the preoperative condition, amplification devices had been optimized according to appropriate prescription fitting techniques. Additional data were collated for each patient including the etiology of hearing loss (where known), duration of severe/profound hearing loss for each ear, whether there was a prelingual onset of significant bilateral hearing loss (prior to 3 years of age), preoperative pure-tone audiometric results, the electrode type used in the cochlear implant (straight or precurved), the signal coding scheme used in the speech processor (effectively just two possibilities, SPEAK and ACE, which are similar in their presentation of spectral information but use different overall rates of stimulation, higher for ACE), and the date of implant surgery.

Patients for whom English was a second language or where medical or psychiatric conditions prevented participation in testing were not included in this study leaving 400 sets of results. The postoperative speech perception scores were arcsine transformed to equalize variance and subjected to a principal component analysis. This analysis demonstrated that over 85% of the variance in scores was accounted for by a single weighted average component of the four outcome measures. This weighted average, which provided the best overall measure of each subjects' speech perception was then used as the dependent variable in a series of multiple regression analyses to assess the potential of individual characteristics in predicting outcomes. Five variables were shown to have a significant association with improved speech perception outcomes for this group of adult cochlear implant users. These are listed in order of importance in terms of the amount of variance accounted for.

First, postlingual onset of significant hearing loss was associated with better outcomes ($p < 0.001$) and the overall influence of this factor on the speech perception scores is illustrated in Figure 7–5. Second, shorter duration of severe hearing loss in the implanted ear was associated with better outcomes ($p < 0.001$, see Fig. 7–6). Third,

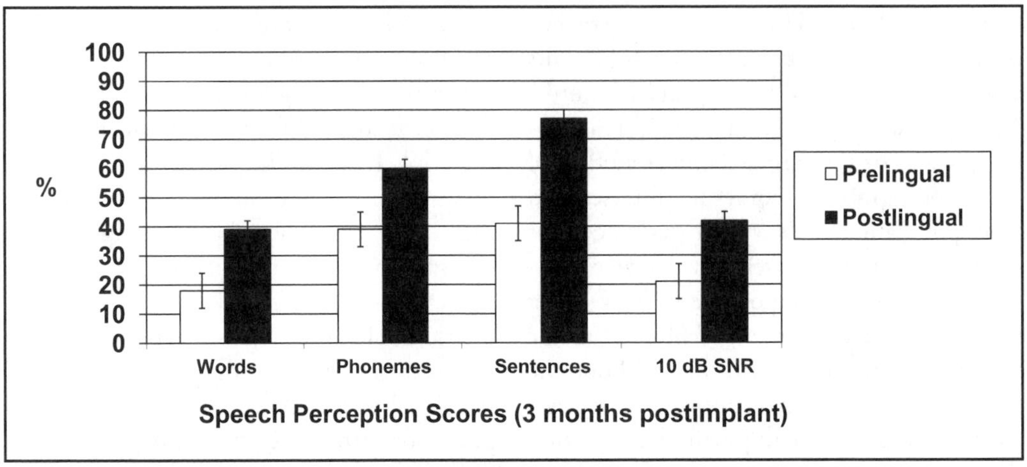

Figure 7–5. *The effect of onset of significant hearing loss on speech perception outcomes for adult cochlear implant recipients. Mean scores are significantly better for subjects with a postlingual compared with a prelingual onset of significant bilateral hearing loss. Results were obtained for a consecutive group of 400 adults implanted in Melbourne between 1994 and 2006.*

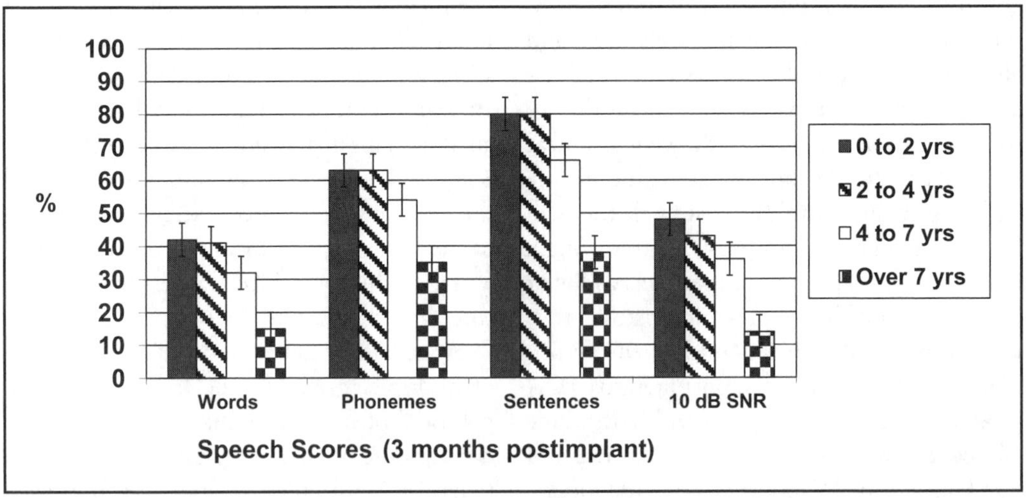

Figure 7–6. *The effect of duration of significant hearing loss on speech perception outcomes for adult cochlear implant recipients. Mean scores are significantly better for subjects with a shorter duration of significant bilateral hearing loss. Results were obtained for a consecutive group of 400 adults implanted in Melbourne between 1994 and 2006.*

younger subjects showed better outcomes ($p < 0.001$, see Fig. 7–7). Fourth, the use of the curved perimodiolar electrode array was associated with better outcomes ($p < 0.002$, see Fig. 7–8) and, finally, better preoperative speech perception skills in the best aided

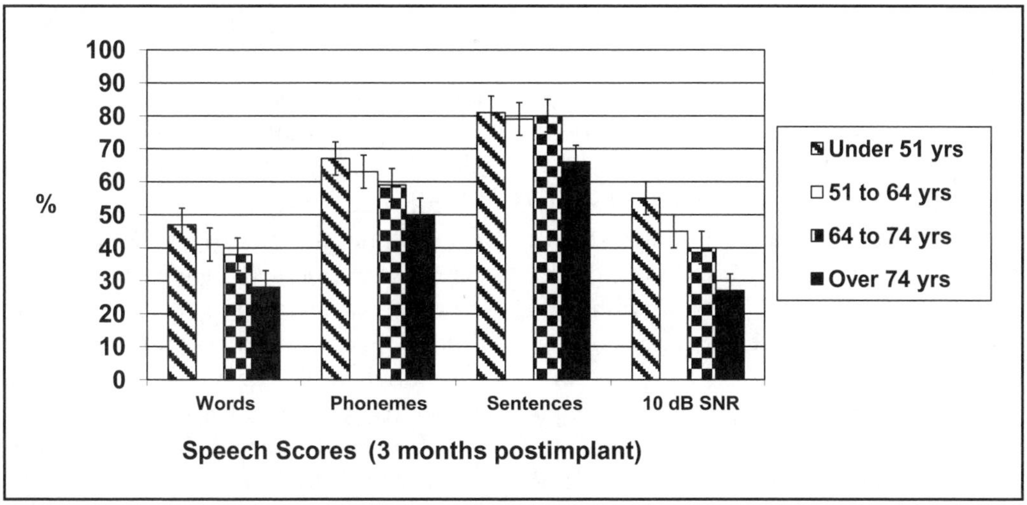

Figure 7–7. *The effect of age at the time of cochlear implant surgery on speech perception outcomes for adult cochlear implant recipients. Mean scores are significantly better for younger subjects particularly for those under 74 years of age. Results were obtained for a consecutive group of 400 adults implanted in Melbourne between 1994 and 2006.*

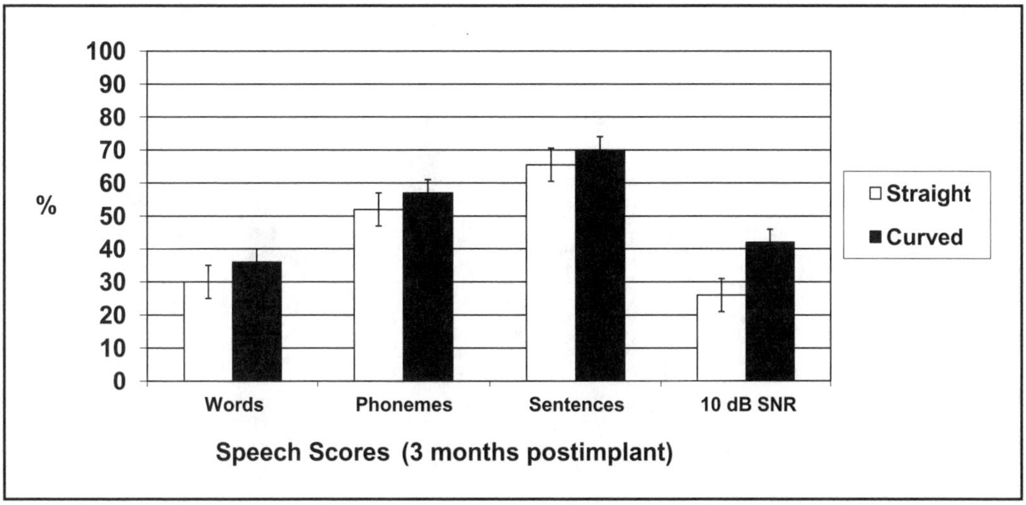

Figure 7–8. *The effect of the curved perimodiolar electrode array on speech perception outcomes for adult cochlear implant recipients. Mean scores are significantly better for subjects implanted with the curved array. The effect is more prominent for sentence perception in background noise. Results were obtained for a consecutive group of 400 adults implanted in Melbourne between 1994 and 2006.*

condition were associated with better outcomes ($p < 0.005$, see Fig. 7–9)

Approximately 30% of the variance in speech perception outcomes was accounted for by these five significant factors. The results were consistent with many previous studies which have shown similar effects for postlingual onset of hearing loss, duration of hearing loss, age, and preoperative auditory skills, but the result for the curved electrode array represents a new finding. Although the perimodiolar electrode had been designed with the aim of reducing electrical thresholds and providing more precise stimulation within the cochlea, there has not been a clear demonstration of a benefit to speech perception until this study. It appears likely that the multiple factors influencing results have obscured this finding until an adequate sample size could be analyzed that took these factors into account.

The etiology of hearing loss was investigated in this study in a separate analysis of variance. Although it seems likely that etiology does have an influence on outcomes in individual cases, an analysis in a large group of implanted subjects is hampered by the lack of a known etiology in over 50% of cases and a relatively small number of cases for some groups. For instance, deafness due to head trauma brings with it the possibility of temporal bone fracture affecting the auditory nerve or brain trauma affecting central auditory and/or language skills. There is no doubt in individual cases that this can have an effect on outcomes, but the relatively small number of cases makes establishing significance difficult. The analysis showed no significant effects for etiology, except for an association between birth complications as a cause for hearing loss and poorer outcomes. Clearly, this etiology has a close correlation with prelingual hearing loss, already identified as a strong predictor.

Of interest are some of the factors that did not show any significant effects. Apart from the etiology of hearing loss, as discussed above, the preimplant audiometric thresh-

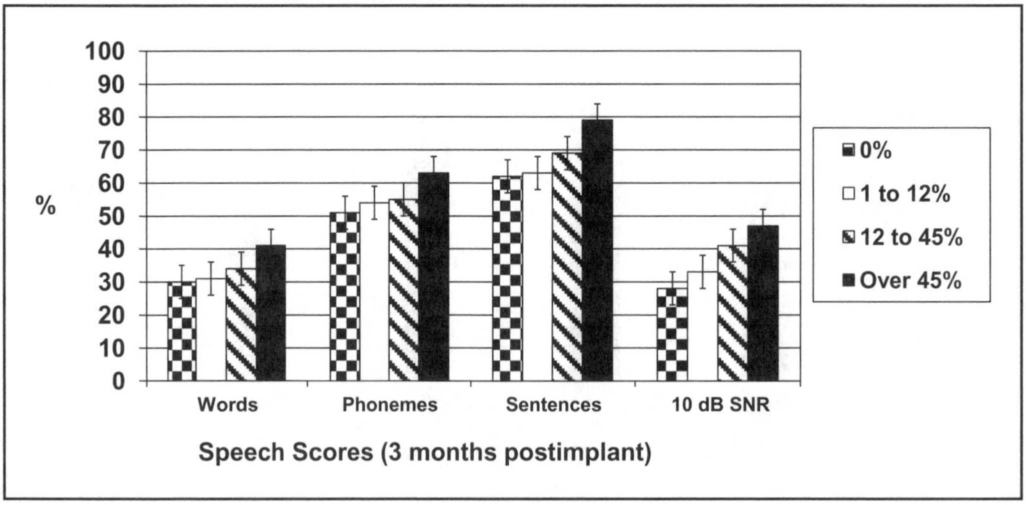

Figure 7–9. *The effect of preoperative auditory skills using optimized amplification on speech perception outcomes for adult cochlear implant recipients. Subjects are grouped based on their preoperative open set sentence score. Mean scores are significantly better for subjects with better preimplant speech perception. Results were obtained for a consecutive group of 400 adults implanted in Melbourne between 1994 and 2006.*

olds showed no relationship with outcomes. This suggests that audiometric information in the severe to profound deafness range does not provide a reliable indication of the state of neural elements at the cochlear level and higher in the auditory pathway. The speech perception ability, however, gives an indication of higher level processing and is associated with cochlear implant outcomes. In addition, there was no significant trend in results over time (1994 to 2006) for this group despite advances in both the implant electronics and signal coding for the cochlear implant system. In particular, no significant effect was seen for the change in speech coding from SPEAK to ACE, nor for the change from the original 22 electrode cochlear prosthesis used between 1982 and 1997, to the 24 electrode design used from 1998 onward. This contrasts with the results summarized previously that showed significant improvements in speech perception for cochlear implant users as signal coding was improved between 1982 and 1994. Figure 7–10 shows the results for the 400 subjects divided into 2-year intervals from 1994 to 2006. It would be harsh to suggest that none of the technological improvements in implants systems over the last 15 years have improved outcomes for the users. The usability of implant systems has improved due to the reduced size of processors, directional microphones, improved compression systems, and noise reduction algorithms. These improvements have been assessed by specific studies that target particular acoustic environments where the features become relevant. It is probable that the standard test battery described in this study, although adequate for an overall measure of performance, does not provide a comprehensive measure of auditory skills under the variable acoustic conditions encountered in real life. We need to consider the relevance and face validity of our assessment tools and modify them when there is evidence that they do not reflect the quality of communication benefit for patients. An example of this issue within cochlear implant work is the use of standard speech perception assessments presented in quiet conditions in a sound-treated environment. It became clear

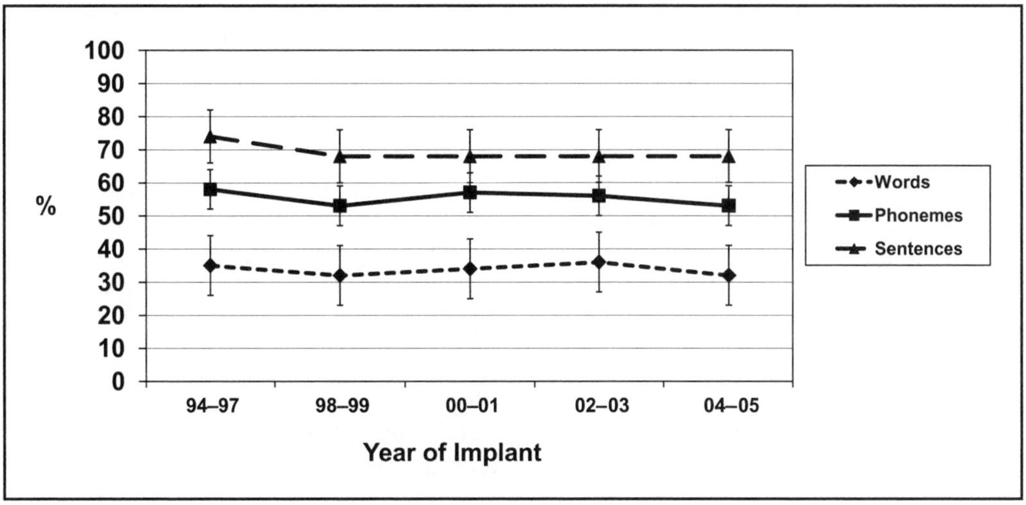

Figure 7–10. *Mean speech perception scores over the period from 1994 to 2006 for 400 consecutive adult cochlear implant patients who received their implant in Melbourne. No significant trend is evident over this time period in contrast to Figure 7–2.*

in the late 1980s that, although some cochlear implant users performed well on these standard tests, they struggled with communication as soon as they walked out of the clinic. If we wish to know about real-world benefit, the assessments need to include background noise or competing signals that may or may not be spatially separated.

It is possible that there are some subtle interactions occurring within this data set that could misrepresent the changes in performance over time. As the criteria for cochlear implantation have broadened to include more prelingual patients, older patients, and those with anatomical anomalies of the inner ear, there may have been a tendency for average outcomes to decrease if the technology had stayed the same. There may well be some improvement over time that has been masked by these gradual changes in the patient population.

INTERPRETING THE EVIDENCE ON OUTCOMES FOR ADULT COCHLEAR IMPLANT USERS

Having presented some of the studies that have guided an evidence-based approach to cochlear implantation, it seems appropriate to summarize the key findings in the context of the information transmission model introduced early in this chapter. The factors affecting the overall quality of outcome for cochlear implant users (which are equated with speech perception abilities here) fall into two main categories: those that affect the presentation of auditory information to the central auditory system, and those that affect the ability of an individual to use that information to aid communication (Dowell, Blamey, & Clark, 1995).

The first category includes many of the technical aspects of the design of cochlear implant systems including microphones, acoustic signal processing, coding of the signal for electrical stimulation within the cochlea, and the electrode array interface to the auditory nerve. It also includes the quality of the surgical result and the viability of auditory neurons within the cochlea. Any of these factors could affect the transfer of information prior to processing within the patient's auditory system. We have seen that improvements in signal coding strategies, derived from an understanding of speech science and rapid improvements in technology, resulted in rapid improvements in speech perception for cochlear implant users between 1982 and 1994. Similar improvements have not been evident in recent years, but the study described above has identified small but significant improvements associated with the curved perimodiolar electrode array introduced for the Cochlear Ltd. cochlear implant system in 1999. This result suggests that the next major step forward for cochlear implant systems may require new electrode technology that can improve the information transmission capacity of the electroneural interface.

The second set of factors relates to the ability of patients to use information, evident in the effects of prelingual hearing loss, duration of deafness and age. Clearly, the lack of good quality auditory input during the first years of life is likely to have a profound effect on the development of central auditory processing and its interaction with language and communication. The deterioration of the central auditory system when deprived of input is well documented in animal studies and the consistent finding that longer auditory deprivation can compromise results for cochlear implant users fits with our understanding of the physiology. Central auditory function has been demonstrated to deteriorate with age and thus, it is no surprise to observe similar effects for cochlear implant users. Despite all the factors that can get in the way of effective information transmission, the overall picture is very positive. Cochlear implant systems have developed to a level of sophistication and reliability that provides vastly improved auditory skills for profoundly deaf patients and significantly improved skills for most severely deaf patients.

It is now possible to use the evidence from outcome studies to provide reliable information to patients about the likelihood of success. This approach does not reduce the importance of the individual consideration of each patient by the audiologist and surgeon, where aspects of the patients' history, medical and otological issues, the patient's communication needs, and personality play a part in making recommendations. It is clear, for instance, that expectations for prelingually deaf adults need to be lower than for those with an acquired loss. Other factors such as duration of deafness, age, and preoperative auditory skills, although significant, have relatively weak effects on overall outcomes and should not play a strong part in making recommendations. The statistical approach based on existing outcomes provides a supportable way of predicting success while we are still searching for the factors that contribute over 50% of the variance. In providing guidance to patients, it is somewhat daunting to discuss all of the factors that might influence their individual result, particularly as many of the factors have weak and unpredictable effects. The average person can, however, understand the concept of the chances or odds of success. The collection of data in studies such as the ones described above, place us in a position today to provide estimates of the chances of improving speech perception for individuals. The discussion can be along the following lines:

> Having measured your ability to understand speech with your hearing aids, we can say that about 80% of people like you who are using a cochlear implant are doing better. That gives you a pretty good chance of success if you decided to have the procedure, but you have to remember that 20% of the implant users are not doing as well as you are now.

There will be other factors to discuss including age, medical and otological conditions, duration of hearing loss, use of hearing aids, which ear to implant, and, of course, the actual hearing goals for the individual, but factual information based on the scientific evidence provided in an appropriate way (as in the above example) gives a good starting point for the informed consent process.

CONCLUSIONS AND FUTURE WORK

Cochlear implantation has developed into one of the more successful medical/surgical treatments available in modern health care. It is a multidisciplinary field with audiologists playing the key case management role in the clinical application. Scientific skepticism, the risks of a surgical procedure, and the cost of cochlear implant systems have mandated an evidence-based approach in both the development and clinical application. Audiologists are well suited to the assessment and rehabilitation of adults undergoing cochlear implantation as the role requires good technical knowledge of auditory physiology, acoustic phonetics, and acoustic signal processing, careful integration of audiological findings, and the ability to provide effective counseling and advice to patients with compromised communication ability. The analysis of outcomes for adult cochlear implant users has demonstrated that factors related to the presentation of information to the auditory system, and others related to the ability of individuals to use this information, play a part in the overall result. Statistical analysis of the distribution of speech perception scores has provided solid evidence to guide recommendations for patients who are considering cochlear implantation. Studies have identified multiple factors that play a significant part in individual outcomes and inform the direction for future development of cochlear implant systems and auditory rehabilitation. Work needs to continue to refine the assessment tools used in the field in the light of improving auditory skills, changing patient populations, and the need to increase the validity of measurements for everyday communication.

Future research needs to focus on optimizing the use of binaural hearing for cochlear implant recipients whether by the use of bilateral implants (Dowell, Galvin, Dettman, Leigh, Hughes, & van Hoesel, 2011) or the combination of amplification in the contralateral ear (Mok, Grayden, Dowell, & Lawrence, 2006). The preservation of residual hearing for the implanted ear is now more of a reality with new designs for electrode arrays that minimize trauma to the cochlea, and surgical techniques and pharmaceutical intervention that reduces the inflammatory response within the inner ear. This allows the use of amplification in some cases on the implanted side as well as the contralateral ear (Gantz, Turner, Gfeller, & Lowder, 2005; Lenarz, Stover, Buechner, Lesinski-Shiedat, Patrick, & Pesch, 2009; Simpson, McDermott, & Dowell, 2005). Current work is evaluating the way that residual hearing (usually in the low frequencies) can be combined with electrical stimulation to provide improved speech perception in competing noise, localization and music appreciation. The careful assessment and optimization of the auditory skills essential to a full appreciation of modern life will continue to challenge hearing researchers and audiologists into the future. The clinical application of cochlear implants has maintained a strong evidence-based approach beginning with very small-scale studies that demonstrated feasibility, to studies in small groups of subjects that helped to enhance the quality of the cochlear implant designs, to larger scale prospective studies that have helped to expand the application of cochlear implants and provide better guidance to those considering the procedure.

REFERENCES

Atlas, L. E., Herndon, M. K., Simmon, F. B., Dent, L. J., & White, R. L. (1983). Results of stimulus and speech-coding schemes applied to mutlichannel electrodes. Cochlear prostheses, an international symposium. *Annals of the New York Academy of Sciences*, *405*, 377–386.

Bilger, R. C., Black, F. O., & Hopkinson, N. T. (1977). Evaluation of subjects presently fitted with implanted auditory prostheses. *Annals of Otology, Rhinology and Laryngology*, *86* (Suppl. 38), 1–176.

Blamey, P., Arndt, P., Bergeron, F., Bredberg, G., Brimacombe, J., Facer, G., . . . Whitford, L. (1996). Factors affecting auditory performance of postlinguistically deaf adults using cochlear implants. *Audiology Neurotology*, *1*, 293–306.

Clark, G. M. (1969). Hearing due to electrical stimulation of the auditory system. *Medical Journal of Australia*, *1*, 1346–1348.

Clark, G. M. (2003). *Cochlear implants: Fundamentals and applications.* New York, NY: Springer-Verlag.

Clark, G. M., Black, R. C., Forster, I. C., Patrick, J. F., & Tong, Y. C. (1978). Design criteria of a multiple-electrode cochlear implant hearing prosthesis. *Journal of the Acoustical Society of America*, *63*, 631–633.

Clark, G. M., Crosby, P. A., Dowell, R. C., Kuzma, J. A., Money, D. K., Patrick, J. F., Seligman, P.M., & Tong, Y.C. (1983). The preliminary clinical trial of a multichannel cochlear implant hearing prosthesis. *Journal of the Acoustical Society of America*, *74*, 1911–1913.

Clark, G. M., Tong, Y. C., & Dowell, R. C. (1982). Single versus multiple channel electrical stimulation of the auditory nerve in speech processing for a totally deaf patient. *Proceedings of the Australian Physiological and Pharmacological Society, 13*, 212.

Cumming, G., & Finch, S. (2001). A primer on the understanding, use, and calculation of confidence intervals that are based on central and noncentral distributions. *Educational and Psychological Measurement, 61*, 530–572.

Djourno, A., & Eyries, C. (1957). Prosthes auditive par excitation electrique a distance du nerf sensoriel a l'aide d'un bobnage include a demeure. *Presse medicale, 35*, 14–17.

Dowell, R. (2005). Evaluating cochlear implant candidacy: Recent developments. *Hearing Journal, 58*(11), 9–23.

Dowell, R. C., Blamey, P. J. & Clark, G. M. (1995). The potential and limitations of cochlear implants in children. *Annals of Otology, Rhinology and Laryngology, 104* (Suppl. 166), 324–327.

Dowell, R. C., Blamey, P. J., & Clark, G. M. (1997). Rehabilitation strategies for adult cochlear implant users. In G. M. Clark (Ed.), *Cochlear implants* (pp. 33–40). Bologna, Italy: Monduzzi Editore.

Dowell, R. C., Fellows, J., & Hollow, R. (2007). *Recent developments in predicting outcomes for adult cochlear implant recipients.* Proceedings of the 6th Asia Pacific Symposium on Cochlear Implants and Related Sciences. Sydney, Australia.

Dowell, R. C., Galvin, K. G., Dettman, S. J., Leigh, J. R., Hughes, K. C., & van Hoesel, R(2011). Bilateral implants in children. *Seminars in Hearing, 32*(1), 53–72

Dowell, R. C., Hollow, R., & Winton, E. (2004). Outcomes for cochlear implant users with significant residual hearing: Implications for selection criteria in children. *Archives of Otolaryngology, Head and Neck Surgery, 130*, 575–581.

Dowell, R. C., Martin, L. F. A., Clark, G. M., & Brown, A. M. (1985). Results of a preliminary clinical trial on a multiple channel cochlear prosthesis. *Annals of Otology, Rhinology and Laryngology, 94*, 244–250.

Dowell, R. C., Martin, L. F. A., Tong, Y. C., Clark, G. M., Seligman, P. M., & Patrick, J. F. (1982). A 12-consonant confusion study on a multiple channel cochlear implant patient. *Journal of Speech and Hearing Research, 25*, 509–516.

Dowell, R. C., Seligman, P. M., Blamey, P. J., & Clark, G. M. (1987). Speech perception using a two-formant 22-electrode cochlear prosthesis in and quiet and in noise. *Acta Otolaryngologica, 104*, 439–446.

Eddington, D. K., Dobelle, W. H., & Brackmann, D. E. (1978). Auditory prostheses research with multiple channel intracochlear stimulation in man. *Annals of Otology, 87*, 1–39.

Fourcin, A. J., Rosen, S. M., & Moore, B. C. J. (1979). External electrical stimulation of the cochlea: Clinical, psychophysical, speech-perceptual and histopathological findings. *British Journal of Audiology, 13*(3), 85–107.

Gantz, B. J., McCabe, B. F., Tyler R. S., & Preece, J. P. (1987). Evaluation of four cochlear implant designs. *Annals of Otology, Rhinology and Laryngology, 96*, 145–147.

Gantz, B. J., Turner, C. W., Gfeller, K. E., & Lowder, M. (2005). Preservation of hearing in cochlear implant surgery: Advantages of combined electrical and acoustical speech processing. *Laryngoscope, 115*, 796–802.

Fields, W. S., & Leavitt, L. A. (Eds.). *Neural organization and its relevance to prosthetics.* New York, NY: Intercontinental Medical Books.

Hawthorne, G., Hogan A., Giles, E., Stewart, M., Kethel L., White K., . . . Taylor, A.(2004). Evaluating the health-related quality of life effects of cochlear implants: A prospective study of an adult cochlear implant program. *International Journal of Audiology, 43*(4), 183–192.

Henry, B. A., McKay, C. M., McDermott, H. J., & Clark, G. M. (2000). The relationship between speech perception and electrode discrimination in cochlear implantees. *Journal of Acoustical Society of America, 108*, 1269–1280.

Hochmair, E. S., Hochmair-Desoyer, I. J., & Burian, K. (1979). Investigations towards an artificial cochlea. *International Journal of Artificial Organs, 2*(5), 255–261.

Hochmair-Desoyer, I. J., Hochmair, E. S., Fischer, R. E., & Burian, K. (1980). Cochlear prostheses in use: Recent speech comprehension results. *Archives of Otolaryngology, 229*, 81–98.

Hollow, R. D., Plant, K., Larratt, M., Skok, M., Whitford, L., Dowell, R., & Clark, G. M. (1997). Current speech perception benefits for adults using the Nucleus 22-channel cochlear implant. In G. M. Clark (Ed.), *Cochlear implants* (pp. 249–254). Bologna, Italy: Monduzzi Editore.

House, W. F., Berliner, K. I., Eisenberg, L. S., Edgerton, B. J., & Thielemier, M. A. (1981). The cochlear implant: 1980 update. *Acta Otolaryngologica, 91*, 457–462.

House, W. F., & Urban, J. (1973). Long-term results of electrode implantation and electronic stimulation of the cochlea in man. *Annals of Otology, Rhinology, and Laryngology, 82*(4), 504–517

Kerr, A., & Schuknecht H. F. (1968). The spiral ganglion in profound deafness. *Acta Otolaryngologica, 65*(6), 586–598.

Lawrence, M. (1964). Direct stimulation of the auditory nerve fibres. *Archives of Otolarygology, 80*, 367–368.

Leigh, J. R., Dettman, S. J., Dowell, R. C. & Sarant, J. Z. (2011). Evidence based approach for making cochlear implant recommendations for infants with significant residual hearing. *Ear and Hearing, 32*(3), 313–322.

Lenarz, T., Stover, T., Buechner, A., Lesinski-Schiedat, A., Patrick J., & Pesch, J. (2009). Hearing conservation surgery using the Hybrid-L electrode. *Audiology and Neurotology, 14*(Suppl. 1), 22–31.

Liberman, A. M., Delattre, P. C., Gerstman, L. J., & Cooper, F. S. (1954). The role of consonant-vowel transitions in the perception of stop and nasal consonants. *Psychological Monographs, 8*, 1–13.

McDermott, H. J., McKay, C. M., & Vandali, A. (1992). A new portable sound processor for the University of Melbourne/Nucleus Limited multi-electrode cochlear implant. *Journal of the Acoustical Society of America, 91*, 3367–3371.

Michelson, R. P. (1971). Electrical stimulation of the human cochlea—a preliminary report. *Archives of Otolaryngology, 93*, 317–323.

Mok, M., Grayden, D., Dowell, R. C., & Lawrence, D. (2006). Speech perception for adults who use hearing aids in conjunction with cochlear implants in opposite ears. *Journal of Speech, Language and Hearing Research, 49(2)* 338–351.

Pialoux, P., Chouard, C. H., & Meyer, B. (1979). Indications and results of the multichannel cochlear implant. *Acta Otolaryngologica, 87*, 185–189.

Rose, J. E., Brugge, J. F., Anderson, D. J., & Hind, J. E. (1971). Some effects of stimulus intensity on the response of the auditory nerve fibres in the squirrel monkey. *Journal of Neurophysiology, 34*, 685–699.

Sek, A., & Moore, B. C. J. (1995). Frequency discrimination as a function of frequency measured in several ways. *Journal of the Acoustical Society of America, 97*, 2479–2486.

Shannon, R. V. (1983). Multichannel electrical stimulation of the auditory nerve in man. I. Basic psychophysics. *Hearing Research, 11*, 157–189.

Shepherd, R. K., Franz, B. K. H., & Clark, G. M. (1990). The biocompatibility and safety of cochlear prostheses. In G. M. Clark, Y. C. Tong, & J. F. Patrick (Eds.), *Cochlear prostheses* (pp. 69–98). London, UK: Churchill Livingstone.

Simmons, F. B. (1966). Electrical stimulation of the auditory nerve in man. *Archives of Otolaryngology, 84*, 2–54.

Simpson, A., McDermott, H. J., & Dowell, R. C. (2005). Benefits of audibility for listeners with severe high-frequency hearing loss. *Hearing Research, 210*, 42–52.

Skinner, M., Fourakis, M., Holden, T., Holden, L., & Demorest, M. (1996). Identification of speech by cochlear implant recipients with the Multipeak (MPEAK) and Spectral Peak (SPEAK) speech coding strategies. *Ear and Hearing, 17*, 182–197.

Skinner, M. W., Holden, L. K., Holden, T. A., Dowell, R. C., Seligman, P. M., Brimacombe, J. A., & Beiter, A. L. (1991). Performance of postlinguistically deaf adults with the wearable speech processor (WSP III) and mini speech processor (MSP) of the Nucleus multi-electrode cochlear implant. *Ear and Hearing, 12*(1), 3–22.

Skinner, M. W., Holden, L. K., Whitford, L. A., Plant, K. L., Psarros, C., & Holden, T. A. (2002). Speech recognition in the Nucleus 24 SPEAK, ACE and CIS speech coding strategies in newly implanted adults. *Ear and Hearing, 23*, 207–223.

Tong, Y. C., Blamey, P. J., Dowell, R. C., & Clark, G. M. (1983). Psychophysical studies evaluating the feasibility of a speech processing strategy for a multiple-channel cochlear prosthesis. *Journal of the Acoustical Society of America, 74*, 73–80.

Tong, Y. C., Clark, G. M, Blamey, P. J., Busby, P. A., & Dowell, R. C. (1982). Psychophysical studies for two multiple channel cochlear implant patients. *Journal of the Acoustical Society of America, 71*, 153–160.

Tong, Y. C., Dowell, R. C., Blamey, P. J., & Clark, G. M. (1983). Two component hearing sensations produced by two electrode stimulation in the cochlea of a totally deaf patient. *Science, 219*, 993–994.

Wever, E. V., & Bray, C. W. (1930). Auditory nerve impulses. *Science, 71*, 215.

Wilson, B. S. (2000). Strategies for representing speech information with cochlear implants. In J. K. Niparko (Ed.), *Cochlear implants* (pp. 129–170). Philadelphia, PA: Lipincott Williams & Wilkins.

CHAPTER 8

Evidence About the Effectiveness of Cochlear Implants for Children: Open-Set Speech Recognition

Emily A. Tobey, Andrea Warner-Czyz, Lana Britt, Olga Peskova, and Kenneth C. Pugh

INTRODUCTION

Cochlear implantation is often sought by families as a lifelong intervention program for young children with severe to profound sensorineural hearing losses (SNHL). However, a wide variety of performance levels are observed following implantation, ranging from children relying on speech and hearing for communication to children who rely on simultaneous communication using both speech and sign techniques. Audiologists perform many roles, as shown in Table 8–1.

Clearly, evidence-based decisions need to be made by audiologists in every one of these domains of their clinical practice. In this chapter, we focus on the importance of evaluating the published literature regarding the acquisition of speech perception skills in young children receiving cochlear implants. More importantly, we focus on a narrower question pertaining to parents' desire to know what they should expect in terms of speech perception/recognition when their child receives a cochlear implant. Namely, what levels of open-set speech recognition in quiet listening conditions are associated with pediatric cochlear implantation for children between the ages of 2 and 12 years wearing either one or two cochlear implants?

In the mid- to late 1990s, several investigators argued the evidence for widespread use of cochlear implants as a treatment plan for severe to profound SNHL in children was limited (Carlson et al., 2010; Lane, 1995; Lane & Bahan, 1998; Lane & Grodin, 1997; McJunkin & Jeyakumar, 2010). Although many investigators heralded the efficacy and safety of cochlear implant surgery (Clark, 2000, 2008), many remained concerned regarding the levels of speech recognition abilities reported in the literature for individuals receiving cochlear implants. For example, Lane and Bahan (1998, p. 229) noted, "Con-

Table 8–1. Roles of the Audiologist

Role	*Specific Examples*
Diagnostic observation and evaluation of the child's hearing loss	• Detection and evaluation of the hearing loss through behavioral and physiological assessment (Jakubikova, Kabatova, Pavlovcinova, & Profant, 2009)
Selection and fitting of appropriate auditory prostheses	• Facilitation of decisions regarding amplification versus cochlear implantation (Eisenberg, Martinez, Sennaroglu, & Osberger, 2000; Ramsden, Papaioannou, Gordon, James, & Papsin, 2009) • Determination of candidacy for implantation (Cohen, 2004; Cosetti & Roland, Jr., 2010; Osberger, 1997; Osberger, Zimmerman-Phillips, & Koch, 2002; Wiley & Meinzen-Derr, 2009) • Observation and monitoring in surgical situations (Shapiro, Huang, Shaw, Roland, Jr., & Lalwani, 2008; Zhang et al., 2010)
Regular maintenance and monitoring of device settings and function	• Regulation and setting of the cochlear implant device settings (mapping) (Jethanamest, Tan, Fitzgerald, & Svirsky, 2010) • Tracking progress and the need for mapping adjustments (Osberger et al., 1991; Sarant, Blamey, Dowell, Clark, & Gibson, 2001) • Establishment of routine schedules for monitoring progress or maintenance of the device(s) (Peters, Litovsky, Parkinson, & Lake, 2007; Tajudeen, Waltzman, Jethanamest, & Svirsky, 2010; Wang et al., 2008) • Application of troubleshooting techniques when routine problems (such as poor sound quality due to a cable or battery needing replacement) or more complex problems involving the internal processor and electrode array occur (Carlson et al., 2010; McJunkin & Jeyakumar, 2010) • Cognizance of a rapidly changing field requiring knowledge of both hardware and software upgrades as they become available (Buechner, Frohne-Buechner, Boyle, Battmer, & Lenarz, 2009; Jethanamest et al., 2010; Qian, Loizou, & Dorman, 2003)
Active participation and interaction with the cochlear implant team	• Audiological assessment to determine how much benefit the children experience (Geers, Brenner, & Davidson, 2003; Holt, Kirk, Eisenberg, Martinez, & Campbell, 2005; Peters et al., 2007; Waltzman et al., 1997; Zimmerman-Phillips, Robbins, & Osberger, 2000) • Consultation with speech-language pathologists and other professionals involved in the long-term care of the communication needs of the children (Moog & Geers, 2010) • Interaction with teachers and other educators involved in the child's progress through the school years (Moog & Geers, 2010; Osberger et al., 1991; Ramsden et al., 2009)

Table 8–1. *continued*

Role	*Specific Examples*
Ongoing evaluation and counseling of the child and family	• Determination of the efficacy of bimodal auditory inputs (a combination of a hearing aid on one ear and cochlear implant on the other ear) versus bilateral cochlear implantation (providing cochlear implants to two ears) (Ching, Psarros, Hill, Dillon, & Incerti, 2001; Galvin, Hughes, & Mok, 2010) • Provision of creative solutions for active children (such as how to provide a listening system for children actively involved in sports) (Kompis, Vibert, Senn, Vischer, & Hausler, 2003) • Provision of counseling, guidance, and assistance to family members in adjusting and providing environments conducive to promoting their child's ability to communicate (in whatever manner they elect) (Hardonk et al., 2010) • Answering the most frequent question asked by parents, "What will my child be able to do?"

genitally Deaf children do very poorly on tests of unprompted (open-set) word recognition, even after many years of implant use and habilitative therapy." In one of the earliest applications of an evidence-based approach for evaluating the literature in cochlear implantation, they reviewed 12 studies conducted between 1991 and 1997 (Cowan et al., 1997; Fryauf-Bertschy, Tyler, Kelsay, Gantz, & Woodworth, 1997; Miyamoto, Osberger, Robbins, Myres, & Kessler, 1993; Osberger et al., 1991; Osberger, Fisher, Zimmerman-Phillips, Geier, & Barker, 1998; Waltzman et al., 1994; Waltzman et al., 1997). Lane and Bahan concluded children receiving cochlear implants demonstrated poor speech recognition of phonetically balanced stimuli. The limitations of scientific evidence regarding open-set speech recognition performance reported by Lane and Bahan fostered intense debates regarding ethical considerations associated with cochlear implantation in pediatric populations. Debates focused on who should be a candidate; how to evaluate and account for conflicting value sets between families of normal hearing and families identifying with Deaf culture; what educational methods provide the best results for young children; and whether a representative from Deaf culture should weigh in on the decisions of whether a child should receive a cochlear implant (Haimowitz, 1999; Lane & Bahan, 1998; Lane & Grodin, 1997; Tucker, 1998). However, since this early debate, many changes in the field of cochlear implantation for pediatric populations have occurred. These changes include advances in hardware and software technology, thoughtful development of speech recognition measures for pediatric populations, longitudinal studies of speech recognition performance in children receiving cochlear implants, and systematic descriptions regarding how to conduct evidence-based research and interpret the results. Thus, it seems entirely appropriate in this chapter to carefully consider the status of open-set speech recognition in pediatric users of multichannel cochlear implants more than 20 years after the U.S. Food and Drug Administration and other regulatory agencies issued approval for use in children ages 2 to 17 years.

Using evidence-based practice principles reviewed in the early chapters of this book, we consider the state of speech recognition abilities in children using cochlear implants reported over the past 10 years. The principle question we are interested in addressing is, what levels of open-set speech recognition in quiet listening conditions are associated with pediatric cochlear implantation for children between the ages of 2 and 12 years wearing either one or two cochlear implants? The literature regarding speech recognition/perception outcomes in children with cochlear implants has grown exponentially over the last 10 years with nearly 352 publications reported in PubMed alone for "cochlear implants" in 2010. To address our question, we accessed several electronic databases (e.g., PubMed, Scopus, Medline, Academic Search Complete, Turning Research Into Practice [TRIP], Cumulative Index to Nursing, and Allied Health Literature [CINAHL]) using stringent criteria and limiting our search to peer-reviewed articles published between 2000 and 2010. We carefully considered articles that adhered to the following criteria: (a) Inclusion of subjects using one or two cochlear implants; (b) inclusion of at least 5 participants to address the widespread variability in speech perception performance in pediatric cochlear implant users; (c) inclusion of subjects between the ages of 2 and 12 years, who were chronologically old enough to meet the final criteria; and (d) administration of open-set speech perception testing. Open-set speech recognition measures included the Glendonald Auditory Screening Procedure (GASP) (Erber, 1982), Multisyllabic Lexical Neighborhood Test (MLNT) (Kirk, Pisoni, & Osberger, 1995), the Lexical Neighborhood Test (LNT) (Kirk et al., 1995), the Phonetically Balanced Kindergarten Word (PBK) List (Haskins, 1949), the Bamford-Kowal-Bench Sentence (BKB) Test (Bench, Kowal, & Bamford, 1979), and the Hearing in Noise Test for Children (HINT-C) (Nilsson, Soli, & Gelnett, 1995).

Table 8–2 designates the raw numbers of articles obtained in our initial search as a function of the databases explored and the type of information discovered. A total of 101 peer-reviewed articles were considered. No studies used a blinded randomized controlled design. Forty-one studies were excluded from the analysis because stimuli were not presented to English-learning or English-speaking participants. Twenty-four additional studies were eliminated from exploration because open-set speech recognition measures were not used (n = 14) or numerical data from participants was not reported (n = 10). An additional 21 studies failed to meet study selection criteria because the articles were off-topic. The remaining 20 studies included children between the chronologic ages of 2 and 12 years who use at least one cochlear implant and who completed open-set speech perception testing to meet our four criteria outlined in the previous paragraph to assess critically the evidence for open-set speech perception testing in children using cochlear implants (Buchman et al., 2004; Cullen et al., 2004; Davidson, 2006; Dolan-Ash, Hodges, Butts, & Balkany, 2000; Dowell, Dettman, Blamey, Barker, & Clark, 2002; Dowell, Dettman, Hill et al., 2002; Eisenberg, Martinez, Holowecky, & Pogorelsky, 2002; Eisenberg, Kirk, Martinez, Ying, & Miyamoto, 2004; Gantz et al., 2000; Geers, Brenner, & Davidson, 2003; Harrison et al., 2001; Holt, Kirk, Eisenberg, Martinez, & Campbell, 2005; Kirk et al., 2007; Peters, Litovsky, Parkinson, & Lake, 2007; Sarant, Blamey, Dowell, Clark, & Gibson, 2001;

Table 8–2. Sources of the Identified Studies

Electronic Databases Searched	*Total Hits (Non-duplicate)*[a]	*Non-English*	*Not Open-Set*	*Individual Scores Not Reported*	*Off-Topic*	*On-Topic Articles*
PubMed	55 (N/A)	26	10	3	10	6
Scopus	89 (46)	15	4	7	11	6
Academic Search Complete[b]	52 (0)					
speechBITE	29 (1)	0	0	0	0	1
ASHA Compendium of Evidence-Based Practice Guidelines and Systematic Reviews	5 (1)	0	0	0	0	1
CINAHL	9 (0)	0	0	0	0	0
TRIP	13 (0)	0	0	0	0	0
Additional search procedures						
Manual search of topical articles						6
Total hits	**101**	**41**	**14**	**10**	**21**	**20**

Note: The following search terms were used: speech perception and cochlear implant and "open set." Limits included language (English), age (child: 2 to 5 years; child: 6 to 12 years), and publication date (2000–2010). Abbreviations: CINAHL—Cumulative Index to Nursing and Allied Health Literature; TRIP—Turning Research Into Practice.

[a] Total hits refers to the total number of references meeting search criteria in each electronic database. Nonduplicate indicates the number of new references not accounted for in other electronic databases.

[b] Academic Search Complete simultaneously searches four electronic databases: MEDLINE, PsycARTICLES, Psychology and Behavioral Sciences Collection, and PsycINFO.

Staller, Parkinson, Arcaroli, & Arndt, 2002; Teagle et al., 2010; Waltzman, Scalchunes, & Cohen, 2000; Waltzman, Roland, Jr., & Cohen, 2002; Wang et al., 2008). In order to set the stage for our evaluation of the literature, let us first turn our attention to the principles and measurements of open-set speech recognition.

OUTCOME DOMAINS: OPEN-SET SPEECH RECOGNITION

Open-set speech recognition involves verbal responses, gesturing or signing when necessary, to auditory-only stimuli without relying on any additional visual or lip reading cues (Thibodeau, 2007). Responses typically are scored as the percentage of phonemes, words, or sentences correctly identified. When data are collected from a test battery at pre- and postimplant intervals, indices of open-set skill at the phoneme, word, or sentence levels provide useful metrics because they represent best-case outcome measures of speech perception with cochlear implants in everyday listening conditions. Open-set recognition scores are based on several factors associated with the child being tested, the examiner, the task the child is asked to complete, and environmental factors influencing the child's performance or the task presentation.

Open-set speech recognition in children is typically measured by a relatively small set of measures. The most common open-set word lists used to determine speech recognition of pediatric recipients of cochlear implants are the PBK word lists (Haskins, 1949). The original version of the PBK test consisted of four phonetically balanced lists of 50 words each. However, lists 1, 3, and 4 produce equivalent performance levels and are recommended for use in clinical practice. The PBK test is administered in quiet via monitored live-voice or with recorded materials. It assesses speech recognition at word and phoneme levels and is appropriate for children ages 5 years and older.

The LNT consists of two monosyllabic word lists, each containing 25 "easy" words (e.g., good, juice) and 25 "hard" words (e.g., hi, ear) (Kirk et al., 1995). The MLNT also has two separate word lists, but each list contains 24 two- or three-syllable words, 12 of which are "easy" (e.g., banana, children) and 12 of which are "hard" (e.g., butter, puppy). Development of the LNT and the MLNT are based on the neighborhood activation model of spoken word recognition where the "easy" component is represented by words that contain few phonemic similarities while the "hard" component is based on words that have many phonemic similarities (Luce & Pisoni, 1998). Both LNT and MLNT stimuli are presented auditory-alone in quiet and are scored according to the number of words and phonemes repeated correctly. Both lists are used for assessing children between the ages of 3 to 5 years.

The HINT-C examines open-set speech recognition of children ages 5 years or older at the sentence level (Nilsson et al., 1995). Because there is no carrier phrase, cueing is often used for children below age 5. The HINT-C contains 13 equivalent lists of 10 phonetically balanced sentences. The test can be administered with recorded materials in quiet, by using an adaptive procedure to vary the signal-to-noise ratio, or by presenting sentence lists with a fixed signal-to-noise ratio. Scoring is based on the number of words in each sentence repeated correctly.

The BKB test consists of 16 sentence lists with 3 to 4 words per sentence; each sentence list contains 50 key words (Bench et al., 1979). Practice lists are also available to familiarize children with the test. The BKB test is administered auditory-only in quiet via monitored live voice or with recorded materials and speech recognition performance is determined by the percentage of words correctly repeated. This test is used routinely to assess children aged 5 years and older.

The GASP was initially designed as a closed-set measure but has been also administered as an open-set speech recognition task by using presentations of 10 sentences commonly used every day (Erber, 1982). It also measures word recognition of monosyllables, trochees, spondees, and polysyllables. Scores are based on total correct sentences and total correct words.

Open-set measures differ from closed-set measures of speech recognition in terms of both the stimuli and response required for the stimuli (Clopper, Pisoni, & Tierney, 2006). Closed-set recognition tasks provide a pre-determined set of alternative choices from which a child selects a response after listening to the stimulus. Closed-set measures focus on different aspects of recognition and often control for word frequencies. In the field of cochlear implantation, several closed-set measures are used in conjunction with open-set measures to document performance. Closed-set measures include the Word Intelligibility by Picture Identification (WIPI; Ross & Lerman, 1970) test which is appropriate for children between the ages of 5 years and 10 years, 11 months. The WIPI is composed of four lists of 25 words with children selecting a response from the six pictures placed on a page. The Northwestern University Children's Perception of Speech (NU-CHIPS: Elliott & Katz, 1980) uses 50 monosyllable words that are in the vocabulary of children older than 2.5 years. The words are presented and children respond by pointing to a four-alternative picture set. The Early Speech Perception Test (ESP; Moog & Geers, 1990) was designed to be used with young children. Children select an answer from a set of four objects rather than a page of pictures for response. The Video Speech Pattern Contrast (VIDSPAC; Boothroyd, 1997) test requires children to indicate when a phonetic change is detected in a series of syllables. The Pediatric Speech Intelligibility (PSI; Jerger & Jerger, 1984) includes 20 monosyllabic words and 10 sentences. Children respond to either the vocabulary or sentences. PSI testing may be accomplished with children as young as 2.5 or 3 years of age. The Test of Auditory Comprehension (TAC; Trammell, 1976) evaluates environmental sounds and speech. Children select their answers by pointing to pictures. Although this chapter does not focus on closed-set measures, we describe them here because they often appear in conjunction with open-set measures within the audiological battery.

IMPORTANT SPEECH RECOGNITION TEST BATTERY CONSIDERATIONS

Researchers use commercially available open-set speech recognition measures to evaluate the listening skills of children using cochlear implants; however, comparison across studies remains difficult because of differences in test administration and how the results are reported. Differences are evident regarding when various test measures are administered following implantation, what intensities are used to assess the measures, and whether to extend speech recognition testing to include both quiet and signal-to-noise test conditions. For example, Cullen and colleagues (2004) report results from participants at annual intervals following implantation, whereas Holt and colleagues (2005) report on baseline measures acquired prior to implantation and semi-annually for the next 1 to 2 years following implantation. Open-set speech perception abilities of pediatric cochlear implant users increase over time regardless of the testing intervals used (Gantz et al., 2000; Staller et al., 2002). Dowell and his colleagues report the greatest changes in speech recognition accuracy occur within 3 to 4 years after implantation (Dowell, Dettman, Blamey, et al., 2002; Dowell, Dettman, Hill, et al., 2002). Higher levels of recognition performance also are attributed to newer, more flexible speech coding strategies which increase the dynamic range and sampling rate of the signals delivered by the implants (Buechner, Frohne-

Buechner, Boyle, Battmer, & Lenarz, 2009; Davidson, 2006).

A hallmark characteristic of speech recognition performance reported across different clinical sites is the consistent report of variability in performance. Children with cochlear implants demonstrate a wide range of levels in their speech perception abilities, even among users deemed as "better" candidates prior to implantation (Waltzman et al., 2000; Waltzman et al., 2002). For example, Kirk and colleagues (1995) report performance on the LNT and MLNT ranged from 4 to 82% and 6 to 84%, respectively. Individual variability occurs in children's abilities to tell the difference between two unfamiliar talkers, regardless of the children's chronological age or experience listening with the devices (Kovacic & Balaban, 2009). Large standard deviations on the GASP, LNT, and HINT-C were reported at baseline and at 3- and 6-months postimplantation for a group of children involved in the Nucleus 24 Contour clinical trial (Staller et al., 2002). Word recognition scores improve with additional sensory information available from access to both auditory and visual cues during testing but performance remains highly variable (Kirk et al., 2007). Wide variability results in clinicians applying renewed vigor to the methodologies. For example, practice effects are observed for the recorded LNT, reinforcing the need to alternate test lists if re-administration of the test occurs in relatively short periods of time (Kirk et al., 1995). The PBK word lists are one of the most common open-set pediatric measures used clinically and in research to document speech recognition performance (Buchman et al., 2004; Cullen et al., 2004; Dolan-Ash et al., 2000; Dowell, Dettman, Blamey, et al., 2002; Eisenberg et al., 2004; Gantz et al., 2000; Geers et al., 2003; Harrison et al., 2001; Holt et al., 2005; Sarant et al., 2001; Teagle et al., 2010; Waltzman et al., 2000; Waltzman et al., 2002; Wang et al., 2008). Children with cochlear implants often achieve higher phoneme scores than word scores (Eisenberg et al., 2004).

Kirk and colleagues (1995) first called attention to the discrepancy observed between many pediatric cochlear implant users' real-world performance and relatively low PBK scores. They theorized that the PBK, although phonetically balanced, is not representative of the words usually found in the discourse of children with severe to profound SNHL. The MLNT and LNT were created in response to this concern and consist of multisyllabic and monosyllabic words based on words commonly used in conversation by normal-hearing 3- to 5-year old children. Test development indicates children with cochlear implants: (a) organize, store, and access words in their lexicons similarly to their normally hearing peers; (b) use word length as a cue in word recognition; and (c) perceive words within the context of other words in their vocabularies. All 19 children in the Kirk et al. (1995) study achieved poorer word and phoneme recognition on the PBK than on the LNT, suggesting the PBK was underestimating pediatric implant users' open-set auditory abilities.

Several general patterns of performance are evident across children using cochlear implants. Monosyllabic stimuli, such as in the LNT or the PBK, are more difficult and result in lower scores than multisyllabic stimuli (Kirk et al., 1995). Lexically easy words are recognized more readily than their lexically hard counterparts. Sentence scores, as in the Lexical Neighborhood Sentence Test (LSNT; Eisenberg et al., 2002), BKB, or HINT-C, are significantly higher than word scores (Eisenberg et al., 2002). Sentence scores also provide insight into how children with cochlear implants use context to assist their word recognition. Eisenberg's results (2002) enabled assignment of children using cochlear implants to either "high- or "low-performing" groups. Low performers process sentences as individual words strung together, resulting in increased stress on short-term memory and reduced scores. High performers and normal-hearing children showed similar patterns of performance for easy and hard stimuli suggesting they are using similar strategies of linguistically "chunking" concepts. Kirk and her colleagues (2007) duplicated these results and further showed an increase in speech recognition scores with audiovisual presentations as opposed to auditory-only testing. Audiovisual testing is recommended by many clinicians to provide a better representation of children's functional word recognition in the real world, where both auditory and visual information are presented simultaneously.

CRITIQUE OF OPEN-SET RECOGNITION EVIDENCE IN PEDIATRIC COCHLEAR IMPLANTATION

Table 8–3 illustrates information regarding methodologies from each study meeting the inclusion criteria necessary to address our question of what levels of open-set speech recognition in quiet listening conditions are associated with pediatric cochlear implantation for children between the ages of 2 and 12 years wearing either one or two cochlear implants. Open-set speech recognition data were reported for children using cochlear implants once in the years 2003, 2005, 2006, 2008, and 2010; three times in 2004; twice in 2000, 2001, and 2007; and 6 times in 2002. The population sizes discussed in the papers ranged from 6 to 181 children. As Table 8–3 indicates, different studies used different speech recognition test measures, often in combination with the closed-set measures briefly described above. A key point to notice is that these studies do not completely focus their investigations on our question, nor do they frame their investigation to answer this question. Below, we review key issues associated with open-set speech recognition the investigators have considered closely and then discuss how we might apply this information to address our question. Following this description, we address how further studies may contribute to the evidence-based literature associated with speech recognition in pediatric populations receiving cochlear implants.

Influence of Age of Implantation on Open-Set Speech Recognition

One of the chief concerns for audiologists and families of children with severe to profound SNHL is associated with "when should cochlear implantation occur?" Over the last decade, investigators probed the impact of "early" versus "later" cochlear implantation with the presumed argument that the earlier the intervention, the more successful the outcomes and the higher the levels of open-speech recognition. To a large extent, this argument is based on the considerable literature regarding brain plasticity, the explosion of language capabilities in young children and landmark studies by Yoshinaga-Itano and colleagues (Yoshinaga-Itano & Apuzzo, 1998; Yoshinaga-Itano, Sedey, Coulter, & Mehl, 1998; Yoshinaga-Itano, 1999) demonstrating that by age 3 years significant differences occurred in children with severe to profound SNHL depending on whether they received services before 6 months of age or between 6 and 12 months of age. However, comparisons of different ages of implantation are often complicated by the heterogeneity of the children receiving cochlear implants.

Table 8–3. Summary of Testing Parameters and Results from the Evidence-Based Literature Regarding Children with Cochlear Implants

	Buchman et al. (2004)	*Cullen et al. (2004)*		*Davidson (2006)*	*Dolan-Ash et al. (2000)*
Participants (*n*)	28	21 GJB2+	27 GJB2–	26	13
Testing Materials	ESP, PBK	ESP, PBK	ESP, PBK	LNT	PBK, GASP, CP
Stimuli				**Recorded**	**MLV**
		70 dB SPL	70 dB SPL		65–70 dB SPL
	0° azimuth	0° azimuth	0° azimuth		0° azimuth
Statistics	Analysis of Variance (ANOVA)	Wilcoxon signed rank test	Wilcoxon signed rank test	Multiple regression analysis/Principal Components Analysis	Mixed model
Results (Quiet)	Children with inner ear malformations obtain open-set speech perception but more slowly than without malformations.	No significant differences between the GJB2+ and GJB2– groups at 12, 24, or 36 months postimplantation. Most participants had some open-set speech perception at 12 and 24 months postimplant and scored 40–50% correct on words at 36 months.	Children exhibited higher perception scores with greater intensity (70 vs. 50 dB SPL). Children with CI performed similarly to children wearing digital hearing aids.	"Borderline" candidates improved significantly post-CI. Children with greater experience achieved higher scores on the PBK (6 to 12 months: 55%; 12 to 24 months: 63%; 24 to 48 months: 76%).	

	Dowell, Dettman, Blamey, et al. (2002a)	*Dowell, Dettman, Hill, et al. (2002b)*	*Eisenberg et al. (2004)*	*Eisenberg et al. (2002)*
Participants (*n*)	102	25	117	12
Testing Materials	Closed-set tests, PBK, NU-CHIPs, BKB	BKB	LNT, PBK, HINT-C (+5 SNR)	Lexically controlled words & sentences
Stimuli	**Recorded & MLV**		**Recorded**	**Recorded**
		70 dB SPL	70 dB SPL	70 dB SPL
Statistics	Student *t*-test	Stepwise multiple linear regression	Paired *t*-tests; Student's *t*-tests; Spearman correlations	ANOVA
Results (Quiet)	Phoneme scores were higher for SPEAK vs. MPEAK, oral vs. total communication, and shorter duration of deafness (<2 yrs). Significant improvement in the first 3 to 4 years post-CI.	A positive association exists between open-set speech perception pre- and post-CI. A negative association exists between duration of deafness and postoperative speech perception.	Children with profound hearing loss perform similarly to children with severe loss after 5 to 6 years of device experience. Scores highest for phonemes vs. words; lexically easy vs. hard words; and oral vs. total communication.	Performance scores improved with increases in intensity level. Scores were higher for easy versus hard words and for words in sentences versus words in isolation.

continues

Table 8–3. *continued*

	Gantz et al. (2000)		*Geers et al.* (2003)	*Harrison et al.* (2001)	*Holt et al.* (2005)	
Participants (*n*)	7	6	181	69	10 CI + HA	12
Testing Materials	PBK	PBK	ESP, VIDSPAC, CAVET, BKB, LNT, WIPI	TAC, GASP, WIPI, PBK	PBK, HINT-C	PBK, HINT-C
Stimuli	**Recorded**	**Recorded**	**Recorded**		**Recorded & MLV**	**Recorded & MLV**
			70 dB SPL	70 dB SPL	70 dB SPL	70 dB SPL
Statistics			Multiple regression analysis; *t*-tests	Stepwise linear regression, multiple regression analysis	Z-scores, mean scores only	
Results (Quiet)	Children with residual hearing and limited functional use with HA achieved open set word recognition with a CI (M = 52% and 75% after 6 and 24 months of CI experience, respectively). Scores were similar to a group of children with moderate hearing loss (71 dB HL) using hearing aids.	Children achieved 44 to 56% words correct with 4 to 7 years of CI experience. Early age of implant (between 22 and 64 months) and later age at onset of deafness (<36 months) did not contribute significantly to levels measured at ages 8 to 9.	Age at implantation distinguishes differences in performance based on the test used. Closed-set tasks: younger partitioning age and open-set tasks: older partitioning ages.	Children using CI alone or CI + HA attained approximately 40% and 60% correct on words at 1 and 2 years postimplantation. After 2 years of CI experience, children using CI + HA perform better than HA alone and 5 to 16% better than CI alone on PBK lists		

	Kirk et al. (2007)	*Peters et al. (2007)*			*Sarant et al. (2001)*
Participants (*n*)	15	7	10	13	167
Testing Materials	LNT, AVLNST	MLNT	LNT	LNT, HINT-C in quiet	BKB, PBK, CNC
Stimuli	**Recorded**				**MLV**
	65–70 dB SPL	70 dB SPL	70 dB SPL		70 dB A
					0° azimuth
Statistics	Mixed model, Pearson correlation coefficients	Paired *t*-tests			ANOVA
Results (Quiet)	Children are sensitive to the acoustic-phonetic similarity of words and organize words into similarity neighborhoods and use this structure in open-set speech recognition tasks. Both auditory and visual cues are useful to children with CIs.	Speech perception in the second ear (CI2) improves between 6 and 12 months postactivation of CI2. Bilateral improvement was not statistically significant for any of the groups for speech perception testing in quiet conditions.			Shorter duration of deafness, more implant experience, and oral communication result in higher scores on phoneme, word, and sentence perception. The largest improvements occurred on sentence-level tasks followed by phonemes and words.

continues

Table 8–3. *continued*

	Staller et al. (2002)			*Teagle et al. (2010)*		
Participants (*n*)	83	75	98	11	15	26
Testing Materials	IT-MAIS	ESP, GASP, MLNT, MAIS	ESP, GASP, MLNT, MAIS		ITMAIS/MAIS, ESP	IT-MAIS/MAIS, PBK, MLNT, LNT
Stimuli		**Recorded**	**Recorded & MLV**		**Recorded & MLV**	**Recorded & MLV**
		70 dB SPL	70 dB SPL		70 dB SPL	70 dB SPL
Statistics	ANOVA, when possible	Mann Whitney U	ANOVA		ANOVA	Binary partitioning
Results (Quiet)	Mean performance for children older than 5 years improved significantly on all measures after 3 months device use (GASP, LNT, HINT-C). Mean LNT score after 3 months for children with preoperative open-set abilities was 44.9% (28.1) vs. 22.0% (29.8) for children w/o open set. At 6 months post: LNT = 58.4% (26.8) and 25.8% (36.9) for children with better and poorer preoperative hearing, respectively. These differences were significant for both intervals.					Children with ANSD and >24 months of CI experience attained mean scores of 76% and 54% on PBK phonemes and words, but one-third of children scored <30% correct. Significant score differences emerge based on ECAP, MRI, and medical comorbidities.

	Waltzman et al. (2000)	*Waltzman et al. (2002)*	*Wang et al. (2008)*
Participants (*n*)	29	35	181
Testing Materials	ESP, NU-CHIPS, GASP, PBK, MLNT, LNT, CP	PBK, MLNT, LNT, CP, BKB	ITMAIS, MAIS, ESP, PSI, MLNT, LNT
Stimuli	**MLV**	**Recorded**	**Recorded**
	70 dB SPL	70 dB SPL	
			0° azimuth
Statistics	Chi-square, Pearson Pairwise Correlation, ANCOVA	Paired *t*-tests, Student's *t*-tests	Regressions, Descriptive, Growth trajectories.
Results (Quiet)		Speech perception is higher with increased experience and short duration of deafness. Scores similar among speech processing strategies, although ACE users tended toward greater improvement.	Speech recognition index in quiet (SRI-Q) scores for children with CI were more variable than 97 peers with typical hearing. Earlier implanted children exhibited growth patterns similar to that of typically hearing peers.

Notes: Empty cells indicate that information was not available in the published article. Abbreviations: N = Number; GJB2+ = positive for gap junction β2, a mutation in the Connexin 26 gene; GJB2- = negative for gap junction β2; ESP = Early Speech Perception Tests (Moog & Geers, 1990); PBK = Phonetically Balanced Kindergarten Word List (Haskins, 1949); LNT = Lexical Neighborhood Test (Kirk et al., 1995); GASP = Glendonald Auditory Screening Procedure (Erber, 1982); CP = Common Phrases test (Robbins, Renshaw, & Osberger, 1995); CI = Cochlear Implant; MLV = Monitored Live Voice; NU-Chips = Northwestern University Children's Perception of Speech (Elliott & Katz, 1980); BKB = Bamford-Kowal-Bench Sentence Test (Bench, Kowal, & Bamford, 1979); HINT-C = Hearing in Noise Test for Children (Nilsson, Soli, & Gelnett, 1995); CI+HA = bimodal cochlear implant + hearing aid; VIDSPAC = Video Speech Pattern Contrast (VIDSPAC; Boothroyd, 1997); CAVET = Children's Audio-Visual Enhancement Test (Tye-Murray & Geers, 2001); WIPI = Word Intelligibility by Picture Identification (WIPI; Ross & Lerman, 1970); TAC = Test of Auditory Comprehension (TAC; Trammell, 1976); HA = Hearing Aid; AVLNST = Audiovisual Lexical Neighborhood Sentence Test (Holt, Kirk, Pisoni, Burckhartzmeyer, & Lin, 2005); MLNT = Multisyllabic Lexical Neighborhood Test (Kirk, Pisoni, & Osberger, 1995); CNC = Consonant-Nucleus-Consonant test (Peterson & Lehiste, 1962); IT-MAIS = Infant-Toddler Meaningful Auditory Integration Scale (Zimmerman-Phillips, Osberger, & Robbins, 1997); MAIS = Meaningful Auditory Integration Scale (Robbins, Renshaw & Berry, 1991); PSI = Pediatric Speech Intelligibility (PSI; Jerger & Jerger, 1984).

Age of implantation becomes an important issue in considering speech perception outcomes in children using cochlear implants. Although it seems age of implantation should be a relatively simple variable to account for in the performance of cochlear implant children, its influence on performance is often confounded with the effects of duration of deafness and duration of hearing following cochlear implantation (Davidson, Geers, & Brenner, 2010; Geers et al., 2003; Nicholas & Geers, 2007). The issue is more straightforward for children with congenital SNHL since the age of implantation and duration of hearing represent equivalent values. However, the situation is less straightforward when children experience a period of normal hearing followed by the onset of SNHL and cochlear implantation (Niparko et al., 2010). Children with congenital deafness who experience shorter periods of deafness and earlier ages of implantation outperform children with congenital deafness that experience longer periods of deafness and later ages of implantation (Cohen, 2004; Dowell, Dettman, Hill, et al., 2002; Fryauf-Bertschy et al., 1997; Geers et al., 2003; Harrison et al., 2001; Kirk et al., 2007; Sarant et al., 2001; Waltzman et al., 1994; Waltzman et al., 1997; Wang et al., 2008). Such observations pose serious dilemmas for clinical audiologists since prolonged periods of hearing aid use prior to implantation also postpone the age of implantation. Prolonged use of hearing aids, in conjunction with later ages of implantation, results in poorer receptive and expressive language performance relative to children who receive shorter periods of hearing aid use and earlier implantation (Niparko et al., 2010). Better speech recognition performance is associated with earlier implantation on a number of measures (Davidson et al., 2010).

Steady decreases in age of implantation reflect the surgical and technological safety of cochlear implantation as determined by Food and Drug Administration trials conducted in the United States and by regulatory agencies in other countries. However, the moving landscape of performance outcomes as a function of age of implantation is increasingly difficult to assess because of these relatively rapid and fluid changes in candidacy requirements. Harrison and colleagues (2001) report the optimum age of implantation is not easily answered by performance on single measures but rather appears dependent on the demands of the outcome measure as they relate to task difficulty and linguistic knowledge. Children implanted prior to 4.4 years of age achieved higher performance on closed-set measures of speech recognition than those children implanted at later ages. For more demanding open-set measures, Harrison and colleagues also determined children implanted at earlier years demonstrated higher performance at age 8.4 years for the PBK words and age 5.6 years for the GASP words. Children with shorter durations of deafness and earlier ages of implantation achieved higher scores on PBK and BKB tests than children with longer periods of deafness or earlier implantation (Dowell, Dettman, Blamey, et al., 2002; Sarant et al., 2001; Waltzman et al., 2002). Children implanted before age 6 years achieved higher scores on the LNT (mean 56%) than children implanted at later years (mean 18%) (Davidson, 2006). In addition, Davidson demonstrated a correlation ($r = -0.57$, $p = 0.002$) between the age of implantation and LNT scores.

Age of implantation, in combination with bilateral cochlear implantation, also is examined in the speech recognition performance of pediatric cochlear implantation populations. Bilateral cochlear implantation is either performed in a single surgical procedure (referred to as simultaneous bilateral implantation) or as two procedures separated in time (referred to as sequential bilateral implantation) (Galvin, Hughes, & Mok, 2010; Peters et al., 2007). Speech recognition performance is influenced by the age of implantation of the second, sequential implant. Children who receive their first implant before the age of 5 years and subsequently receive a second cochlear implant at varying times after this (3 to 5 years; 5 years, one month to 8 years; or 8 years, one month to 13 years) show varying rates of speech recognition performance with higher levels occurring for the youngest group, who received their second device between 3 and 5 years of age (Peters et al., 2007). Although one might argue that sequential implantation should only occur in the youngest pediatric populations, bilateral, sequential implantation appears to significantly aid even older children in noisy conditions. Peters and colleagues (2007) report word recognition scores of 44% for children performing with their first implant and 89% after the second implant using HINT-C measures. Chapter 9 in this book also contains a review of the evidence on bilateral implantation.

Influence of Residual Hearing on Open-Set Speech Recognition

Residual hearing also plays a role in guiding clinical decisions for referring patients as candidates for cochlear implants (Fitzpatrick, Olds, et al., 2009). Audiologists with and without experience with cochlear implants often do not agree as to who should receive cochlear implants. The largest disagreements occur with borderline candidates. Audiologists experienced with cochlear implants rate approximately a quarter of the cases designated as "borderline" by audiologists without implant experience as "definite" candidates and around 20% as "definitely not" candidates (Wiley & Meinzen-Derr, 2009). Definite candidates demonstrated audiometric thresholds of 90 dB HL or higher bilaterally, with limited open-set capabilities. Borderline candidates demonstrated greater degrees of residual hearing and wider degrees of open-set speech recognition capabilities.

Preoperative residual hearing predicts speech perception performance in children using cochlear implants. Children with higher levels of residual hearing often receive greater benefit from cochlear implants than they received from more traditional amplification. Dolan-Ash and colleagues (2000) investigated the improvement achieved through cochlear implantation for a group of children with pre-implantation pure-tone averages (PTA) of 96 dB HL (unaided) and 41 dB HL (aided) with average aided word recognition levels below chance level. After nearly 2 years of implant experience, the average aided PTAs were reduced (28 dB HL) and open-set speech recognition scores improved to 61% correct on word tests and 92% on sentence tests. Children with severe SNHL also achieved significantly higher open-set word recognition scores on the PBK after implantation, with continued improvement with longer durations of device experience. Clinical trials in North America for Cochlear Corporation's N24 Contour device showed the children with open-set word recognition above chance levels prior to implantation also achieve the highest levels of speech recognition postimplantation (Staller et al., 2002). Collectively, these observations suggest expansion of candidacy criteria to include children with more residual hearing.

Clinicians providing habilitation for children with severe to profound SNHL need to question when hearing aid performance indicates cochlear implantation may be a better clinical intervention. Children with severe to profound SNHL using either cochlear implants or hearing aids respond similarly to LNT words presented at loud intensity levels (70 dB SPL); however, the cochlear implant users outperformed hearing aid users when the stimuli were presented at lower intensity 50 dB SPL presentation levels (Davidson,

2006). Eisenberg and colleagues (2004) recommend implantation in children with significant residual hearing when their hearing aids no longer permit performance levels comparable to those of average cochlear implant users. They failed to find statistically significant differences in performance on the LNT, PBK, and HINT-C in quiet between comparable groups of children using hearing aids or cochlear implants. However, the cochlear implant users showed a greater discrepancy between their HINT-C scores in quiet and those obtained using a +5 dB SNR, indicating the implant group had more difficulty with sentence recognition in noise and possibly required a larger signal-to-noise ratio than the hearing aid users. Assessing speech recognition in the presence of background noise has been proposed as a way to determine if a child with a hearing aid might be a cochlear implant candidate (Eisenberg et al., 2004).

For many cochlear implant centers, bilateral cochlear implantation is considered when a child meets candidacy criteria for both ears. For a variety of reasons, a child may be implanted unilaterally, and bimodal stimulation may be pursued (Ching, Psarros, Hill, Dillon, & Incerti, 2001; Fitzpatrick, Seguin, Schramm, Chenier, & Armstrong, 2009; Galvin et al., 2010). In this instance, a hearing aid is fitted to the ear contralateral to the cochlear implanted ear to take advantage of residual hearing in the non-implanted ear. Children using bimodal stimulation performed better on speech recognition testing in noise compared to peers with only hearing aids or unilateral-only cochlear implants (Holt et al., 2005).

Although the literature appears to indicate open-set speech recognition improves postimplantation, it is not entirely clear what levels of performance should be expected. That is, are the levels of improvement observed postimplant clinically relevant? Levels of performance will be influenced by the chronological age of the child, the listening age of the child, and the language age of the child. These various ages are important clinical considerations as one plans what open-set test measures are appropriate for a given child. Test measures need to be carefully selected to represent the language and developmental skill levels of child. One approach used by many clinical groups is to consider a child's "listening" age rather than chronological age for establishing appropriate expectations and placing open-set speech recognition performance into perspective (Flexer & Madell, 2009). Listening age refers to the period of time a child is able to hear. However, listening age is generally a simple concept that is fraught with complexity associated with when technology is given to a child, the audibility of the hearing provided by the technology, how long per day the child wears the technology and how effectively those in the child's communication environment interact with the child (Flexer & Madell, 2009).

Additional Factors Influencing Open-Set Speech Recognition

Several studies also evaluate how mode of communication influences open-set speech perception after cochlear implantation. Children using communication relying on speaking and listening achieve significantly higher open-set speech perception scores than those children relying on modes of communication emphasizing sign components (Gantz et al., 2000; Geers et al., 2003). Higher levels of open-set speech recognition appear to be associated with children who include listening and speaking in their communication; however, substantial open-set speech perception skills also are evident in children using total communication who also incorporate signs (Gantz et al., 2000; Geers et al., 2003; Staller et al., 2002; Waltzman et al., 1997). Mode of communication and age of implantation often confound the easy assessment of open-set performance postimplantation, particularly if children are implanted at older ages. Dowell and colleagues failed to find a significant mode of communication effect on PBK scores for children aged 8 to 18 years implanted at later ages (Dowell, Dettman, Hill, et al., 2002).

Cochlear implant candidacy currently includes children 12 months old and younger. Many medical conditions, communication disorders, and developmental delays cannot be accurately diagnosed in toddlers and very young children. Very young children are at risk for language and motor delays, genetic syndromes, autism spectrum disorders, and cerebral palsy (Waltzman et al., 2000). Children with cochlear implants often are found to have concomitant medical conditions that alter expectations for their performance postimplantation. Developmental delays, identified prior to cochlear implantation, are significant predictors of open-set speech perception scores on PBK word and BKB sentence lists at 5 years postimplantation (Dowell, Dettman, Blamey, et al., 2002). Children with multiple handicaps receive significant benefit from their cochlear implants but score more poorly than children with fewer handicaps (Waltzman et al., 2000). Significant improvements in performance occurred even though their auditory skill development was slower, more erratic, and more likely to be supplemented with visual cues and/or manual communication than for their peers with fewer additional handicapping conditions. Children with multiple handicapping conditions experienced improved auditory access, better communication skills, more social interaction, and a "connectedness" to their environments. Thus, it appears additional handicapping conditions should not preclude cochlear implantation, as improved access to auditory stimulation may provide additional strengths for the child.

Children with auditory neuropathy spectrum disorder (ANSD) represent a relatively new population of pediatric cochlear implant candidates and users. Diagnosis of ANSD relies on normal outer hair cell function indicated by otoacoustic emissions or cochlear microphonics, abnormal auditory brainstem testing, fluctuating hearing loss, varying degrees of hearing loss, and difficulties listening in noisy environments. The recommended course of habilitation is determined on an individual basis, and there is no consensus as to what type of amplification works best. Of 140 children with ANSD, those children with open-set speech perception abilities showed great variability in their performance on the PBK, with 73% scoring over 30% and 27% scoring under 30% (Teagle et al., 2010). The typically accepted characteristics, including age at testing, implant experience, duration of hearing aid use before implantation, and others, were found to be poor predictors of postimplantation outcomes for children with ANSD. Better predictors of implant performance for those with ANSD were found to be: (1) presence of robust electrical-elicited compound action potentials (ECAP), and (2) magnetic resonance imaging (MRI) findings with no obvious structural abnormalities or central nervous system pathology. For example, mean PBK word scores were 62% (SD = 24%) for those with robust ECAP responses and 17% (SD = 9%) for those with absent or atypical ECAP responses. The authors suggest that, with more supporting evidence from other studies, MRI and ECAP abnormalities might prove to be predictors of poor open-set performance following cochlear implantation (Teagle et al., 2010).

Hearing loss etiology does not diminish a child's benefit from a cochlear implant. For example, speech perception scores of pediatric cochlear implant users with the GJB2 genetic mutation did not differ from a group of users without the mutation (Cullen et al., 2004). As such, expectations must be formed on a case-by-case basis. Because no outcome can be guaranteed, it is warranted that a guarded yet cautiously optimistic clinical approach to counseling is taken and that changes are made as new information becomes available.

CRITIQUE OF EVIDENCE FOR OPEN-SET RECOGNITION IN CHILDREN WITH COCHLEAR IMPLANTS

As the brief review above demonstrates, the evaluation of open-set speech recognition in children with cochlear implants requires careful consideration of multiple factors. Below, we carefully consider and apply the evidence-based principles described in the early chapters of this publication as a means of assisting readers in learning how to apply such principles to their own work.

Uniformity of Reporting of Demographic Factors

All publications report some collection of demographic variables, but which variables are reported in studies of speech perception in pediatric cochlear implant users are not uniform, as shown in Table 8–4. Relationships between speech perception outcomes and variables such as age at cochlear implant activation, duration of cochlear implant experience and chronological age at time of testing leads to relatively consistent reporting of these factors. However, other participant characteristics such as age at onset of hearing loss, age at hearing aid fitting, and duration of deafness also impact open-set speech perception in pediatric implant users and often are not reported. An additional factor that has gained importance as cochlear implant candidacy has changed is the duration of time between activation of the first and second devices. The lack of standardization in reporting of demographic factors in studies of speech perception in children who use cochlear implants creates difficulties in comparing across studies.

Age at Implantation

The single most frequently reported demographic characteristic is age at implantation, with 18 of 20 studies reporting on this variable (Buchman et al., 2004; Cullen et al., 2004; Davidson, 2006; Dolan-Ash et al., 2000; Dowell, Dettman, Blamey, et al., 2002; Dowell, Dettman, Hill, et al., 2002; Eisenberg et al., 2002; Eisenberg et al., 2004; Gantz et al., 2000; Geers et al., 2003; Kirk et al., 2007; Sarant et al., 2001; Teagle et al., 2010; Waltzman et al., 2000; Waltzman et al., 2002; Wang et al., 2008). In the two studies not directly reporting this variable, one used age at implantation as an inclusion criteria (Peters et al., 2007) and the other study used it as an outcome variable in a binary partitioning analysis (Harrison et al., 2001). Age at implantation is not delineated specifically as age at implant surgery or age at implant activation. Six studies defined "age at cochlear implantation" unequivocally. Four studies referred to the age at device fit or stimulation as age at first mapping (Cullen et al., 2004), age fit with cochlear implant (Sarant et al., 2001), mean age when fitted (Eisenberg et al., 2004), or age at initial implant stimulation (Eisenberg, Martinez, Sennaroglu, & Osberger, 2000). One study referenced the congenital onset of hearing loss (i.e., mean age at cochlear implantation and mean length of deafness) (Waltzman et al., 2002) and another reported the age at surgery (Dolan-Ash et al., 2000). The remaining 13 studies fail to specify age at implantation as the date of surgery or the date of device activation. The average age at implantation across studies was just over 5 years (M = 5.6 years, SD = 3.0 years) with nine studies reporting a mean age younger than 5 years and ten studies reporting a mean older than 5 years.

Table 8–4. Demographic Information from the Evidence-Based Literature Regarding Open-Set Speech Recognition in Children with Cochlear Implants

		Buchman et al. (2004)	*Cullen et al. (2004)*		*Davidson (2006)*	*Dolan-Ash et al. (2000)*	*Dowell , Dettman, Blamey, et al. (2002)*	*Dowell, Dettman, Hill, et al. (2002)*	*Eisenberg et al. (2004)*
Participants (*n*)		28	21 GJB2+	27 GJB2–	26	13	102	25	117
Age at HL Onset (Months)	***Mean***				15.5	21	16.8		1.5
	SD				8.9	40.8	39.6		
	Range				3–36	0–108	0–202.8		0–29
Duration of Deafness (Months)	***Mean***					78.6	55.2	105.6	
	SD					53.9	49.2		
	Range					0–108	4.8–211.2	4.8–211.2	
Age at HA Fitting (Months)	***Mean***				16.6			26.4	
	SD				8.8				
	Range				3–36			8.4–84	
Age at CI Stimulation (Months)	***Mean***	66.8	39	38	59.6	8.3	70.8	147.6	31.4
	SD	59.7	35	32	37.1	3.47	52.8		
	Range	17–212			19–168	1.3–14	18–211	97–211	7–58

continues

Table 8–4. *continued*

		Buchman et al. (2004)	*Cullen et al. (2004)*		*Davidson (2006)*	*Dolan-Ash et al. (2000)*	*Dowell , Dettman, Blamey, et al. (2002)*	*Dowell, Dettman, Hill, et al. (2002)*	*Eisenberg et al. (2004)*
Duration of CI Use (Months)	***Mean***	29.1	39	25	43.5	21.7	48	32.4	LNT: 58.8; PBK: 57.6; HINT-C: 66
	SD	25.1	20	10	15.5	14.6	32.4		
	Range	3–86			17–71	3–48	3.6–123.6	6–90	
Age at Testing (Months)	***Mean***	96.0	76.8	62.4	102.7	121.3			LNT: 92.4; PBK: 92.4; HINT-C: 98.4
	SD	63.7	39.6	33.6	33.1	41.2			
	Range	25–269			59–185	27.6–192	>48	96–216	

		Eisenberg et al. (2002)	*Gantz et al. (2000)*		*Geers et al. (2003)*	*Harrison et al. (2001)*	*Holt et al. (2005)*	
Participants (*n*)		12	7	6	181	69	10 CI+HA	12
Age at HL Onset (Months)	***Mean***	26.3			4		4.4	0.3
	SD	26.4			8		9.3	1.2
	Range	0–74			0–36	Congenital	<36	<36
Duration of Deafness (Months)	***Mean***							
	SD							
	Range							
Age at HA Fitting (Months)	***Mean***				15			
	SD				7			
	Range				1–36			
Age at CI Stimulation (Months)	***Mean***	132.6		100	40		83.5	49.1
	SD	241.1	26.7	38.3	10		37.0	25.8
	Range	24–889	24–108	42–138	20–64			
Duration of CI Use (Months)	***Mean***	41.3	24	6	66			
	SD	19.3			4			
	Range	8–68			45–90	≤50	0–24	0–24
Age at Testing (Months)	***Mean***	103.8	77.1	106	107			
	SD	30.9	26.7	38.3	6			
	Range	65–172	48–132	48–144	95–119	24–180		

continues

Table 8–4. *continued*

		Kirk et al. (2007)	*Peters et al. (2007)*			*Sarant et al. (2001)*	*Staller et al. (2002)*		
Participants (*n*)		15	7	10	13	167	83	75	98
Age at HL Onset (Months)	***Mean***								
	SD								
	Range	Prelingual							
Duration of Deafness (Months)	***Mean***					54, 57.6	15.6	33.6	79.2
	SD					38.4, 40.8	15.6	15.6	54.0
	Range					2.4–164.4			
Age at HA Fitting (Months)	***Mean***								
	SD								
	Range								
Age at CI Stimulation (Months)	***Mean***	23.0	CI1: <60; CI2: 36–60	CI1: <60; CI2: 61–96	CI1: <60; CI2: 97–156	63.6, 67.2			
	SD	7.9				37.2, 39.6			
	Range	10.3–35.8				14–186	<24; 25–24	25–59	≥60
Duration of CI Use (Months)	***Mean***	47.3				46.8, 51.6			
	SD	22.0				25.2, 25.2			
	Range	11.9–83.2	3, 6, 12	3, 6, 12	3, 6, 12	1.2–127.2	3 or 6	3 or 6	3 or 6
Age at Testing (Months)	***Mean***	70.3				110.4, 118.8	18.0	40.8	116.4
	SD	20.9				42, 40.8	61.2	12	43.2
	Range	45.5–107.5				33.6–237.6			

		Teagle et al. (2010)			*Waltzman et al. (2000)*	*Waltzman et al. (2002)*	*Wang et al. (2008)*
Participants (*n*)		11	15	26	29	35	188
Age at HL Onset (Months)	***Mean***						10.6
	SD						10.5
	Range				Congenital	Congenital	<60
Duration of Deafness (Months)	***Mean***					139.8	10.1
	SD					34.1	8.4
	Range					97–201	
Age at HA Fitting (Months)	***Mean***		11.3				
	SD		5.3				
	Range		4–21				
Age at CI Stimulation (Months)	***Mean***		30		50.6	139.8	29.4
	SD		18.2		29.6	34.1	14.4
	Range		16–90		21–144	97–201	<60

continues

Table 8–4. *continued*

		Teagle et al. (2010)			*Waltzman et al. (2000)*	*Waltzman et al. (2002)*	*Wang et al. (2008)*
Duration of CI Use (Months)	***Mean***		19.7	49.6			
	SD		13.9	25.8			
	Range	<6	6–44	17–113	12–96	6–36	6–36
Age at Testing (Months)	***Mean***				50.7		46.4
	SD				29.6		14.4
	Range				21–144		0–90

Note: Empty cells indicate that information was not available in the published article. Abbreviations: N = Number. GJB2+ = positive for gap junction β2, a mutation in the Connexin 26 gene; GJB2- = negative for gap junction β2; HL = hearing loss; HA = hearing aid; CI = cochlear implant; LNT = Lexical Neighborhood Test (Kirk, Pisoni, & Osberger, 1995); PBK = Phonetically Balanced Kindergarten Word List (Haskins, 1949); HINT-C = Hearing in Noise Test for Children (Nilsson, Soli, & Gelnett, 1995); CI1 = first CI device; CI2 = second CI device.

Duration of Cochlear Implant Experience

Duration of cochlear implant experience is the second most frequently reported characteristic, reported by 55% (11/20) of the studies and shown in the components of Figure 8–1. Two additional studies used cochlear implant experience as inclusion criteria (Cullen et al., 2004; Waltzman et al., 2000). Test administration differed as a function of duration of cochlear implant experience. The MLNT was selected as an early measure (<24 months) of open-set speech perception (Fig. 8–1A) whereas the LNT, PBK, and HINT-C were administered across a broader range of cochlear implant experience from 0 to 72 months postimplantation, as shown in Figures 8–1B, 8–1C, and 8–1D, respectively. A positive relationship exists between duration of cochlear implant use and speech perception scores: individuals with more experience demonstrate higher performance levels. Overall duration of implant experience ranged from 0.3 to 10.3 years across all studies. Nine studies reported on outcomes in children who have used the implant for an average of less than 4 years. Five articles reported an average duration of device use between 4 and 6 years.

Chronological Age

As shown in Figure 8–2, chronological age of the child impacts the test administered. The design of this figure highlights the overall range of ages of children assessed by different measures of speech perception. Within each shaded bar lie vertical lines denoting the mean chronological ages reported for each of the measures by the various studies. For example, the MLNT was administered to children as young as 21 months and as old as 144 months (Waltzman et al., 2000), but reported mean age at administration approximated 48 months (M = 41 months (Staller et al., 2002) and 51 months (Waltzman et al., 2000). Older children possess the necessary vocabulary knowledge to complete more tasks with more advanced lexical items such as the PBK, BKB, and HINT-C tests. Additionally, chronologically older children have the maturation and short-term memory skills to repeat back not only words, but also sentences—a task that may be more difficult for chronologically younger children. Nearly half of the studies (9/20, 45%) reported on chronological age at the time of testing (one more used it as inclusion criteria). Most studies included participants over 5 years old and most of the children in the studies exceeded 7 years of age.

Other Important Hearing Variables

Duration of deafness and onset/identification of hearing loss, age at hearing aid fitting, and unaided PTA receive far less attention. Onset or identification of hearing loss was mentioned in only eight articles. Unaided PTA was reported in half the articles. Duration of deafness was reported in six articles. Age at hearing aid fitting was only reported in three articles.

Completeness of Reporting

Understanding the demographic characteristics of a population requires measures of central tendency, variability, and range. The most commonly used measures of central tendency are the mean (or the average across individual participants) and the median (or the midpoint of a distribution). Variability is measured in terms of standard deviations,

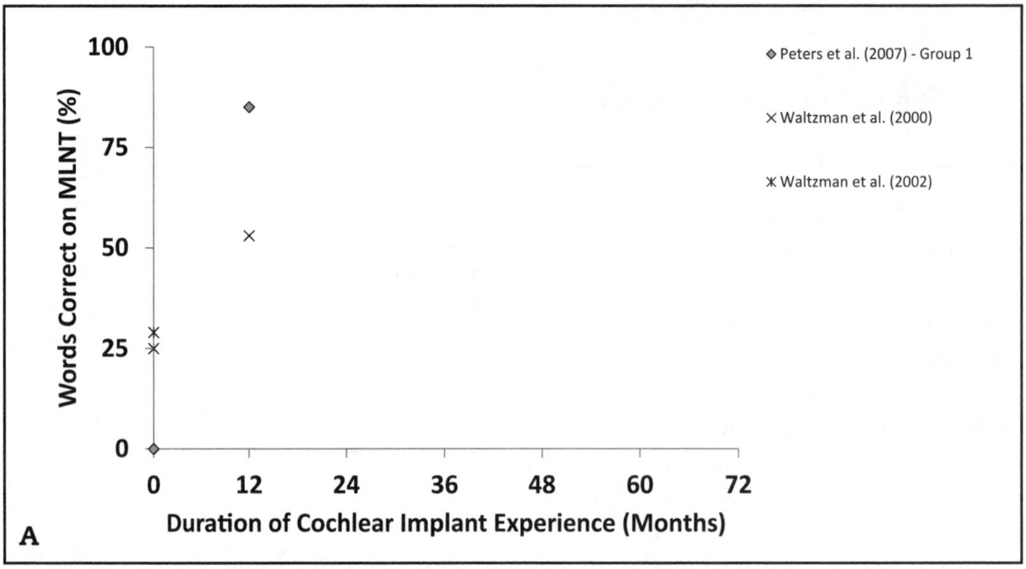

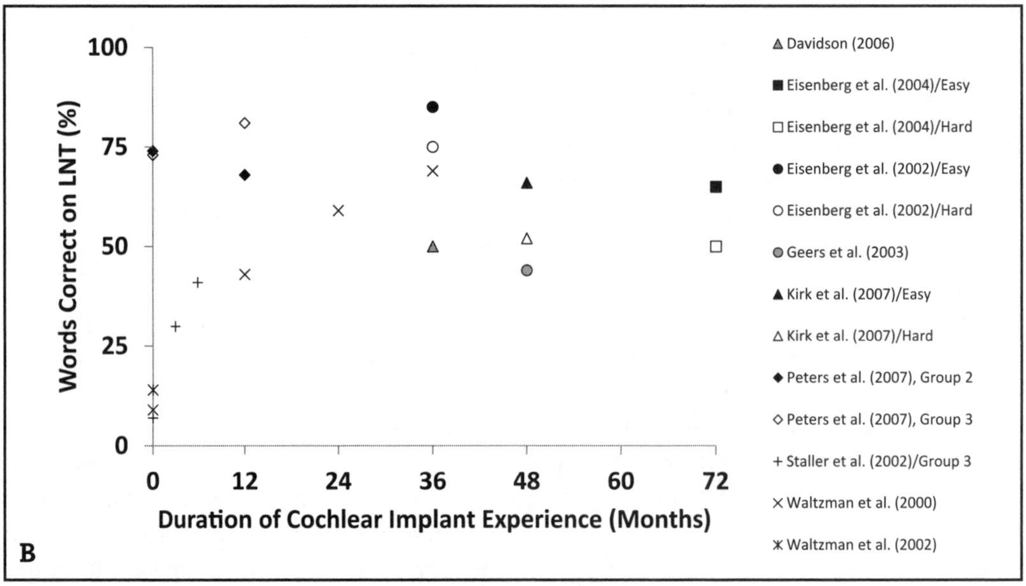

Figure 8–1. **A.** *MLNT word scores by duration of cochlear implant experience. Duration of cochlear implant experience in months is shown on the x-axis. Preimplant scores are represented as zero months of experience. Percent correct for words is shown on the y-axis. Two additional studies administered the MLNT to participants but are excluded because numeric scores or figures were not included in the paper (Staller et al, 2002; Wang et al., 2008). Waltzman et al. (2002) also reported phoneme scores, which are not represented in the figure.* **B.** *LNT word scores by duration of cochlear implant experience. Duration of cochlear implant experience in months is shown on the x-axis. Preimplant scores are represented as zero months of experience. Percent correct for words is shown on the y-axis. A few studies reported separate scores for easy and hard words (Eisenberg et al., 2002; Eisenberg et al., 2004; Kirk et al., 2007) and one study reported scores for two separate groups (Peters et al., 2007). Waltzman et al. (2002) also reported phoneme scores, which are not represented in the figure. Results from one study (Wang et al., 2008) are not included because individual scores were not reported or shown in a figure.* continues

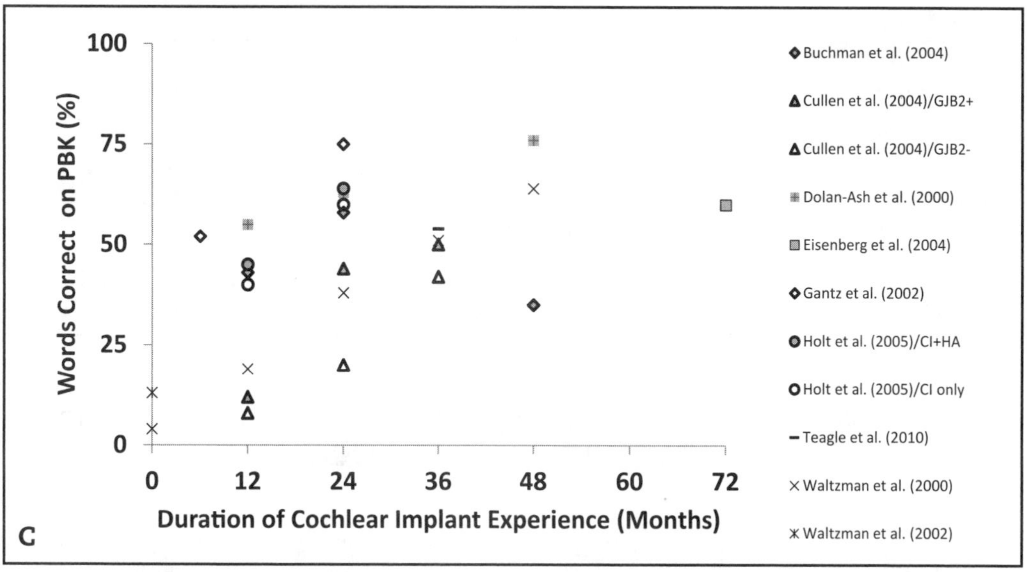

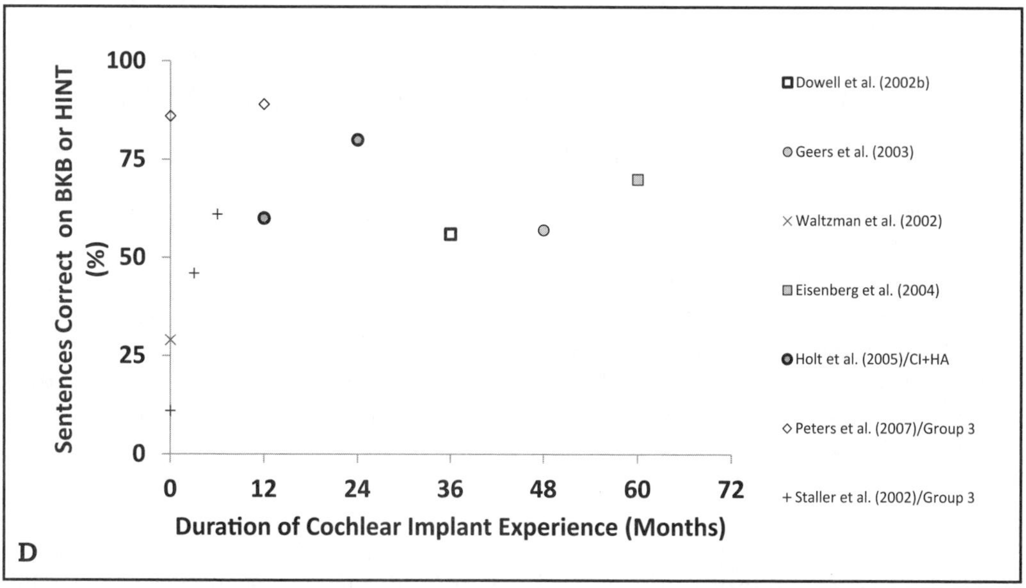

Figure 8–1. continued **C.** *PBK word scores by duration of cochlear implant experience. Duration of cochlear implant experience in months is shown on the x-axis. Preimplant scores are represented as zero months of experience. Percent correct for words is shown on the y-axis. A few studies delineated data by participant group (Cullen et al., 2004; Holt et al., 2005). Four additional studies administered PBK to participants but could not be included because numeric scores were not reported and could not be estimated from published figures (Dowell et al., 2002a; Harrison et al., 2001; Sarant et al., 2001; Wang et al., 2008). Phoneme scores were reported by Waltzman et al. (2000; 2002) but are not represented.* **D.** *Sentence scores on BKB and HINT-C measures by duration of cochlear implant experience. Duration of cochlear implant experience in months is shown on the x-axis. Preimplant scores are represented as zero months of experience. Percent correct for sentences is shown on the y-axis. Three other studies administered a sentence-level test to pediatric cochlear implant participants but numeric results were not reported (BKB: Dowell et al., 2002a; Sarant et al., 2001; HINT-C: Wang et al., 2008).*

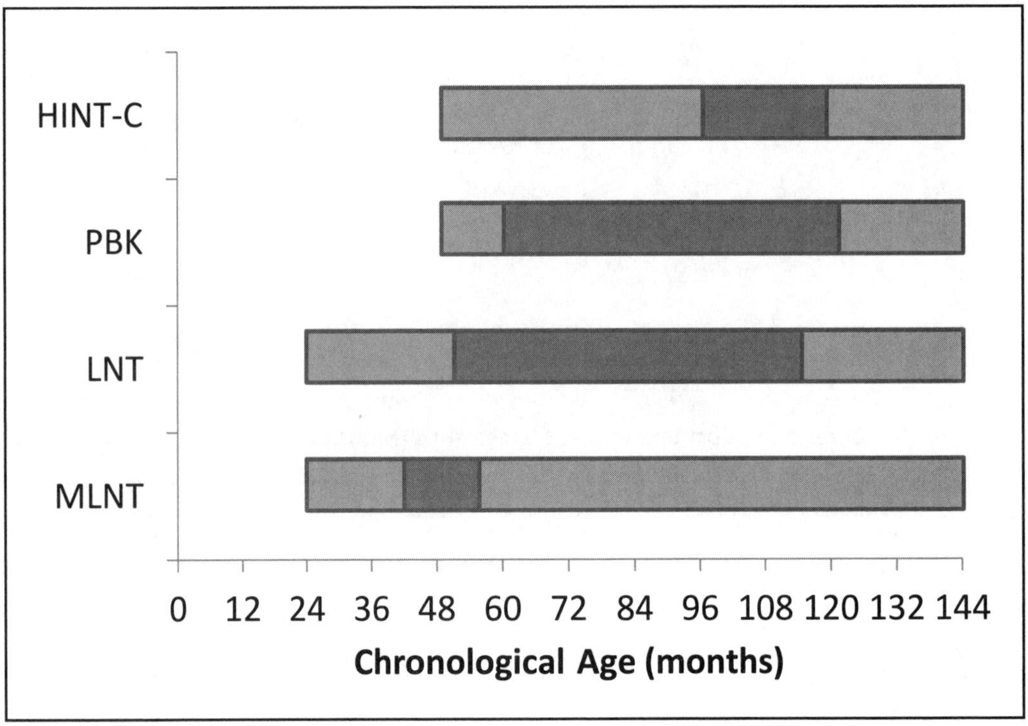

Figure 8–2. *Chronological age of pediatric cochlear implant users at administration of open-set speech perception tests. Chronological age in months is shown on the x-axis. Tests of open-set speech perception are shown on the y-axis. The shaded area represents the range of chronologic ages at which the test was administered as estimated from the age range reported in the participants' description in the methods section of the articles. The dark shaded areas indicate the mean chronologic age at which the tests were administered in individual studies.*

standard errors, or percentiles. Because variability is a hallmark of speech perception outcomes in children with cochlear implants, it is important to evaluate different scores. The range provides knowledge about the upper and lower limits of performance scores. These three measures—central tendency, variability, and range—combine to describe the population at hand. Unfortunately, most studies we reviewed in our evaluation failed to provide comprehensive assessment of demographic variables. Some studies present information without calculating means, standard deviations, and ranges. Other studies report means without divulging variability or ranges. Children using cochlear implants form a heterogeneous cohort with differences in age at identification of hearing loss, age at initial hearing aid fitting, age at cochlear implant fitting, different modes of communication and differing degrees of confounding handicaps. Performance also is confounded by chronological age and general maturational processes, as well. It is important to clearly define terms and variables to allow the most accurate comparisons to clinical populations.

If we consider the three most frequently reported demographic characteristics—age at cochlear implantation stimulation, chronologic age, and duration of cochlear implant experience—only six articles report a measure of central tendency, measure of variability, and range for these variables. Ten studies provide complete reports for age at cochlear implant stimulation, eight studies report duration of cochlear implant experience, and seven studies include chronologic age. Only five articles presented complete information about the onset of hearing loss and only two studies provided complete data on age of hearing aid fitting.

Open-Set Speech Recognition

The most common open-set speech recognition test used across studies was the PBK word lists. Seventy-five percent of the studies report average PBK scores. The next most common open-set tests administered are the LNT (reported in eight studies) and the MLNT (reported in seven studies). BKB sentences and HINT-C sentences were assessed in five and two studies, respectively. Eighteen of the studies presented stimuli at 70 dB SPL with 14 studies reporting they used recorded stimuli. Eleven of the studies represent cohort and cross-sectional studies with level 4 evidence. The remaining studies provided weaker levels of evidence in their case control or uncontrolled descriptive designs. Seven studies provided retrospective analyses and 13 studies engaged in prospective designs. Cohort comparisons occurred across normal-hearing children in two studies and with children using hearing aids in an additional three studies.

As shown in Figure 8–1C, percent correct average scores for PBK words as a function of duration of cochlear implant experience range from a low of 8 to 55% 1 year following implantation. PBK scores continue to increase with 24 months of experience to ranges of 20% to approximately 75%. Remarkably, the range of variability associated with PBK performance at 12 and 24 months postoperatively is similar. Striking reductions in PBK performance variability across studies is evident at 36 months postimplant. Performance continues to rise to 60 to 70% with 48 months experience. Of course, interpretation of individual study data requires a penetrating evaluation of all factors within the study including the number and age of subjects, particularly implants used and other demographic variables. Even with such a caveat, it is clear from the LNT performance levels contained in Figure 8–1B that steady increases in LNT performance occur within the first year postimplantation and remain evident through the first 3 years of implant experience. Fewer studies are available to assess MLNT performance; however, the data again support substantial improvements in MLNT performance with only 12 months listening experience (see Fig. 8–1A). Figure 8–1D shows that open-set sentence recognition with BKB sentences falls within the range of performance for open-set word recognition with 1 year's worth of experience listening. BKB sentence recognition appears slightly higher than HINT-C performance measured at 48 months but these minor differences may be related to test measure constructs as discussed early in this chapter.

Following the guidelines established in earlier chapters and summarized in Table 8–5, the studies were evaluated on their methods, internal validity, and external validity to provide overall judgments. All of the studies were rated plausible and pertinent. Five studies were rated as descriptive and 15 studies were rated analytic. In eight studies, we were unable to determine if bias, confounding or chance values had been carefully considered. Statistical treatment of the data was deemed appropriate and evident in only nine of the studies. In most studies, internal validity measures suggested the evidence produced by the articles was compelling.

Table 8–5. Summary of Evidence-Based Practice Queries Applied to Selected Articles on Open-Set Speech Recognition with Cochlear Implants in Children

		Buchman et al. (2004)	***Cullen et al. (2004)***	***Davidson (2006)***	***Dolan-Ash et al. (2000)***
	Level of Evidence	4	5	4	4
	Type of Analytic Study	Case-control	Case-control	Cohort	Cohort
Introduction	***Aim of study***	Assess audiological and surgical outcomes in children with inner ear malformations	Compare speech perception scores of children with & without GJB2-related deafness	Evaluate predictive value of unaided PTA on open-set word recognition	Evaluate open-set speech perception outcomes in borderline candidates
Methods	***Type of study***	Descriptive	Descriptive	Analytic	Analytic
	Control group	No	Yes	No	Yes
	Outcome measurement	Retrospective	Retrospective	Prospective	Retrospective
	Group comparison		Groups Similar	Groups Different	Groups Similar
	Attrition	Not rated	Not rated	<20% drop out	Not rated
	Intervention per group	N/A	Same	N/A	N/A
	Were bias, confounding, chance considered?	No	Unable to rate	No	Unable to rate
	Interventions	CI	CI	CI, HA	CI
	Valid, reliable intervention?	Yes—Qualified	Yes	Yes—Qualified	Yes
	Statistics	No	Yes	Yes	Yes
	Justifiable statistics	N/A	No	Yes	Yes—Qualified

		Buchman et al. (2004)	*Cullen et al. (2004)*	*Davidson (2006)*	*Dolan-Ash et al. (2000)*
Internal validity		Equivocal	Suggestive	Compelling	Compelling
	Statistically significant?	Unable to rate	No	Yes	Yes
	Reliable findings	Unable to rate	Yes	Yes	Yes
	Overlooked data?	Unable to rate	Yes	No	Yes
	If NS, was power adequate?	N/A	No	N/A	N/A
	Importance	Yes	Yes—Qualified	Yes	Yes
	Substantial cost-benefit advantage	Unable to rate	Unable to rate	Yes—Qualified	Yes
	Impact	Suggestive	Suggestive	Compelling	Compelling

		Dowell, Dettman, Blamey et al. (2002)	*Dowell, Dettman, Hill et al. (2002b)*	*Eisenberg et al. (2004)*	*Eisenberg et al. (2002)*
	Type of Evidence	3	4	4	4
	Type of Analytic Study	Case-control	Cohort	Case-control	Uncontrolled
Introduction	***Aim of study***	Examine demographic characteristics on speech perception performance	Examine demographic characteristics on speech perception performance	Compare communication outcomes via residual hearing, HA, and CI	Explore word frequency and neighborhood density in typical hearing and CI
Methods	***Type of study***	Analytic	Analytic	Analytic	Analytic
	Control group	No	No	Yes	No

continues

Table 8–5. *continued*

		Dowell, Dettman, Blamey et al. (2002)	*Dowell, Dettman, Hill et al. (2002b)*	*Eisenberg et al. (2004)*	*Eisenberg et al. (2002)*
Methods *continued*	***Outcome measurement***	Prospective	Retrospective	Prospective	Prospective
	Group comparison	N/A	N/A	Different	Different
	Attrition	<20% drop out	Not rated	Not rated	Not rated
	Intervention per group	N/A	N/A	Different	N/A
	Were bias, confounding, chance considered?	Unable to rate	Unable to rate	No	Yes
	Interventions	CI	CI	CI, HA	CI, TH
	Valid, reliable intervention?	Yes	Yes	Yes	Yes
	Statistics	Yes	Yes	Yes	Yes
	Justifiable statistic	Yes	Yes	Yes	Yes
Internal validity		Compelling	Compelling	Compelling	Compelling
	Statistically significant	Yes		No	
	Reliable findings	Yes	Yes	Yes	Yes
	Overlooked data	No		No	
	If NS, was power adequate?	N/A	Unable to rate	N/A	N/A
	Importance	Yes	Yes—Qualified	Yes	Yes
	Substantial cost-benefit advantage				
	Impact	Compelling	Suggestive	Compelling	Compelling

		Gantz et al. (2002)	*Geers et al. (2003)*	*Harrison et al. (2001)*	*Holt et al. (2005)*
	Type of Evidence	4	4	4	4
	Type of Analytic Study	Cohort	Uncontrolled	Uncontrolled	Cohort
Introduction	***Aim of study***	Review speech perception skills after 2 years of experience	Investigate factors underlying speech perception outcomes	Determine age at implantation that partitions outcomes on speech perception	Determine impact of residual hearing and aids on speech perception
Methods	***Type of study***	Descriptive	Analytic	Analytic	Analytic
	Control group	Yes	No	No	No
	Outcome measurement	Prospective	Prospective	Retrospective	Retrospective
	Group comparison	Similar	N/A	N/A	Different
	Attrition	Not rated	Not rated	Not rated	<20% drop out
	Intervention per group	Same	N/A	N/A	N/A
	Were bias, confounding, chance considered?	No	Yes	Yes—Qualified	Unable to rate
	Interventions	CI	CI	CI	CI, CI + HA
	Valid, reliable intervention?	Yes	Yes	Yes	Yes—Qualified
	Statistics	No	Yes	Yes	Yes
	Justifiable statistics	N/A	Yes	Yes	Yes

continues

Table 8–5. *continued*

		Gantz et al. (2002)	*Geers et al. (2003)*	*Harrison et al. (2001)*	*Holt et al. (2005)*
Internal validity			Compelling	Compelling	Suggestive
	Statistically significant?	Unable to rate	Yes	Yes	Yes
	Reliable findings	Yes—Qualified	Yes	Yes	Yes
	Overlooked data?	Yes		Yes	
	If NS, was power adequate?	N/A	N/A	N/A	N/A
	Importance	Yes—Qualified	Yes	Yes	Yes
	Substantial cost-benefit advantage				
	Impact	Suggestive	Compelling	Compelling	Compelling

		Kirk et al. (2007)	*Peters et al. (2007)*	*Sarant et al. (2001)*	*Staller et al. (2002)*
	Type of Evidence	4	4	4	4
	Type of Analytic Study	Cohort	Cohort	Uncontrolled	Cohort
Introduction	***Aim of study***	Examine audiovisual integration and lexical difficulty on speech perception	Measure age and duration of use of second implant on speech perception	Identify factors affecting speech perception scores	Evaluate outcomes in children using the Cochlear Nucleus 24 Contour
Methods	***Type of study***	Analytic	Analytic	Analytic	Analytic
	Control group	No	Yes	No	No

		Kirk et al. (2007)	*Peters et al. (2007)*	*Sarant et al. (2001)*	*Staller et al. (2002)*
Methods *continued*	***Outcome measurement***	Prospective	Prospective	Prospective	Prospective
	Group comparison	N/A	Similar	N/A	N/A
	Attrition	<20% drop out	Not rated	Not rated	Not rated
	Intervention per group	N/A	Same	N/A	N/A
	Were bias, confounding, chance considered	No	Yes—Qualified	Yes	Unable to rate
	Interventions	CI	CI + CI	CI	CI
	Valid, reliable intervention?	No	Yes	Yes	Yes
	Statistics	Yes	Yes	Yes	No
	Justifiable statistics	Yes	Yes	Yes	N/A
Internal validity		Compelling	Compelling	Compelling	Suggestive
	Statistically significant?	Yes	Yes	Yes	Unable to rate
	Reliable findings	Yes	Yes—Qualified	Yes	Yes
	Overlooked data		Yes	No	
	If NS, was power adequate?	N/A	N/A	N/A	N/A
	Importance	Yes	Yes—Qualified	Yes	Yes—Qualified
	Substantial cost-benefit advantage				
	Impact	Compelling	Compelling	Compelling	Suggestive

continues

Table 8–5. *continued*

		Teagle et al. (2010)	*Waltzman et al. (2000)*	*Waltzman et al. (2002)*	*Wang et al. (2008)*
	Type of Evidence	4	4	4	4
	Type of Analytic Study	Cohort	Uncontrolled	Cross-sectional	Cohort
Introduction	***Aim of study***	Report long-term performance for children with auditory neuropathy	Explore CI candidacy guidelines to include children with multiple handicaps	Determine efficacy of later implantation in children and adults	Develop a single metric summarizing speech perception outcomes
Methods	***Type of study***	Analytic	Descriptive	Analytic	Descriptive
	Control group	No	No	No	Yes
	Outcome measurement	Prospective	Retrospective	Prospective	Prospective
	Group comparison	N/A	N/A	N/A	Different
	Attrition	Not rated	<20% drop out	Not rated	Not rated
	Intervention per group	N/A	N/A	N/A	Different
	Were bias, confounding, chance considered?	Unable to rate	No	No	Unable to rate
	Interventions	CI	CI	CI	CI, TH
	Valid, reliable intervention?	Yes	Yes	Yes	Yes
	Statistics	Yes	Yes	Yes	No
	Justifiable statistics	Yes	Yes—Qualified	Yes—Qualified	N/A

		Teagle et al. (2010)	*Waltzman et al. (2000)*	*Waltzman et al. (2002)*	*Wang et al. (2008)*
Internal validity		Suggestive	Compelling	Compelling	Compelling
	Statistically significant?	Yes	Unable to rate	Yes	Unable to rate
	Reliable findings	Unable to rate	Yes	Yes—Qualified	Yes
	Overlooked data?		No	Unable to rate	
	If NS, was power adequate?	N/A	Unable to rate	N/A	N/A
	Importance	Yes	Yes	Yes	Yes
	Substantial cost-benefit advantage		Unable to rate		
	Impact	Compelling	Compelling	Compelling	Compelling

Note. In the *Type of Study* category, descriptive indicates that the study reported participants and outcomes but did not include a comparison group. An analytic study included participants with CI, a comparison group, and outcomes. In the *Group Comparison* category, similar means that participants across groups received the same intervention; different indicates that the comparison group received a different intervention. Abbreviations: PTA = Pure tone average; N/A = not applicable; NR = not rated; CI = cochlear implant; HA = hearing aid; TH = typical hearing; CI + HA = bimodal cochlear implant + hearing aid; CI + CI = bilateral cochlear implants.

Guidelines for Open-Set Speech Recognition Measures

Remarkable consistencies exist across the assessment of children with cochlear implants regarding when to assess (semiannually or annually), intensity levels (usually 70 dB SPL), and stimuli based on a child's language and developmental ages (words and sentences). Based on an evidence-based practice approach, the following general principles apply to the measurement of open-set speech recognition in children between the ages of 2 and 12 years who wear cochlear implants.

Guidelines for how to assess open-set speech perception in children who use cochlear implants:

- Monitoring of open-set performance with words, particularly over the first years of experience with a cochlear implant, documents a child's progression from sound awareness to various levels of closed-set and open-set speech perception.
- Open-set recognition scores may be acquired across a wide range of ages. MLNT is typically administered to the youngest children and HINT-C is typically reserved for older children.
- Based on language and developmental skill levels, selection of open-set speech recognition measures will vary according to multisyllabic words, monosyllabic words, and sentences. Information important for establishing rehabilitation programs and monitoring of progress are established by scoring the open-set speech recognition measures by phoneme, word, and sentence accuracy.
- Carefully controlled, recorded versions of the tests (either auditory alone or auditory-visual presentations) provide more reliable judgments than live voice presentations.
- Open-set speech recognition typically is administered at 70 dB SPL for young preschool-age children using cochlear implants to monitor the development of speech perception skills at suprathreshold levels. As children mature and gain experience listening with the cochlear implant, performance scores may reach maximum levels (90–100%), which creates difficulties documenting skill progression. Therefore, during school-age years, open-set recognition may be assessed in more demanding conditions such as at less intense levels (50 dB SPL) or in the presence of competing background noise for children using cochlear implants.

Expected open-set speech perception findings of children who use cochlear implants:

- Open-set speech recognition in children with cochlear implants is positively influenced by early detection of hearing loss, early implantation, shorter durations of deafness, and greater amounts of residual hearing.
- Levels of open-set recognition are lower for children with multiple handicaps, more involved inner ear malformations, late identification of hearing loss, prolonged hearing aid use, and late ages of implantation. However, steady clinically significant gains are evident in open-set performance over time following cochlear implantation even in these children.

Limitations of Evidence of Open-Set Speech Recognition in Pediatric Cochlear Implantation

Key variables are not consistently reported across studies and this adversely influences the interpretation of research findings. Inconsistently reported key variables include important demographic variables associated with the amount of residual hearing (generally reported as unaided pure tone averages), the length of hearing aid trials, and age of implantation (dates of surgery or initial programming). Central tendencies and variability measures often are incomplete or missing. Consistent information regarding the cochlear implants, themselves, is often missing. Information is needed regarding the processor type, the processing strategies, length of experience and history (particularly, as it may relate to implant failures and periods of auditory deprivation). Information about such variables is critical for understanding how the technology is providing viable audibility to these young developing auditory systems.

In spite of these limitations, the data suggest open-set speech recognition is achievable in young children using cochlear implants. We originally asked what levels of open-set speech recognition in quiet listening conditions are associated with cochlear implantation for children between the ages of 2 and 12 years wearing either one or two cochlear implants. Children with severe to profound hearing loss who undergo cochlear implantation can achieve word and sentence recognition performance above chance levels as early as 12 months after cochlear implant activation. Considerable variability in speech perception scores exists, with differences related to age at cochlear implantation, chronological age at testing, residual hearing before implantation, and duration of cochlear implant experience. The evidence suggests that variability in open-set performance across studies decreases with increased experience listening with the devices. The compelling nature of these observations indicates open-set speech recognition should be an important tool in the assessment and monitoring of performance in children using cochlear implants.

REFERENCES

Bench, J., Kowal, A., & Bamford, J. (1979). The BKB (Bamford-Kowal-Bench) sentence lists for partially-hearing children. *British Journal of Audiology, 13*, 108–112.

Boothroyd, A. (1997). *VIDSPAC 2.0: Video game test of assessing speech pattern contrast perception.* New York, NY: City University of New York Graduate Center.

Buchman, C. A., Copeland, B. J., Yu, K. K., Brown, C. J., Carrasco, V. N., & Pillsbury, H. C., III (2004). Cochlear implantation in children with congenital inner ear malformations. *Laryngoscope, 114*, 309–316.

Buechner, A., Frohne-Buechner, C., Boyle, P., Battmer, R. D., & Lenarz, T. (2009). A high rate n-of-m speech processing strategy for the first generation Clarion cochlear implant. *International Journal of Audiolology, 48*, 868–875.

Carlson, M. L., Archibald, D. J., Dabade, T. S., Gifford, R. H., Neff, B. A., Beatty, C. W., . . . Driscoll, C. W. (2010). Prevalence and timing of individual cochlear implant electrode failures. *Otology and Neurotology, 31*, 893–898.

Ching, T. Y., Psarros, C., Hill, M., Dillon, H., & Incerti, P. (2001). Should children who use cochlear implants wear hearing aids in the opposite ear? *Ear and Hearing, 22*, 365–380.

Clark, G. M. (2000). The cochlear implant: A search for answers. *Cochlear Implants International, 1*, 1–15.

Clark, G. M. (2008). Personal reflections on the multichannel cochlear implant and a view of the future. *Journal of Rehabilitation Research and Development, 45*, 651–693.

Clopper, C. G., Pisoni, D. B., & Tierney, A. T. (2006). Effects of open-set and closed-set task demands on spoken word recognition. *Journal of the American Academy of Audiology, 17*, 331–349.

Cohen, N. L. (2004). Cochlear implant candidacy and surgical considerations. *Audiology and Neurotology, 9*, 197–202.

Cosetti, M., & Roland, J. T., Jr. (2010). Cochlear implantation in the very young child: Issues unique to the under-1 population. *Trends in Amplification, 14*, 46–57.

Cowan, R. S., DelDot, J., Barker, E. J., Sarant, J. Z., Pegg, P., Dettman, S., . . . Clark, G. M. (1997). Speech perception results for children with implants with different levels of preoperative residual hearing. *American Journal of Otology, 18*, S125–S126.

Cullen, R. D., Buchman, C. A., Brown, C. J., Copeland, B. J., Zdanski, C., Pillsbury, H. C., III, & Shores, C. G. (2004). Cochlear implantation for children with GJB2-related deafness. *Laryngoscope, 114*, 1415–1419.

Davidson, L. S. (2006). Effects of stimulus level on the speech perception abilities of children using cochlear implants or digital hearing aids. *Ear and Hearing, 27*, 493–507.

Davidson, L. S., Geers, A. E., & Brenner, C. (2010). Cochlear implant characteristics and speech perception skills of adolescents with long-term device use. *Otology and Neurotology, 31*, 1310–1314.

Dolan-Ash, S., Hodges, A. V., Butts, S. L., & Balkany, T. J. (2000). Borderline pediatric cochlear implant candidates: preoperative and postoperative results. *Annals of Otology, Rhinology, and Laryngology. Supplement, 185*, 36–38.

Dowell, R. C., Dettman, S. J., Blamey, P. J., Barker, E. J., & Clark, G. M. (2002). Speech perception in children using cochlear implants: Prediction of long-term outcomes. *Cochlear Implants International, 3*, 1–18.

Dowell, R. C., Dettman, S. J., Hill, K., Winton, E., Barker, E. J., & Clark, G. M. (2002). Speech perception outcomes in older children who use multichannel cochlear implants: Older is not always poorer. *Annals of Otology, Rhinology, and Laryngology. Supplement, 189*, 97–101.

Eisenberg, L. S., Kirk, K. I., Martinez, A. S., Ying, E. A., & Miyamoto, R. T. (2004). Communication abilities of children with aided residual hearing: Comparison with cochlear implant users. *Archives of Otolaryngology—Head and Neck Surgery, 130*, 563–569.

Eisenberg, L. S., Martinez, A. S., Holowecky, S. R., & Pogorelsky, S. (2002). Recognition of lexically controlled words and sentences by children with normal hearing and children with cochlear implants. *Ear and Hearing, 23*, 450–462.

Eisenberg, L. S., Martinez, A. S., Sennaroglu, G., & Osberger, M. J. (2000). Establishing new criteria in selecting children for a cochlear implant: performance of "platinum" hearing aid users. *Annals of Otology, Rhinology, and Laryngology. Supplement, 185*, 30–33.

Elliott, L., & Katz, D. (1980). *Northwestern University Children's Perception of Speech.* St. Louis, MO: Auditec.

Erber, N. P. (1982). *Auditory training.* Washington, DC: A.G. Bell Association for the Deaf.

Fitzpatrick, E., Olds, J., Durieux-Smith, A., McCrae, R., Schramm, D., & Gaboury, I. (2009). Pediatric cochlear implantation: How much hearing is too much? *International Journal of Audiology, 48*, 91–97.

Fitzpatrick, E. M., Seguin, C., Schramm, D., Chenier, J., & Armstrong, S. (2009). Users' experience of a cochlear implant combined with a hearing aid. *International Journal of Audiology, 48*, 172–182.

Flexer, C., & Madell, J. (2009). The concept of listening age for audiologic management of pediatric hearing loss. *Audiology Today, 21*, 31–35.

Fryauf-Bertschy, H., Tyler, R. S., Kelsay, D. M., Gantz, B. J., & Woodworth, G. G. (1997). Cochlear implant use by prelingually deafened children: The influences of age at implant and length of device use. *Journal of Speech, Language, and Hearing Research, 40*, 183–199.

Galvin, K. L., Hughes, K. C., & Mok, M. (2010). Can adolescents and young adults with prelingual hearing loss benefit from a second, sequential cochlear implant? *International Journal of Audiology, 49*, 368–377.

Gantz, B. J., Rubinstein, J. T., Tyler, R. S., Teagle, H. F., Cohen, N. L., Waltzman, S. B., . . . Kirk, K. I. (2000). Long-term results of cochlear implants in children with residual hearing. *Annals of Otology, Rhinology, and Laryngology. Supplement, 185*, 33–36.

Geers, A., Brenner, C., & Davidson, L. (2003). Factors associated with development of speech perception skills in children implanted by age five. *Ear and Hearing, 24*, 24S–35S.

Haimowitz, S. (1999). Deaf culture. *Hastings Center Report, 29*, 5.

Hardonk, S., Bosteels, S., Desnerck, G., Loots, G., Van Hove, G., Van Kerschaver, E., . . . Louckx, F. (2010). Pediatric cochlear implantation: A qualitative study of parental decision-making processes in Flanders, Belgium. *American Annals of the Deaf, 155*, 339–352.

Harrison, R. V., Panesar, J., El-Hakim, H., Abdolell, M., Mount, R. J., & Papsin, B. (2001). The effects of age of cochlear implantation on speech perception outcomes in prelingually deaf children. *Scandinavian Audiology, 30*(Suppl. 53), 73–78.

Haskins, H. A. (1949). *A phonetically balanced test of speech discrimination for children.* Master's Thesis, Northwestern University, Evanston, IL.

Holt, R. F., Kirk, K. I., Eisenberg, L. S., Martinez, A. S., & Campbell, W. (2005). Spoken word recognition development in children with residual hearing using cochlear implants and hearing aids in opposite ears. *Ear and Hearing, 26*, 82S–91S.

Holt, R. F., Kirk, K. I., Pisoni, D. B., Burckhartzmeyer, L., & Lin, A. (2005). Lexical and context effects in children's audiovisual speech recognition. In *150th Meeting of the Acoustical Society of America.*

Jakubikova, J., Kabatova, Z., Pavlovcinova, G., & Profant, M. (2009). Newborn hearing screening and strategy for early detection of hearing loss in infants. *International Journal of Pediatric Otorhinolaryngology, 73*, 607–612.

Jerger, S., & Jerger, J. (1984). *Pediatric Speech Intelligibilty Test: Manual for administration.* St. Louis, MO: Auditec.

Jethanamest, D., Tan, C. T., Fitzgerald, M. B., & Svirsky, M. A. (2010). A new software tool to optimize frequency table selection for cochlear implants. *Otology and Neurotology, 31*, 1242–1247.

Kirk, K. I., Hay-McCutcheon, M. J., Holt, R. F., Gao, S., Qi, R., & Gehrlein, B. L. (2007). Audiovisual spoken word recognition by children with cochlear implants. *Audiological Medicine, 5*, 250–261.

Kirk, K. I., Pisoni, D. B., & Osberger, M. J. (1995). Lexical effects on spoken word recognition by pediatric cochlear implant users. *Ear and Hearing, 16*, 470–481.

Kompis, M., Vibert, D., Senn, P., Vischer, M. W., & Hausler, R. (2003). Scuba diving with cochlear implants. *Annals of Otology Rhinology Laryngology, 112*, 425–427.

Kovacic, D., & Balaban, E. (2009). Voice gender perception by cochlear implantees. *Journal of the Acoustical Society of America, 126*, 762–775.

Lane, H. (1995). The dispute concerning the benefits to be expected from cochlear implantation of young deaf children. *American Journal of Otology, 16*, 393–399.

Lane, H., & Bahan, B. (1998). Ethics of cochlear implantation in young children: A review and reply from a Deaf-World perspective. *Otolaryngology—Head and Neck Surgery, 119*, 297–313.

Lane, H., & Grodin, M. (1997). Ethical issues in cochlear implant surgery: An exploration into disease, disability, and the best interests of the child. *Kennedy Institute of Ethics Journal, 7*, 231–251.

Luce, P. A., & Pisoni, D. B. (1998). Recognizing spoken words: The neighborhood activation model. *Ear and Hearing, 19*, 1–36.

McJunkin, J., & Jeyakumar, A. (2010). Complications in pediatric cochlear implants. *American Journal of Otolaryngology, 31*, 110–113.

Miyamoto, R. T., Osberger, M. J., Robbins, A. M., Myres, W. A., & Kessler, K. (1993). Prelingually deafened children's performance with the nucleus multichannel cochlear implant. *American Journal of Otology, 14*, 437–445.

Moog, J., & Geers, A. (1990). *Early Speech Perception Test for Profoundly Deaf Children.* St. Louis, MO: Central Institute for the Deaf.

Moog, J. S. ,& Geers, A. E. (2010). Early educational placement and later language outcomes for children with cochlear implants. *Otology and Neurotology, 31*, 1315–1319.

Nicholas, J. G., & Geers, A. E. (2007). Will they catch up? The role of age at cochlear implantation in the spoken language development of children with severe to profound hearing loss. *Journal of Speech, Language, and Hearing Research, 50*, 1048–1062.

Nilsson, M., Soli, S., & Gelnett, D. (1995). *Development of the Hearing in Noise Test for Children (HINT-C).* Los Angeles, CA: House Ear Institute.

Niparko, J. K., Tobey, E. A., Thal, D. J., Eisenberg, L. S., Wang, N. Y., Quittner, A. L., & Fink, N. E. (2010). Spoken language development in children following cochlear implantation. *Journal of the American Medical Association, 303*, 1498–1506.

Osberger, M. J. (1997). Cochlear implantation in children under the age of two years: Candidacy considerations. *Otolaryngology—Head and Neck Surgery, 117,* 145–149.

Osberger, M. J., Dettman, S. J., Daniel, K., Moog, J. S., Sieber, R., Stone, P. et al. (1991). Rehabilitation and education issues with implanted children: perspectives from a panel of clinicians and educators. *American Journal of Otology, 12*(Suppl.), 205–212.

Osberger, M. J., Fisher, L., Zimmerman-Phillips, S., Geier, L., & Barker, M. J. (1998). Speech recognition performance of older children with cochlear implants. *American Journal of Otology, 19,* 152–157.

Osberger, M. J., Miyamoto, R. T., Zimmerman-Phillips, S., Kemink, J. L., Stroer, B. S., Firszt, J. B., . . . Novak, M. A. (1991). Independent evaluation of the speech perception abilities of children with the Nucleus 22-channel cochlear implant system. *Ear and Hearing, 12,* 66S–80S.

Osberger, M. J., Zimmerman-Phillips, S., & Koch, D. B. (2002). Cochlear implant candidacy and performance trends in children. *Annals of Otology Rhinology and Laryngology Supplement, 189,* 62–65.

Peters, B. R., Litovsky, R., Parkinson, A., & Lake, J. (2007). Importance of age and post-implantation experience on speech perception measures in children with sequential bilateral cochlear implants. *Otology and Neurotology, 28,* 649–657.

Peterson, G. E., & Lehiste, I. (1962). Revised CNC lists for auditory tests. *Journal of Speech and Hearing Disorders, 27,* 62–70.

Qian, H., Loizou, P. C., & Dorman, M. F. (2003). A phone-assistive device based on Bluetooth technology for cochlear implant users. *IEEE Transactions on Neural Systems and Rehabilitation Engineering, 11,* 282–287.

Ramsden, J. D., Papaioannou, V., Gordon, K. A., James, A. L., & Papsin, B. C. (2009). Parental and program's decision making in paediatric simultaneous bilateral cochlear implantation: Who says no and why? *International Journal of Pediatric Otorhinolaryngology, 73,* 1325–1328.

Robbins, A. M., Renshaw, J. J., & Berry, S. W. (1991). Evaluating meaningful auditory integration in profoundly hearing-impaired children. *American Journal of Otology, 12,* 144–150.

Robbins, A. M., Renshaw, J. J., & Osberger, M. J. (1995). *Common Phrases Test.* Indianapolis, IN: Indiana School of Medicine.

Ross, M., & Lerman, J. (1970). *Word intelligibility by picture identification.* Pittsburgh, PA: Stanwix House.

Sarant, J. Z., Blamey, P. J., Dowell, R. C., Clark, G. M., & Gibson, W. P. (2001). Variation in speech perception scores among children with cochlear implants. *Ear and Hearing, 22,* 18–28.

Shapiro, W. H., Huang, T., Shaw, T., Roland, J. T., Jr., & Lalwani, A. K. (2008). Remote intraoperative monitoring during cochlear implant surgery is feasible and efficient. *Otology and Neurotology, 29,* 495–498.

Staller, S., Parkinson, A., Arcaroli, J., & Arndt, P. (2002). Pediatric outcomes with the nucleus 24 contour: North American clinical trial. *Annals of Otology, Rhinology, and Laryngology. Supplement, 189,* 56–61.

Tajudeen, B. A., Waltzman, S. B., Jethanamest, D., & Svirsky, M. A. (2010). Speech perception in congenitally deaf children receiving cochlear implants in the first year of life. *Otology and Neurotology, 31,* 1254–1260.

Teagle, H. F., Roush, P. A., Woodard, J. S., Hatch, D. R., Zdanski, C. J., Buss, E., . . . Buchman, C. A. (2010). Cochlear implantation in children with auditory neuropathy spectrum disorder. *Ear and Hearing, 31,* 325–335.

Thibodeau, L. (2007). Speech audiometry. In R. J. Roeser, M. Valente, & H. Hosford-Dunn (Eds.), *Audiology: Diagnosis* (2nd ed., pp. 288–295). New York, NY: Thieme.

Trammell, J. (1976). *Test of Auditory Comprehension.* North Hollywood, CA: Foreworks.

Tucker, B. P. (1998). Deaf culture, cochlear implants, and elective disability. *Hastings Center Report, 28,* 6–14.

Tye-Murray, N., & Geers, A. (2001). *Children's Audio-Visual Enhancement Test.* St. Louis, MO: Central Institute for the Deaf.

Waltzman, S. B., Cohen, N. L., Gomolin, R. H., Green, J. E., Shapiro, W. H., Hoffman, R. A., . . . Roland, J. T. (1997). Open-set speech perception in congenitally deaf children using cochlear implants. *American Journal of Otology, 18,* 342–349.

Waltzman, S. B., Cohen, N. L., Gomolin, R. H., Shapiro, W. H., Ozdamar, S. R., & Hoffman, R. A. (1994). Long-term results of early cochlear implantation in congenitally and prelingually deafened children. *American Journal of Otology, 15*(Suppl. 2), 9–13.

Waltzman, S. B., Roland, J. T., Jr., & Cohen, N. L. (2002). Delayed implantation in congenitally deaf children and adults. *Otology and Neurotology, 23*, 333–340.

Waltzman, S. B., Scalchunes, V., & Cohen, N. L. (2000). Performance of multiply handicapped children using cochlear implants. *American Journal of Otology, 21*, 329–335.

Wang, N. Y., Eisenberg, L. S., Johnson, K. C., Fink, N. E., Tobey, E. A., Quittner, A. L., . . . Niparko, J. (2008). Tracking development of speech recognition: Longitudinal data from hierarchical assessments in the Childhood Development after Cochlear Implantation Study. *Otology and Neurotology, 29*, 240–245.

Wiley, S., & Meinzen-Derr, J. (2009). Access to cochlear implant candidacy evaluations: Who is not making it to the team evaluations? *International Journal of Audiology, 48*, 74–79.

Yoshinaga-Itano, C. (1999). Benefits of early intervention for children with hearing loss. *Otolaryngologic Clinics of North America, 32*, 1089–1102.

Yoshinaga-Itano, C., & Apuzzo, M. L. (1998). Identification of hearing loss after age 18 months is not early enough. *American Annals of the Deaf, 143*, 380–387.

Yoshinaga-Itano, C., Sedey, A. L., Coulter, D. K., & Mehl, A. L. (1998). Language of early- and later-identified children with hearing loss. *Pediatrics, 102*, 1161–1171.

Zhang, J., Wei, W., Ding, J., Roland, J. T., Jr., Manolidis, S., & Simaan, N. (2010). Inroads toward robot-assisted cochlear implant surgery using steerable electrode arrays. *Otology and Neurotology, 31*, 1199–1206.

Zimmerman-Phillips, S., Osberger, M. J., & Robbins, A. M. (1997). *Infant-Toddler Meaningful Auditory Integration Scale*. Sylmar, CA: Advanced Bionics Corp.

CHAPTER 9

Bimodal Fitting or Bilateral Cochlear Implantation?

Teresa Y. C. Ching and Paola Incerti

INTRODUCTION

It is widely accepted that listening with two ears is better than one. For people with bilateral severe or profound hearing loss, binaural hearing is possible by either combining electric and acoustic hearing in opposite ears (bimodal fitting) or using electric hearing in both ears (bilateral cochlear implantation). In this chapter, a brief description of binaural effects is first provided, followed by an examination of the scientific evidence on the extent to which the respective methods of bilateral stimulation leads to improvements in listeners' hearing functions and ability to participate in activities in real life. The goal is to provide recommendations for best practice in the provision of audiological management of people with bilateral severe or profound hearing loss. Finally, studies that compared bimodal fitting with bilateral implantation are evaluated to address the question of whether one provides a better option than the other. This chapter does not address treatment with bimodal stimulation in the same ear.

The evidence is reviewed under three broad categories: bimodal fitting relative to unilateral implants; bilateral implants relative to unilateral implants; and bimodal fitting compared to bilateral implantation. The schemes for rating evidence (see Table 1–5) and the grading recommendation (see Table 1–6) of the American Academy of Audiology are adopted for classifying evidence in each area. The evidence is also categorized according to whether assessments were carried out under laboratory/ ideal conditions (Efficacious, EF) or in the real world (Effectiveness, EV).

WHAT BENEFITS ARE POSSIBLE WITH BINAURAL HEARING?

When we listen to sounds in the environment, we extract information from the audible signal to help us understand what we hear and determine where the sounds come from (Blauert, 1997). People with normal hearing can achieve these tasks by using acoustic cues that arise from listening with two ears. The acoustic cues relate to differences in time and level of sounds arriving at each of the two ears. These cues are commonly referred to as interaural time difference (ITD) and interaural level difference (ILD) cues. Due to the physical size of the head and the position of the two ears, a sound originating from one side of the head reaches the near ear a bit sooner than the farther ear. It will also be higher in level at the near than at the farther ear. For instance, a sound that originates at 90° azimuth reaches the left ear 0.7 milliseconds after it reaches the right ear, whereas a sound that is directly in front at 0° azimuth arrives at the two ears at the same time. Interaural time difference cues are carried most efficiently in the low frequencies, up to about 1500 Hz (Moore, 2003). Furthermore, the head acts as an acoustic barrier and causes a level difference between ears. For a sound originating from one side, head diffraction produces an attenuation of sound on the far side of the head and this is usually referred to as head shadow. Head diffraction also produces a boost on the near side of the head. These effects have the greatest magnitude in the high frequencies, due to the short wavelengths of high-frequency sounds compared to the size of the head. The resulting ILD is therefore more pronounced in the high frequencies, reaching up to 20 dB for sounds that are located at 90° azimuth. The binaural auditory system relies on information about ITD and ILD to determine sound source locations (Dillon, 2001; Middlebrooks & Green, 1991; Stern & Ttrahiotis, 1996).

Listening with two ears also helps normal-hearing listeners extract speech from competing noise. When a target sound comes from one location and a competing sound from a different spatial location, the signal-to-noise ratio (SNR) will be higher in one ear than the other due to the "head shadow" effect. Speech intelligibility can be improved through selective attention to the ear with the more favorable SNR. Even when the two competing sounds are not spatially separated, there is benefit when the auditory system can extract speech information from the signal reaching each of the ears. This benefit arises from "redundancy" of information (Bronkhorst, 2000; Durlach & Colburn, 1978). Furthermore, comparisons of information from both ears by the auditory system, that is, the use of ITD and ILD cues, contribute to grouping sounds into auditory streams (Culling, Hawley, & Litovsky, 2004). This binaural "squelch" effect assists with improving speech intelligibility in noisy backgrounds.

Head shadow and redundancy are possible for people with hearing loss when sounds are audible in both ears, irrespective of whether audibility is provided via bimodal fitting or bilateral implantation (Ching, van Wanrooy, & Dillon, 2007). An additional advantage is possible with bimodal fitting but not with bilateral implantation. This relates to the way in which low-frequency information provided by acoustic amplification complements high-frequency information provided by electric stimulation. Because cochlear implants are unable to convey sufficient information about pitch to their users (McDermott, 2004), bimodal fitting for listeners with sufficient hearing functions in the low frequencies is likely to enhance transmission of pitch information. The effect has been referred to as "complementarity" (Ching et al., 2007). In the following sections, the evidence on the effects of bilateral stimulation using either mode is examined with a view to providing recommendations and strategies for audiological management.

Bimodal Fitting

The research on children's performance with bimodal stimulation, relative to unilateral cochlear implantation, is summarized in Table 9–1, and findings in adults are summarized in Table 9–2.

Several studies have documented the added benefit of a hearing aid to a cochlear implant for localization by comparing performance under monaural (with an implant alone) and binaural (an implant and a hearing aid in opposite ears) listening conditions.

Table 9–1. Evidence of Bimodal Stimulation (a hearing aid in one ear and a cochlear implant in the other ear) Compared with Unilateral Cochlear Implantation in Children*

Evidence	*Source*	*Level*	*Grade*	*EFficacy/ EffectiVeness*
Horizontal localization was better with bimodal stimulation.	Ching et al, 2001; Ching et al, 2005; Litovsky et al, 2006a, 2006b	3	B	EF
Speech perception in quiet was better with bimodal stimulation due to binaural redundancy.	Beijin et al., 2008; Ching et al, 2000, 2001; Dettman et al, 2004; Holt et al., 2005	3	B	EF
Speech perception in noise was better with bimodal stimulation due to binaural redundancy.	Ching et al., 2001; Ching et al., 2006; Lee et al., 2008.	3	B	EF
Speech perception in noise was better with bimodal stimulation, due to effects of head shadow, binaural redundancy, and squelch.	Beijin et al., 2008; Ching et al,, 2005; Litovsky et al., 2006a; Yuen et al., 2009.	3	B	EF
Children with bimodal stimulation did not obtain benefits from interaural timing cues for speech perception in noise.	Ching et al., 2005.	3	B	EF
Acoustic information about voice pitch provided by bimodal stimulation improved consonant perception.	Ching et al, 2001; Ching et al., 2007	3	B	EF
Children's functional performance in real life improved with bimodal stimulation, as perceived by parents.	Ching et al., 2001	3	B	EV
Children with severe hearing loss in low frequencies obtained benefits from bimodal stimulation.	Ching et al., 2004b, 2007	3	B	EF/EV
Children with better residual hearing in low frequencies (better aided thresholds) and poorer high frequencies obtained greatest bimodal bilateral advantage.	Mok et al., 2010	3	B	EF

continues

Table 9–1. *continued*

Evidence	*Source*	*Level*	*Grade*	*EFficacy/ EffectiVeness*
Loudness balance and optimized hearing aid frequency response with cochlear implants led to increased benefits with bimodal stimulation in children.	Ching et al., 2004a; Ching 2005; Ching et al., 2007; Huart & Sammeth, 2008	3	B	EF/EV

*The quality of evidence is rated on a scale from 1 (high-quality studies) to 6 (expert opinion) (see Table 1–5). The grade of recommendation is rated on a scale from A (level 1 or 2 studies with consistent conclusions) to D (level 6 evidence or inconclusive studies) (see Table 1–6). The evidence is also categorized according to whether assessments were carried out under laboratory/ ideal conditions (Efficacy, EF) or in the real world (Effectiveness, EV).

Table 9–2. Evidence of Bimodal Stimulation (a hearing aid in one ear and a cochlear implant in the other ear) Compared with Unilateral Cochlear Implantation in Adults*

Evidence	*Source*	*Level*	*Grade*	*EFficacy/ EffectiVeness*
With bimodal fitting, adults who had moderate hearing loss in the ear that used acoustic hearing localized nearly as well as normal-hearing listeners.	Seeber et al, 2004	3	B	EF
Horizontal localization was significantly better with bimodal stimulation.	Ching et al, 2004c; Potts et al., 2009; Seeber et al., 2004	3/4	B/C	EF
Speech perception in quiet was better with bimodal stimulation, due to effects of binaural redundancy.	Armstrong et al., 1997; Berretini et al.2010;.Ching et al., 2004a; Gifford et al., 2007; Iwaki et al, 2004; Kong et al., 2005; Mok et al., 2006	3/4	B/C	EF

Table 9–2. *continued*

Evidence	*Source*	*Level*	*Grade*	*EFficacy/ EffectiVeness*
Speech perception in noise was better with bimodal stimulation, due to combined effects of binaural redundancy and squelch.	Dunn et al., 2005; Morera et al., 2005	3	B	EF
Speech perception in noise was better with bimodal stimulation, due to combined effects of head shadow, binaural redundancy, and squelch.	Berretini et al., 2010; Ching et al., 2004; Dunn et al., 2005; Gifford et al., 2007; Luntz et al., 2007; Morera et al, 2005; Tyler et al., 2002.	3/4	B/C	EF
Unaided thresholds and speech perception in the nonimplanted ear were significantly related to performance with bimodal stimulation.	Potts et al., 2009	3	B	EF
Acoustic information about voice pitch provided via bimodal stimulation improved consonant perception.	Incerti et al., 2011	3	B	EF
Acoustic information below 150 Hz provided via bimodal stimulation improved speech perception.	Zhang et al., 2010	3	B	EF
Recognition of melodies was significantly better with bimodal stimulation.	Dorman et al., 2008; El Fata et al., 2009; Kong et al., 2005; Sucher & Mcdermott, 2009	3	B	EF
Loudness balance between ears with bimodal stimulation improved performance.	Ching et al., 2004a	3	B	EF

*The quality of evidence is rated on a scale from 1 (high-quality studies) to 6 (expert opinion) (see Table 1–5). The grade of recommendation is rated on a scale from A (level 1 or 2 studies with consistent conclusions) to D (level 6 evidence or inconclusive studies) (see Table 1–6). The evidence is also categorized according to whether assessments were carried out under laboratory/ ideal conditions (Efficacy, EF) or in the real world (Effectiveness, EV).

Under relatively nonchallenging situations (e.g., Tyler et al., 2002) in controlled laboratory environments, such as identifying whether the sound originated from one of two loudspeakers located to the left or right of the listener, some users of bimodal hearing were able to localize almost as well as normal-hearing listeners. But in more challenging situations (e.g. Ching, Incerti, & Hill, 2004a; Seeber, Baumann, & Fastl, 2004) when there were larger numbers of loudspeakers in a test room, localization performance was poorer than normal. Across studies, localization improved (i.e., participants made fewer errors) for about half of the listeners when using bimodal stimulation compared to using a cochlear implant alone, with the remaining ones showing no significant difference between the two listening conditions.

There is also evidence to demonstrate significant speech intelligibility benefits due to head shadow and binaural redundancy effects, both in children (see Table 9–1) and adults (see Table 9–2). However, when binaural cues were limited to only ITDs, these did not assist with improving speech perception (Ching, van Wanrooy, Hill, & Dillon, 2005). It is likely that the timing information presented by the cochlear implant and the hearing aid was too distorted to be useful to the listeners. In all studies that investigated speech intelligibility, the largest benefit is associated with experimental conditions in which combined effects of head shadow, redundancy, and complementarity contribute to speech intelligibility.

In addition to improved performance for word and sentence recognition due to binaural effects, bimodal fitting also led to improved perception of voicing contrasts in identification of consonants by children (Ching, 2011) and adults (Incerti, Ching, & Hill, 2011). These findings are consistent with recent evidence on adults showing that binaural speech perceptual benefits were possible even when acoustic amplification bandwidth was restricted to frequencies below 150 Hz (Cullington & Zeng, 2010; Zhang, Dorman, & Spahr, 2010). The research suggests that speech perception benefits with bimodal stimulation can be explained largely in terms of the increase in transmission of voice-pitch information via acoustic amplification. Not only is voice pitch information important for linguistic contrasts relating to lexical tones and intonation, information about the onset and duration of voicing as well as the presence or absence of voicing contribute to identification of consonants (Faulkner & Rosen, 1999) and facilitate lexical access (Spitzer, Liss, Spahr, & Landsford, 2009; Zue, 1985). Also, the low-frequency speech signal provides prosodic information and assists with perceptual organization of the speech signal in marking syllable structures and word boundaries, thereby facilitating speech perception especially in noisy situations.

The availability of enhanced voice-pitch cues via bimodal stimulation has also been associated with improved language development in young children. A recent report on language development of 26 children who received bilateral cochlear implants revealed significant advantages relating to mean length of utterance and use of pronouns in generative language samples for children who had some period of bimodal stimulation (Nittrouer & Chapman, 2009). Recent evidence from a longitudinal study on outcomes of children also indicated that experience with bimodal hearing was associated with better auditory comprehension and expressive communication skills as well as auditory functional performance for children who received cochlear implants (Ching, 2010a).

Furthermore, the use of acoustic with electrical stimulation via bimodal fitting in opposite ears has been shown to improve music perception in adults (McDermott, 2004, 2011). Listeners whose ability to recognize melodies with a cochlear implant alone was at chance level improved significantly when they used hearing aids alone, or hearing aids with cochlear implants. Adult listeners also reported improved sound quality and clarity and enhanced functional performance in real life when they used bimodal fitting, compared to unilateral implantation (Berrettini, Passetti, Giannarelli, & Forli, 2009; Ching et al., 2004a; Fitzpatrick et al., 2010; Potts, Skinner, Litovsky, Strube, & Kuk, 2009). The listeners also indicated strong preferences for bimodal fitting across a range of real-world environments, including listening to music, and listening to speech in noisy and reverberant situations.

Although there are no published data on children's music perception with bimodal stimulation, there are parent reports solicited using structured interviews that indicate a significant improvement in children's functional performance in real life, including awareness of environmental sounds, music perception, and listening in noisy situations (Ching, Psarros, Hill, Dillon, & Incerti, 2001).

These data support the provision of bimodal fitting over the use of a cochlear implant alone as the standard care for children and adults. Recent evidence linking the amount of residual hearing with bimodal benefits suggest that even though greater benefits may be associated with more residual hearing (e.g., Seeber et al., 2004), major benefits are obtainable even when acoustic amplification is restricted to very low frequencies (Ching, 2005; Cullington & Zeng, 2010; Mok, Gavin, Dowell & McKay, 2010; Zhang et al., 2010).

An important aspect of bimodal fitting is the need to fine-tune a hearing aid with a cochlear implant to maximize performance (Blamey, Dooley, James, & Parisi, 2000; Ching, 2005; Ching et al., 2007; Huart & Sammeth, 2008). The studies are in agreement that the loudness of sounds heard simultaneously through each device should be similar. Although the relationship between the input signal level and the loudness perceived by the device user differs between devices (McDermott & Varsavsky, 2009), balancing of loudness between ears, albeit imperfect, results in improved performance. For this reason, it is recommended that bimodal fittings be optimized using a procedure that has been validated, such as that described in Ching et al. (2004b).

To summarize, the research evidence indicates that there is:

1. Significantly better speech perception with bimodal stimulation than with unilateral cochlear implantation for children and adults, which is attributable to the effects of head shadow, redundancy, and complementarity,
2. A larger effect size for improved speech understanding with bimodal stimulation occurs in noise than in quiet.
3. Significant improvement in horizontal localization in the bimodal condition for children and adults, relative to unilateral cochlear implants.
4. Significant improvement in music perception in the bimodal condition for adults.
5. Overall significant improvement in functional performance in real life with bimodal stimulation, relative to unilateral cochlear implants.
6. Maximum benefit with bimodal stimulation is obtainable if hearing aid settings are optimized for use with cochlear implants using a validated procedure.
7. Better language development and speech production in young children with cochlear implants who have previous experience with bimodal hearing.

Recommendation: Fit an acoustic hearing aid to the nonimplanted ear when there is residual hearing usable with acoustic amplification in that ear.

The hearing aid should be fine-tuned with the cochlear implant using a systematic approach to balance loudness between ears. Evaluation of performance with bimodal stimulation should form part of standard clinical management.

Bilateral Cochlear Implantation

The research comparing unilateral with bilateral cochlear implants is summarized in Table 9–3 for children and Table 9–4 for adults.

Findings on localization for children are mixed, with measured advantages in relatively nonchallenging situations (Galvin, Mok, Dowell, & Briggs, 2008; Litovsky, Johnstone, & Godar, 2006a; Steffens et al., 2008) but much variability in more challenging conditions (Galvin, Mok, & Dowell, 2007; Litovsky et al., 2004). Studies on children with bilateral implants revealed that about one-third to one-half of the children tested were not able to localize sounds significantly above chance (Grieco-Calub & Litovsky, 2010; Van Deun et al., 2010). Nonetheless, there is some evidence to indicate that some children developed spatial hearing abilities over time (Litovsky et al., 2006a; Grieco-Calub & Litovsky, 2010). Better performance was associated with implantation before 2 years of age, and use of a hearing aid prior to implantation for 18 months or more (Van Deun et al., 2010).

Findings on localization ability of adults with bilateral cochlear implants are also mixed, with some reports showing advantages in conditions that involved arrays of more than eight loudspeakers (Nopp, Schleich, & D'Haese, 2004; Seeber et al., 2004; Van Hoesel & Tyler, 2003) whereas other studies reporting no significant difference between monaural and binaural conditions (Litovsky et al., 2004; Seeber et al., 2004). There is some evidence to suggest that users of bilateral cochlear implants who were younger than 60 years of age obtained greater benefits than those who were older (Noble, Tyler, Dunn, & Bhullar, 2009).

Speech perception improvements due to binaural effects of head shadow and redundancy have been reported for children (see Table 9–3) and adults (see Table 9–4). The evidence on binaural advantages for speech perception in quiet is mixed, with some showing a significant difference between binaural and monaural conditions for children (e.g., Gordon & Papsin, 2009; Kuhn-Inacker, Shehata-Dieler, Muller, & Helms, 2004) whereas others did not find a significant effect (Peters, Litovsky, Parkinson, & Lake, 2007). In a similar vein, benefits were reported in some studies on adults (e.g., Schön, Müller, & Helms, 2002) but not in others (e.g. Senn, Kompis, Vischer, & Hausler, 2005; Stark et al., 2002).

Many studies on adults with bilateral implants have also shown improved speech perception in noise with bilateral implants compared to unilateral implants, especially when the sound sources are spatially separated (for reviews, see Dorman, Yost, Wilson, & Gifford, 2011; Murphy & O'Donoghue, 2007; Sammeth, Bundy, & Miller, 2011). These benefits were largely due to the effect of head shadow. A few studies have also shown limited benefit in some adults from binaural redundancy (e.g., Ramsden et al., 2005; Schleich, Nopp, & D'Haese, 2004) and binaural squelch (e.g., Eapen, Buss, Adunka, Pillsbury, & Buchman, 2009; Müller, Schön, & Helms, 2002). There does not appear to be a difference between those who received their implants simultaneously or sequentially. When speech and noise are collocated in front of the subject during testing, findings on effects of binaural redundancy and squelch are mixed (see Tables 9–3 and 9–4).

Table 9–3. Evidence of Bilateral Cochlear Implantation Compared with Unilateral Cochlear Implantation in Children*

Evidence	*Source*	*Level*	*Grade*	*EFficacy/ EffectiVeness*
No benefit in sound localization for children measured at 3 and 9 months after bilateral implantation.	Litovsky et al, 2004	3	B	EF
Sound localization in children was better with two implants than with one, for children who have more than 13 months' experience with bilateral experience.	Litovsky et al, 2006a, 2006b	3	B	EF
Sound localization of children measured at 2 years after implantation was better with two implants than with one.	Senn et al, 2005	3	B	EF
Mean lateralization ability (left vs. right) with two implants was significantly better than with either the first or the second implant.	Steffens et al., 2008	3	B	EF
Between-group comparisons indicated that the bilateral implant group localized sounds better (3 loudspeaker array) than the unilateral implant group.	Lovett et al., 2010	3	B	EF
Sound localization was better in the bilateral than in the unilateral listening condition for 11 of 21 children tested. The remaining children did not show a difference between conditions.	Grieco-Calub & Litovsky, 2010	3	B	EF
Testing with bilateral mode only, about 63% of 30 children with sequential bilateral cochlear implants localized significantly better than chance.	Van Deun et al., 2010	3	B	EF
Speech scores in quiet did not differ between unilateral and bilateral implant conditions.	Peters et al., 2007	3	B	EF
Speech scores in noise were significantly better with bilateral implants showing effects of head shadow and redundancy.	Peters et al., 2007	3	B	EF
Speech perception in quiet and in noise was significantly better with bilateral implants than with unilateral implants.	Gordon & Papsin, 2009	3	B	EF

continues

Table 9–3. *continued*

Evidence	*Source*	*Level*	*Grade*	*EFficacy/ EffectiVeness*
Between-group comparisons, with the bilateral group demonstrating benefits from head shadow. Performance was poorer than normal hearing children.	Lovett et al., 2010	3	B	EF
Spatial hearing and communication of children in the bilateral implant condition were rated to be better by parents, compared to the children's performance prior to receiving their second implants.	Galvin et al., 2007	3	B	EV
Between-group comparisons, showing better spatial hearing and communication as rated by parents of children with bilateral implants, compared to ratings of parents of children with unilateral implants.	Lovett et al., 2010	3	B	EV
Between group comparisons, showing no significant difference in quality of life between the bilateral implant group and the unilateral implant group.	Lovett et al., 2010	3	B	EV
Parents' rating of spatial hearing and communication of children with bilateral implants was correlated with localization performance of children.	Van Deun et al., 2010	3	B	EF/EV
Children with bilateral cochlear implants who had bimodal listening experience developed better language than those who did not have bimodal experience.	Nittrouer & Chapman, 2009	3	B	EF/EV
Children with bilateral cochlear implants who had bimodal experience obtained greater speech perception and localization benefits than those who did not have bimodal experience.	Van Deun et al., 2010	3	B	EF

*The quality of evidence is rated on a scale from 1 (high-quality studies) to 6 (expert opinion) (see Table 1–5). The grade of recommendation is rated on a scale from A (level 1 or 2 studies with consistent conclusions) to D (level 6 evidence or inconclusive studies) (see Table 1–6). The evidence is also categorized according to whether assessments were carried out under laboratory/ ideal conditions (Efficacy, EF) or in the real world (Effectiveness, EV). As performance with each of the two implants differs (e.g. Wolfe et al., 2007), an advantage is defined by comparing the binaural scores to the better monaural score. Evidence is drawn from within-group comparisons, unless otherwise stated.

Table 9–4. Evidence of Bilateral Cochlear Implantation Compared with Unilateral Cochlear Implantation in Adults*

Evidence	*Source*	*Level*	*Grade*	*EFficacy/ EffectiVeness*
Adults localized sounds better with two implants than with one in controlled laboratory conditions.	Grantham et al, 2007; Van Hoesel and Tyler, 2003; Schön et al, 2002; Neumann et al., 2007	4/3	B/C	EF
Lateralization ability (left vs. right) improved with bilateral implantation at 3 months postimplantation.	Litovsky et al., 2009	4	B	EF
Mean localization ability was better with bilateral implants than with unilateral implants.	Mosnier et al., 2009	3	B	EF
Between-group comparisons showed better speech perception in quiet for the group with bilateral implants compared to the group with unilateral implants.	Dunn et al., 2008	3	B	EF
Speech perception in quiet was better with bilateral implants than with unilateral implants, showing effects of redundancy.	Dunn et al., 2008	3	B	EF
No significant difference in speech perception in quiet or in noise between the bilateral implant condition and the better unilateral implant condition for the same listeners.	Zeitler et al., 2008	3	B	EF
Speech perception in noise showing significant head shadow and redundancy effects in adults with simultaneous bilateral implants 6 months after implantation.	Litovsky et al., 2006a	3	B	EF
Speech perception in noise was better with bilateral implants than with unilateral implants, showing effects of head shadow and redundancy.	Litovsky et al., 2009; Ramsden et al., 2005; Schleich et al., 2004	3	B	EF
Self-rated communication was better with bilateral implants than with unilateral implants.	Litovsky et al., 2006	3	B	EV

continues

Table 9–4. *continued*

Evidence	*Source*	*Level*	*Grade*	*EFficacy/ EffectiVeness*
Between-group comparisons did not reveal significant differences in self-rated spatial hearing and communication between the bilateral implant group and the unilateral implant group.	Laske et al., 2009	3	B	EV

*The quality of evidence is rated on a scale from 1 (high-quality studies) to 6 (expert opinion) (see Table 1–5). The grade of recommendation is rated on a scale from A (level 1 or 2 studies with consistent conclusions) to D (level 6 evidence or inconclusive studies) (see Table 1–6). The evidence is also categorized according to whether assessments were carried out under laboratory/ ideal conditions (Efficacy, EF) or in the real world (Effectiveness, EV). As performance with each of the two implants differs (e.g., Wolfe et al., 2007), an advantage is defined by comparing the binaural scores to the better monaural score. Evidence is drawn from within-group comparisons, unless otherwise stated.

In children who received two implants sequentially, there is research to suggest that the age at which the second implant was received and the time lag between two implants affected performance of children. Significant differences in speech perception in quiet, for instance, were found between the first and the second implant in a group of children who received their second implant at an age older than 4 years, but the same was not found in a second group who received both implants before 4 years of age (Wolfe et al., 2007). There is also some evidence to suggest that greater speech perception advantages were obtained when the time lag between the first and second implants was within 2 years (Gordon & Papsin, 2009).

Furthermore, parents of children who received two cochlear implants sequentially have reported improvements in spatial hearing and communication in real life (Galvin et al., 2007). Although bilateral implants may be expected to improve quality of life if they were more successful than unilateral implants in alleviating activity limitations and participation restrictions related to communication, this is not borne out by research that compared quality of life estimates for children with bilateral implants and those with unilateral implants (Lovett, Kitterick, Hewitt, & Summerfield, 2010).

Indeed, the National Institute for Health and Clinical Excellence in the United Kingdom conducted a systematic review on the clinical and cost-effectiveness of unilateral and bilateral cochlear implantation in children in 2007 (Bond et al., 2007) and reported neutral findings. This review was updated in 2010 (Sparreboom et al., 2010) with the conclusion that "no robust conclusions could be drawn about the clinical effectiveness of bilateral cochlear implants (for children) from the present body of evidence" (p. 1069).

Recommendation: The evidence is insufficient to recommend for or against bilateral cochlear implantation for children and adults.

BIMODAL FITTING OR BILATERAL COCHLEAR IMPLANTATION?

The research summarized in the previous sections support the provision of hearing in both ears. In people with unilateral cochlear implants who have residual hearing in one ear, the question of whether bimodal fitting or bilateral implantation provides greater benefits needs to be addressed. The published evidence that compares these two modes of stimulation in children is summarized in Table 9–5, and findings in adults are shown in Table 9–6.

Three approaches have been used in comparison studies. The first draws on meta-analysis methods to examine results from peer-reviewed publications relating to performance of users of bimodal fitting or bilateral cochlear implantation. One review concluded from an analysis of publications related to speech recognition in noise at fixed signal-to-noise ratios (SNRs) that there was no significant difference between the two modes of stimulation (Schafer, Amlani, Seibold, & Shattuck, 2007). Three recent reviews of the literature on bimodal and bilateral stimulation literature concluded that there was insufficient evidence to guide decisions on which of the two stimulation modes was better (Ching et al., 2007; Sammeth et al., 2011; Sparrelboom et al., 2010).

The second approach compares performance of a group of users of bimodal fitting with a group of users of bilateral implants. The evidence reveals no significant difference in mean localization ability (Litovsky et al, 2006a) or in speech unmasking in noise (Mok, Galvin, Dowell, & McKay, 2007) between groups of children who used different stimulation modes. The findings in these studies are limited by the extent to which the comparison groups were matched. For children with bilateral cochlear implants, there is some evidence to suggest that those who had bimodal listening experience prior to receiving a second cochlear implant developed better generative language (Nittrouer & Chapman, 2009). For adults, a recent study compared self-perceived handicaps in groups who had unilateral cochlear implants, or bimodal fitting or bilateral cochlear implants. The findings

Table 9–5. Evidence of Comparisons Between Bilateral Cochlear Implantation and Bimodal Fitting in Children*

Evidence	*Source*	*Level*	*Grade*	*EFficacy/ EffectiVeness*
Between-group comparisons revealed no significant difference in sound localization.	Litovsky et al., 2006a	3	B	EF
Between-group comparisons revealed no significant difference in speech perception in noise between children with bimodal fitting and children with bilateral implants.	Litovsky et al., 2006a; Schafer & Thibodeau, 2006	3	B	EF
Between-group comparisons revealed that children with bilateral implants demonstrated greater head shadow effect than those with bimodal fitting.	Mok et al., 2007	3	B	EF

*The quality of evidence is rated on a scale from 1 (high-quality studies) to 6 (expert opinion) (see Table 1–5). The grade of recommendation is rated on a scale from A (level 1 or 2 studies with consistent conclusions) to D (level 6 evidence or inconclusive studies) (see Table 1–6). The evidence is also categorized according to whether assessments were carried out under laboratory/ ideal conditions (Efficacy, EF) or in the real world (Effectiveness, EV).

Table 9–6. Evidence of Comparisons Between Bilateral Cochlear Implantation and Bimodal Fitting in Adults*

Evidence	*Source*	*Level*	*Grade*	*EFficacious/ EffectiVeness*
Meta-analysis approach: No significant difference between bimodal and bilateral groups for speech perception.	Schafer et al., 2007	3	B	EF
Between-group comparison: Self-perceived handicap scores were highest (poorest) for bimodal users, lower for unilateral cochlear implant users, and lowest (best) for bilateral cochlear implant users.	Noble et al., 2008	3	B	EV
Between-group comparison: Speech perception benefits and localization benefits for the bimodal group and the bilateral cochlear implant group. In the latter group, younger cohort showed more substantial benefits whereas the older cohort had mixed outcomes.	Noble et al., 2009 (cohorts overlap with those in Noble et al., 2008)	3	B	EF
Between-group comparison: Bimodal fitting group had higher scores for music perception, talker identification, affective prosody discrimination, and speech recognition than the bilateral implant group.	Cullington & Zeng, 2011	3	B	EF
Cross-over comparison: Voice pitch information was more effectively transmitted via bimodal fitting than bilateral implants for consonant perception.	Ching et al., 2007	3	B	EF

*The quality of evidence is rated on a scale from 1 (high-quality studies) to 6 (expert opinion) (see Table 1–5). The grade of recommendation is rated on a scale from A (level 1 or 2 studies with consistent conclusions) to D (level 6 evidence or inconclusive studies) (see Table 1–6). The evidence is also categorized according to whether assessments were carried out under laboratory/ ideal conditions (Efficacy, EF) or in the real world (Effectiveness, EV).

indicated that the bimodal group had the poorest self-rated handicap scores, including emotional distress and social restriction, whereas the bilateral cochlear implant group had the best scores (Noble, Tyler, Dunn, & Bhullar, 2008). The authors identified a potential sample bias in the comparison, and noted that the listeners with bimodal fitting were the ones who performed poorly with cochlear implants alone. As a pronounced benefit of bimodal fitting relates to enhanced transmission of pitch information, a recent study (Cullington

& Zeng, 2011) compared pitch perception in a group of adults who used bimodal fitting with a second group who used bilateral implants, matched in terms of speech scores in quiet conditions. The listeners were evaluated using four pitch-related tasks, including music perception, talker identification, affective prosody discrimination, and speech recognition with competing male, female, or child talkers. The mean scores for users of bimodal fitting were on average higher than those for users of bilateral implants on all tasks, but the difference was not statistically significant. The results in these studies are inconclusive with neither configuration proving to be better than the other.

A third approach to addressing the question of whether a listener with a unilateral cochlear implant would benefit more from a contralateral hearing aid or a second cochlear implant is to use a cross-over design whereby listeners start with bimodal stimulation that has been optimized. Evaluations of performance can be carried out after a period of familiarization. The same listeners then receive a second implant, and their performance can be evaluated after they have experience with the bilateral implant condition. This approach was adopted in a pilot study of two adult listeners (Ching et al., 2007). It took 12 months of experience with bilateral implants for the two listeners to achieve the same level of performance attained when they were using bimodal fitting in speech perception tests. Furthermore, tests of nonsense syllables revealed that voice-pitch information was more effectively transmitted in the bimodal than in the bilateral cochlear implant condition. One participant localized sounds better with bilateral cochlear implants than with bimodal fitting, but the other did not. Further research is necessary to identify factors that influence the relative success of bimodal fitting and bilateral cochlear implants for adults and children.

Currently, there is insufficient evidence to answer the question of whether bimodal fitting or bilateral implantation is more beneficial for people who have residual hearing in one ear that can be aided with acoustic amplification. It is recommended that bimodal fitting should be standard care (Ching, 2005; 2011; Offeciers et al., 2005; Olson & Shinn, 2008; Schafer et al., 2007; Tange, Grolman, & Dreschler, 2009), that hearing aids should be optimized using a validated procedure (Ching et al., 2001; Ching et al., 2004b; Huart & Sammeth, 2008), and that effectiveness of bimodal fitting should be evaluated after familiarization. For young children, evaluations can be carried out using a combination of systematic parental observations (e.g., Ching & Hill, 2007; Zimmerman-Phillips, Osberger, & Robbins, 1998) and electrophysiologic tests (e.g., Golding et al., 2007; Sharma, 2011). For older children and adults, a combination of assessments in real life and in clinical settings would assist with establishing the effectiveness and efficacy of the devices.

Recommendation: The evidence is insufficient to recommend bilateral implantation over bimodal fitting for people who have a cochlear implant in one ear and residual hearing that is usable with acoustic amplification in the other ear.

SUMMARY AND DISCUSSION

Binaural hearing is clearly superior to monaural hearing, with measured benefits typically relating to localization of sound sources and speech intelligibility in noisy backgrounds in controlled settings, and improvements in functional performance in real-life situations. Because bimodal stimulation is superior to bilateral implantation in transmission of pitch information, there is added benefit of bimodal experience for language development, speech acquisition, and music perception. There appears to be a link between experience with bimodal stimulation prior to bilateral implantation (e.g., Van Deun et al., 2010) and better performance postimplantation. There is clear evidence to support the provision of binaural hearing as standard care for people who have severe to profound hearing impairment in both ears, whenever it can be provided without significant risks. For people who have residual hearing that can be aided with hearing aids, bimodal stimulation should be the treatment of choice, with systematic procedures for fine-tuning and evaluation in place to optimize performance. Bilateral implantation is the treatment of choice for people who have profound hearing loss in both ears.

REFERENCES

Armstrong, M., Pegg, P., James, C., & Blamey, P. (1997). Speech perception in noise with implant and hearing aid. *American Journal of Otology, 18*, S140–141.

Beijen, J. W., Mylanus, E. A., Leeuw, A. R., & Snik, A. F. (2008). Should a hearing aid in the contralateral ear be recommended for children with a unilateral cochlear implant? *Annals of Otology, Rhinology, and Laryngology, 117*(6), 397–403.

Berrettini, S., Passetti, S., Giannarelli, M., & Forli, F. (2010). Benefit from bimodal hearing in a group of prelingually deafened adult cochlear implant users. *American Journal of Otolaryngology, 31*(5), 332–338.

Blamey, P. J., Dooley, G. J., James, C. J., & Parisi, E. S. (2000). Monaural and binaural loudness measures in cochlear implant users with contralateral residual hearing. *Ear and Hearing, 21*(1), 6–17.

Blauert, J. (1997). *Spatial hearing.* Cambridge, MA: MIT Press.

Bond, M., Mealing, S., Anderson, R., Elston, J. Weiner, G., Taylor, R. S., . . . Stein, K. (2007). *The effectiveness and cost-effectiveness of cochlear implants for severe to profound deafness in children and adults: a systematic review and economic model.* Retrieved from http://www.nice.org.uk/nicemedia/pdf/ACDCochlearImplantsFinalReport.pdf

Bronkhorst, A. (2000). The cocktail party phenomenon: A review of research on speech intelligibility in multiple-talker conditions. *Acta Acustica, 86*, 117–128.

Ching, T. Y. C. (2005). The evidence calls for making binaural-bimodal fittings routine. *Hearing Journal, 58*(11), 32–41.

Ching, T. Y. C. (2010a). Longitudinal outcomes of hearing-impaired children. Keynote address. Phonak Paediatric Amplification Conference, April 23–24, 2010, Stuttgart.

Ching, T. Y. C. (2010b). Binaural hearing with hearing aids and/or cochlear implants in children. *ENT and Audiology News, 18*(6), 88–90.

Ching, T. Y. C. (2011). Acoustic cues for consonant perception with combined acoustic and electric hearing in children. *Seminars in Hearing, 32*(1): 32–41.

Ching, T. Y. C., & Hill, M. (2007). The Parents' Evaluation of Aural/oral performance of Children (PEACH) scale: normative data. *Journal of the American Academy of Audiology, 18*(3), 220–235.

Ching, T. Y. C., Incerti, P. V., & Hill, M. (2004a). Binaural benefits for adults who use hearing aids and cochlear implants in opposite ears. *Ear and Hearing, 25*, 9–21.

Ching, T. Y. C., Incerti, P., Hill, M., & Brew, J. (2004c). Fitting and evaluating a hearing aid for recipients of unilateral cochlear implants: The NAL approach. Part 2. Bimodal hearing should be standard for most cochlear implant users. *Hearing Review, 11*(8), 32, 36–40, 63.

Ching, T. Y. C., Incerti, P., Hill, M., & van Wanrooy, E. (2006) An overview of binaural advantages for children and adults who use binaural/bimodal hearing devices. *Audiology and Neurotology, 11*(Suppl. 1), 6–11.

Ching, T. Y. C., Psarros, C. & Hill, M. (2000) Hearing aid benefit for children who switched from the SPEAK to the ACE Strategy in their contralateral Nucleus 24 Cochlear Implant System. *Australian and New Zealand Journal of Audiology, 22*(2), 123–132.

Ching, T. Y. C., Psarros, C., Hill, M., & Dillon, H. (2004b). Fitting and evaluating a hearing aid for recipients of a unilateral cochlear implant: The NAL approach. Part1. *Hearing Review, 11*(7), 14–22, 58.

Ching, T. Y. C., Psarros, C., Hill, M., Dillon, H., & Incerti, P. (2001). Should children who use cochlear implants wear hearing aids in the opposite ear? *Ear and Hearing, 22*(5), 365–380.

Ching, T. Y. C., van Wanrooy, E., & Dillon, H. (2007). Binaural-bimodal fitting or bilateral implantation for managing severe to profound deafness: A review. *Trends in Amplification, 11*(3), 161–192.

Ching, T. Y. C., van Wanrooy, E., Hill, M., & Dillon, H. (2005). Binaural redundancy and interaural time difference cues for patients wearing a cochlear implant and a hearing aids in opposite ears. *International Journal of Audiology, 25*, 9–21.

Culling, J. F., Hawley, M. L., & Litovsky, R.Y. (2004). The role of head-induced interaural time and level differences in the speech reception threshold for multiple interfering sound sources. *Journal of the Acoustical Society of America, 116*, 1057–1065.

Cullington, H. E., & Zeng, F-G. (2010). Bimodal hearing benefit for speech recognition with competing voice in cochlear implant subject with normal hearing in contralateral ear. *Ear and Hearing, 31*(1), 70–73.

Cullington, H. E., & Zeng, F-G. (2011). Comparison of bimodal and bilateral cochlear implant users on speech recognition with competing talker, music perception, affective prosody discrimination, and talker identification. *Ear and Hearing, 32*(1), 16–30.

Dettman, S. J., D'Costa, W. A., Dowell, R. C., Winton, E. J., Hill, K. L., & Williams, S. S. (2004). Cochlear implants for children with significant residual hearing. *Archives of Otolaryngology—Head and Neck Surgery, 130*, 612–618.

Dillon, H. (2001). *Hearing aids* (pp. 370–388). Turramurrra, Australia: Boomerang Press.

Dorman, M. F., Gifford, R. H., Spahr, A. J., & McKarns, S. A. (2008). The benefits of combining acoustic and electric stimulation for the recognition of speech, voice and melodies. *Audiology and Neurotology, 13*(2), 105–112.

Dorman, M. F., Yost, W. A., Wilson, B. S., & Gifford, R. H. (2011). Speech perception and sound localization by adults with bilateral cochlear implants. *Seminars in Hearing, 32*, 73–89.

Dunn, C., Perreau, A., Gantz, B., & Tyler, R. S. (2010). Benefits of localisation and speech perception with multiple noise sources in listeners with a short-electrode cochlear implant. *Journal of the American Academy of Audiology, 21*(1), 44–51.

Dunn, C., Tyler, R., Oakley, S., Gantz, B. J., & Noble, W. (2008). Comparison of speech recognition and localization performance in bilateral and unilateral cochlear implant users matched on duration of deafness and age at implantation. *Ear and Hearing, 29*(3), 352–359.

Dunn, C. C., Tyler, R. S., & Witt, S. A. (2005). Benefit of wearing a hearing aid on the unimplanted ear in adults users of a cochlear implant. *Journal of Speech, Language, and Hearing Research, 48*, 668–680.

Durlach, N. I., & Colburn, H. S. (1978). Binaural phenomenon. In E. C. Carterette & M. P. Friedman (Eds.), *Handbook of perception* (pp. 365–466). New York, NY: Academic Press.

Eapen, R. J., Buss, E., Adunka, M. C., Pillsbury, H. C. III, & Buchman, C. A. (2009). Hearing-in-noise benefits after bilateral simultaneous cochlear implantation continue to improve 4 years after implantation. *Otology and Neurotology, 30*(2), 153–159.

El Fata, F., James, C. J., Laborde, M. L., & Fraysse, B. (2009). How much residual hearing is "useful" for music perception with cochlear implants? *Audiology and Neurotology, 14*(Suppl. 1), 14–21.

Faulkner, A., & Rosen, S. (1999). Contributions of temporal encodings of voicing, voicelessness, fundamental frequency, and amplitude variation to audio-visual and auditory speech perception. *Journal of the Acoustical Society of America, 106*, 2063–2073.

Fitzpatrick, E. M., Fournier, P., Seguin, C., Armstrong, S., Chenier, J., & Schramm, D. (2010). Users' perspectives on the benefits of FM systems with cochlear implants. *International Journal of Audiology, 49*(1), 44–53.

Galvin, K. L., Hughes, K. C., & Mok, M. (2010). Can adolescents and young adults with prelingual hearing loss benefit from a second, sequential cochlear implant? *International Journal of Audiology, 49*(5), 368–377.

Galvin, K. L., Mok M., & Dowell, R. C. (2007). Perceptual benefit and functional outcomes for children using sequential bilateral cochlear implants. *Ear and Hearing, 28*(4), 470–482.

Galvin, K. L., Mok, M., Dowell, R. C., & Briggs, R. J. (2008). Speech detection and localization results and clinical outcomes for children receiving sequential cochlear implants before four years of age. *International Journal of Audiology*, 47(10), 636–646.

Gfeller, K., Olszewski, C., Turner, C., Gantz, B., & Olson, J. (2006). Music perception with cochlear implants and residual rearing. *Audiology and Neurotology, 11*(Suppl. 1), 12–15.

Gfeller, K., Turner, C., Oleson, J., Zhang, X., Gantz, B., Fromman, R., & Olszewski, C. (2007). Accuracy of cochlear implant recipients on pitch perception, melody recognition, and speech recognition in noise. *Ear and Hearing, 28*, 412–423.

Gifford, R. H. D., Dorman, M. F., McKarns, S. A., & Spahr, A. J. (2007). Combined electric and contralateral acoustic hearing: Word and sentence recognition with bimodal hearing. *Journal of Speech, Language, and Hearing Research, 50*(4), 835–843.

Golding, M., Pearce, W., Seymour, J., Cooper, A., Ching, T., & Dillon, H. (2007). The relationship between obligatory cortical auditory evoked potentials (CAEPs) and functional measures in young infants. *Journal of the American Academy of Audiology, 18*, 117–125.

Gordon, K., & Papsin, B. (2009). Benefits of short interimplant delays in children receiving bilateral cochlear implants. *Otology and Neurotology, 30*, 319–331.

Grantham, D. A., Ricketts, T. A., Labadie, R. F., Haynes, D. S. (2007). Horizontal-plane localization of noise and speech signals by postlingually deafened adults fitted with bilateral cochlear implants. *Ear and Hearing, 28*(4): 524–541.

Grieco-Calub, T. M., & Litovsky, R. Y. (2010). Sound localization skills in children who use bilateral cochlear implants and in children with normal acoustic hearing. *Ear and Hearing, 31*(5), 645–656.

Hamzavi, J., Pok, S., Gstoettner, W., & Baumgartner, W. (2004). Speech perception with a cochlear implant used in conjunction with a hearing aid in the opposite ear. *International Journal of Audiology, 43*, 61–65.

Harris, M. S., & Hay-McCutcheon, M. (2010). An analysis of hearing aid fittings in adults using cochlear implants and contralateral hearing aids. *Laryngoscope, 120*(12): 2484–2488.

Holt, R. F., Kirk, K. I., Eisenberg, L. S., Martinez, A. S., & Campbell, W. (2005). Spoken word recognition development in children with residual hearing using cochlear implants and hearing aids in opposite ears. *Ear and Hearing, 26*, 82–91.

Huart, S. A., & Sammeth, C. A. (2008). Hearing aids plus cochlear implants: Optimizing the bimodal pediatric fitting. *Hearing Journal, 61*(11), 56–58.

Incerti, P. V., Ching, T. Y. C., & Hill, M. (2011). Consonant perception by adults with bimodal fittings. *Seminars in Hearing, 32*(1), 90–102.

Iwaki, T., Matsushiro, N., Mah, S., Sato, T., Yasuoka, E., Yamamoto, K., & Kubo, T. (2004). Comparison of speech perception between monaural and binaural hearing in cochlear implant patients. *Acta Oto-laryngologica, 124*, 358–362.

Kong, Y. Y., Stickney, G. S., & Zeng, F. G. (2005). Speech and melody recognition in binaurally combined acoustic and electric hearing. *Journal of the Acoustical Society of America, 117*(3), 1351–1361.

Kuhn-Inacker, H., Shehata-Dieler, W., Muller, J., & Helms, J. (2004). Bilateral cochlear implants: A way to optimize auditory perception abilities in deaf children. *International Journal of Pediatric Otorhinolaryngology, 68*, 1257–1266.

Laske, R., Veraguth, D., Dillier, N., Binkert, A., Holzmann, D., & Huber, A. M. (2009). Subjective and objective results after cochlear implantation in adults. *Otology and Neurotology, 30*, 313–318.

Lee, S. H., Lee, K. Y., Huh, M. J. H., & Jang, H. S. (2008). Effect of bimodal hearing in Korean children with profound hearing loss. *Acta Oto-laryngologica, 128*(11), 1227–1232.

Lenarz, T., Stöver, T., Buechner, A., Lesinski-Schiedat, A., Patrick, J., & Pesch, J. (2009). Hearing conservation surgery using the Hybrid-L electrode. *Audiology and Neurotology, 14*(Suppl. 1), 22–31.

Litovsky, R.Y., Johnstone, P. M., & Godar, S. P. (2006a) Benefits of bilateral cochlear implants and/or hearing aids in children. *International Journal of Audiology, 45*(Suppl. 1), S78–S91.

Litovsky, R.Y., Johnstone, P., Godar, S., Agrawal, S., Parkinson, A., Peters, R., & Lake, J. (2006b). Bilateral cochlear implants in children: Localization acuity measured with minimum audible angle. *Ear and Hearing, 27*(1), 43–59.

Litovsky, R.Y., Johnstone, P. M., Parkinson, P., Peters, R., & Godar, S. P. (2004). Bilateral cochlear implants and/or hearing aids in children. *International Congress Series, 1273*, 451–454.

Litovsky, R., Parkinson, A., & Arcaroli, J. (2009) Spatial hearing and speech intelligibility in bilateral cochlear implant users. *Ear and Hearing, 30*(4), 419–431.

Lovett, R. E., Kitterick, P. T., Hewitt, C. E., & Summerfield, A. Q. (2010). Bilateral or unilateral cochlear implantation for deaf children: An observational study. *Archives of Disease in Childhood, 95*, 107–112.

Luntz, M., Yehudai, N., & Shpak, T. (2007). Hearing progress and fluctuations in bimodal-binaural hearing users (unilateral cochlear implants and contralateral hearing aid). *Acta Oto-laryngologica, 127*(10), 1045–1050.

McDermott, H. (2004). Music perception with cochlear implants: A review. *Trends in Amplification, 8*(2), 49–82.

McDermott, H. (2011). Benefits of combined acoustic and electric hearing for music and pitch perception. *Seminars in Hearing, 32*(1), 103–114.

McDermott H., & Varsavsky, A. (2009). Better fitting of cochlear implants: modeling loudness for acoustic and electric stimuli. *Journal of Neural Engineering, 6*, 1–8.

Middlebrooks, J. C., & Green, D. M. (1991). Sound localization by human listeners. *Annual Review of Psychology, 42*, 135–159. doi: 10.1146/annurev.ps.42.020191.001031

Mok, M., Galvin, K. L., Dowell, R. C., & McKay, C. M. (2007). Spatial unmasking and binaural advantage for children with normal hearing, a cochlear implant and a hearing aid, and bilateral implants. *Audiology and Neurotology, 12*(5), 295–306.

Mok, M., Galvin, K. L., Dowell, R. C., & McKay, C. M. (2010). Speech perception benefit for children with a cochlear implant and a hearing aid in opposite ears and children with bilateral cochlear implants. *Audiology and Neurotology, 15*(1), 44–56.

Mok, M., Grayden, D., Dowell, R., & Lawrence, D. (2006). Speech perception for adults who use hearing aids in conjunction with cochlear implants in opposite ears. *Journal of Speech, Language, and Hearing Research, 49*, 338–351.

Moore, B. C. (2003). *An introduction to the psychology of hearing* (5th ed.) San Diego, CA: Elsevier Science.

Morera, C., Manrique, M., Ramos, L., Garcia-Ibanex, L., Cavalle, L., Huarte, A., & Estrada, E. (2005). Advantages of binaural hearing provided through bimodal stimulation via a cochlear implant and a conventional hearing aid: A 6-month comparative study. *Acta Oto-laryngologica, 125*, 596–606.

Mosnier, I., Sterkers, O., Bebear, J-P, Godeyg, B., Robierh, A., Deguinei, O., . . . Ferrary, E. (2009). Speech performance and sound localization in a complex noisy environment in bilaterally implanted adult patients. *Audiology and Neurotology, 14*, 106–114.

Müller, J., Schön, F., & Helms, J. (2002). Speech understanding in quiet and noise in bilateral users of the MED-EL Combi 40/40+ cochlear implant system. *Ear and Hearing, 23*, 198–206.

Murphy, J., & O'Donoghue, G. (2007). Bilateral cochlear implantation: An evidence-based medicine evaluation. *Laryngoscope, 117*(8), 1412–1418.

Neumann, A., Haravon, A., Sislian, N., & Waltzman, S. (2007) Sound-direction identification with bilateral cochlear implants. *Ear and Hearing, 28*(1), 73–82.

Nittrouer, S., & Chapman, C. (2009). The effects of bilateral electric and bimodal electric-acoustic stimulation on language development. *Trends in Amplification, 13*(3), 190–205.

Noble, W., Tyler, R., Dunn, C., & Bhullar, N. (2008) Hearing handicap ratings among different profiles of adult cochlear implant users. *Ear and Hearing, 29*(1), 112–120.

Noble, W., Tyler, R., Dunn, C., & Bhullar, N. (2009). Younger- and older-age adults with unilateral and bilateral cochlear implants: Speech and spatial hearing self-ratings and performance. *Otology and Neurotology, 30*(7), 921–929.

Nopp, P., Schleich, P., & D'Haese, P. (2004). Sound localization in bilateral users of MED-EL COMBI 40/40+ cochlear implants. *Ear and Hearing, 25*, 205–214.

Offeciers, E., Morera, C., Müller, J., Huarte, A., Shallop, J., & Cavallé, L. (2005). International consensus on bilateral cochlear implants and bimodal stimulation. *Acta Oto-laryngologia, 125*(9), 918–919.

Olson, A. D., & Shinn, J. B. (2008). A systematic review to determine the effectiveness of using amplification in conjunction with cochlear implantation. *Journal of the American Academy of Audiology, 19*(9), 657–671.

Peters, B. R., Litovsky, R., Parkinson, A., & Lake, J. (2007). Importance of age and postimplantation experience on speech perception measures in children with sequential bilateral cochlear implants. *Otology and Neurotology, 28*(5), 649–657.

Potts, L. G., Skinner, M. W., Litovsky, R. A., Strube, M. J., & Kuk, F. (2009). Recognition and localization of speech by adult cochlear implant recipients wearing a digital hearing aid in the nonimplanted ear (bimodal hearing). *Journal of the American Academy of Audiology, 20*(6), 353–373.

Ramsden, R., Greenham, P., O'Driscoll, M., Mawman, D., Proops, D., Craddock, L., . . . Pickerill, M.. (2005). Evaluation of bilaterally implanted adult subjects with the nucleus 24 cochlear implant system. *Otology and Neurotology, 26*, 988–998.

Sammeth, C. A., Bundy, S. M., & Miller, D. A. (2011). Bimodal hearing or bilateral cochlear implants: A review of the research literature. *Seminars in Hearing, 32*(1), 3–31.

Schafer, E., & Thibodeau, L. (2006). Speech recognition in noise in children with cochlear implants while listening in bilateral, bimodal, and FM-system arrangements. *American Journal of Audiology, 15*, 114–126.

Schafer, E. C., Amlani, A. M., Seibold, A., & Shattuck, P. L. (2007). A meta-analytic comparison of binaural benefits between bilateral cochlear implants and bimodal stimulation. *Journal of the American Academy of Audiology, 18*(9), 760–776.

Schafer, E. C., & Thibodeau, L. M. (2006). Speech recognition in noise in children with cochlear implants while listening in bilateral, bimodal, and FM-system arrangements. *American Journal of Audiology, 15*(2), 114–126.

Schleich, P., Nopp, P., & D'Haese, P. (2004). Head shadow, squelch and summation effects in bilateral users of the MED-EL Combi 40/40+ cochlear implant. *Ear and Hearing, 25*, 197–204.

Schön, F., Müller, J., & Helms, J. (2002). Speech reception thresholds obtained in a symmetrical four-loudspeaker arrangement from bilateral users of MED-EL cochlear implants. *Otology and Neurotology, 23*(5), 710–714.

Seeber, B. U., Baumann, U., & Fastl, H. (2004). Localization ability with bimodal hearing aids and bilateral cochlear implants. *Journal of the Acoustical Society of America, 116*(3), 1698–1709.

Senn, P., Kompis, M., Vischer, M., & Hausler R. (2005). Minimum audible angle, just noticeable interaural differences and speech intelligibility with bilateral cochlear implants using clinical speech processors. *Audiology and Neurotology, 10*, 342–352.

Sharma, A. (2011). Clinical management of children with cochlear implants. *International Journal of Audiology, 50*(2), 106.

Simpson, A., McDermott, H. J., Dowell, R.C., Sucher, C., & Briggs, R. J. S. (2009). Comparison of two frequency-to-electrode maps for acoustic-electric stimulation. *International Journal of Audiology, 8*(2), 63–73.

Sparreboom, M., van Schoonhoven, J., van Zanten, B. G. A., Scholten, R. J. P. M., Mylanus, E. A. M., Grolman, W., & Maat, B. (2010). The effectiveness of bilateral cochlear implants for severe-to-profound deafness in children: A systematic review. *Otology and Neurotology, 31*, 1062–1071.

Spitzer, S., Liss, J., Spahr, A., & Lansford, K. (2009). The use of fundamental frequency for lexical segmentation in listeners with cochlear implants. *Journal of the Acoustical Society of America, 125*(6), 236–241.

Stark, T., Müller, J.,Vischer, M. (2002). Multicenter study on bilateral cochlear implantation. In T. Kubo, Y. Takahashi, & T. Iwaki (Eds.), *Cochlear implants—An update* (pp. 523–526). The Hague, the Netherlands: Kugler Publications.

Steffens, T., Lesinski-Schiedat, A., Strutz, J., Aschendorff, A., Klenzner, T., Rühl, S., & Lenarz, T. (2008). The benefits of sequential bilateral cochlear implantation for hearing-impaired children. *Acta Oto-laryngologica, 128*(2), 164–176.

Stern, R. M., & Ttrahiotis, C. (1996). Models of binaural perception. In R. H. Gilkey, & T. R. Anderson (Eds.), *Binaural and spatial hearing* (pp. 499–531). Hillsdale, NJ: Earlbaum Associates.

Sucher, C. M., & McDermott, H. J. (2009). Bimodal stimulation: benefits for music perception and sound quality. *Cochlear Implants International, 10*(Suppl.), 96–99.

Tange, R. A., Grolman, W., & Dreschler, W. A. (2009). What to do with the other ear after cochlear implantation. *Cochlear Implants International, 10*(1), 19–24.

Tyler, R. S., Parkinson, A. J., Wilson, B. S., Writt, S., Preece, J. P., & Noble, W. (2002). Patients utilising a hearing aid and a cochlear implant: Speech perception and localisation. *Ear and Hearing, 23*(2), 98–105.

Ullauri, A., Crofts, H., Wilson, K., & Titley, S. (2007). Bimodal benefits of cochlear implant and hearing aid (on the non-implanted ear): A pilot study to develop a protocol and a test battery. *Cochlear Implants International, 8*(1), 29–37.

Van Deun, L., van Wieringen, A., Scherf, F., Deggouj, N., Desloovere, C., Offeciers, E., & Wouters, J. (2010). Earlier intervention leads to better sound localization in children with bilateral cochlear implants. *Audiology and Neurotology, 15*, 7–17.

Van Hoesel, R. J., &. Tyler, R. S. (2003). Speech perception, localization, and lateralization with bilateral cochlear implants. *Journal of the Acoustical Society of America, 113*(3), 1617–1630.

Wolfe, J., Baker, S., Caraway, T., Kasulis, H., Mears, A., Smith, J., & Wood, M. (2007). 1-year postactivation results for sequentially implanted bilateral cochlear implant users. *Otology and Neurotology, 28*(5), 589–596.

Yuen, K. C. P., Cao, K. L., Wei, C. G., Luan, L., Li, H., & Zhang, Z. Y. (2009). Lexical tone and word recognition in noise of Mandarin-speaking children who use cochlear implants and hearing aids in opposite ears. *Cochlear Implants International, 10*(Suppl. 1), 120–129.

Zeitler, D. M., Kessler, M. A., Terushkin, V., Roland, J. T., Svirsky, M. A., Lalwani, A. K., & Waltzman, S. B. (2008). Speech perception benefits of sequential bilateral cochlear implantation in children and adults: A retrospective analysis. *Otology and Neurotology, 29*(3), 314–325.

Zhang, T., Dorman, M. F., & Spahr, A. J. (2010). Information from the voice fundamental frequency (F0) region accounts for the majority of the benefit when acoustic stimulation is added to electric stimulation. *Ear and Hearing, 31*(1), 63–69.

Zhang, T., Spahr, A. J., & Dorman, M. F. (2010). Frequency overlap between electric and acoustic stimulation and speech-perception benefit in patients with combined electric and acoustic stimulation. *Ear and Hearing, 31*(2), 195–201.

Zimmerman-Phillips, S., Osberger, M.J., & Robbins, A.M. (1998). Infant-Toddler: Meaningful Auditory Integration Scale (IT-MAIS). In W. Estabrooks (Ed.), *Cochlear implants for kids.* Washington, DC: AG Bell Association for the Deaf.

Zue, V. (1985). The use of speech knowledge in automatic speech recognition. *Proceedings of the Institute of Electrical and Electronic Engineering, 73*, 1602–1615.

PART IV

Other Audiological Interventions

CHAPTER 10

Evidence About the Effectiveness of Aural Rehabilitation Programs for Adults

Theresa Chisolm and Michelle Arnold

INTRODUCTION

When an adult acquires a hearing loss, the primary impact is on the ability to understand speech, particularly in noisy environments. Difficulty in speech understanding can limit meaningful spoken language communication and decrease social connectivity. Ultimately, untreated hearing loss in adults is associated with negative effects on work productivity, access to information sources, cognitive and emotional status and health-related quality of life (HRQoL) (e.g., Dalton, Cruickshanks, Klein, Klein, Wiley, & Nondahl, 2003; Mulrow et al., 1990). According to the World Health Organization (2006), hearing loss ranks third after depression and other unintentional injuries as the leading cause of years lived with disability in adults.

Sensory management, the cornerstone of treatment for adult-onset hearing loss, is aimed at optimizing auditory function through the use of hearing aids, cochlear implants, and/or a variety of hearing-assistive technologies (Boothroyd, 2007). Although there is good evidence that sensory management through device use generally results in significant improvements in the activity of speech understanding (see, for example, Chapters 4 and 7), hearing aids, cochlear implants and hearing-assistive technologies (HATs) do not fully restore a person to his or her preloss state. As sensory management alone cannot fully restore an individual to prehearing loss function there is a need for a holistic approach to adult aural rehabilitation that goes beyond device use.

A holistic approach to adult aural rehabilitation is not a new concept. Many of the processes utilized in a holistic approach were first provided in the military audiology programs established in response to the hearing health care needs of World War II veterans. These programs were comprehensive, including auditory and visual speech perception training and vocational and psychological counseling, in addition to the fitting of hearing aids (Bergman, 2002). Several of the elements of the early military audiology programs provide the basis of contemporary approaches to adult aural rehabilitation. For example, current models of group aural rehabilitation programs for adults focus on provision of information, training, and psychosocial counseling support (Preminger, 2007). Furthermore, as a result of recent neurophysiological, functional magnetic resonance imaging (fMRI), and behavioral studies there is a renewed interest in the potential for the use of auditory and/or visual perceptual training to improve the outcomes of device-based intervention for adults with hearing loss (Pratt, 2005), leading to the development of computerized, cost effective auditory training programs (Taylor & Shrive, 2008).

In current practice, adults with hearing loss who receive an *individual* aural rehabilitation program typically participate in auditory and/or auditory-visual training activities, while those who receive *group* intervention most often will participate in information/counseling-based programs. Recent systematic reviews addressed the evidence for individual auditory training (Sweetow & Palmer, 2005) and counseling-based group aural rehabilitation (Hawkins, 2005). The evidence synthesized in each of these two systematic reviews is presented and updated here to include the results from more recent research and the completion of meta-analyses.

INDIVIDUAL AUDITORY TRAINING

The general goal of auditory training is to increase the listener's ability to compensate for any degradation in the auditory signal due to internal (hearing loss) or external (noise) factors (Sweetow & Palmer, 2005). When a hearing aid, cochlear implant or other hearing assistive device is first used by an individual, he or she must learn how to utilize the auditory sensations that are not only impoverished, but also different from those experienced previously. Formal auditory training, particularly if it occurs in an unthreatening environment, can provide the listener with increased opportunities to engage in perceptual learning, which in turn may lead to higher ultimate speech understanding and improved communication ability (Boothroyd, 2007). Evidence supporting increased speech understanding as a result of auditory training was evaluated and synthesized in Sweetow and Palmer's (2005) systematic review of relevant literature.

Research studies included in the Sweetow and Palmer (2005) systematic review examined the effectiveness of both analytic and synthetic auditory training, as well as combinations of the two. In an analytic training approach, speech is broken down into its component parts, such as vowels and consonants, and training is aimed at improving the discrimination among, and recognition of the parts. In a synthetic approach, exercises typically include sentence-length materials, with a major focus on listening skills and the use of linguistic and situational redundancy. Initially, Sweetow and Palmer identified 213 studies, but only six were found to meet all of the systematic review inclusion criteria. In addition to a focus on auditory training, the following criteria were required: (a) use of a randomized controlled trial (RCT), cohort, or a before/after study design,[1] with or without a control group; (b) adult subjects with hearing loss who were not users of cochlear implants; and (c) the use of either objective or standardized subjective outcome measures assessing communication skills. Sweetow and Palmer identified three RCTs (Kricos, Holmes, & Doyle, 1992; Montgomery, Walden, Schwartz, & Prosek, 1984; Walden, Erdman, Montgomery, Schwartz, & Prosek, 1981); one cohort study with a control group (Kricos & Holmes, 1996); and two cohort studies without control

[1]Sweetow & Palmer's (2005) use of "before/after" designs are classified according to the descriptions in Chapter 1 as "cohort" designs for the purposes of consistency within the chapters in the present text.

groups (Bode & Oyer, 1970; Rubenstein & Boothroyd, 1987) meeting inclusion criteria. The six studies differed in many ways, including: the number of treatment groups; the use of control groups; the type of auditory training (analytic vs. synthetic vs. combination); outcome measures utilized; and, whether or not short- and long-term outcomes were assessed. In addition, the studies were found to have many methodological limitations (e.g., lack of use of power analysis, lack of blinding, etc.). The reviewers elected to complete only a qualitative and not a quantitative synthesis of study results due to the heterogeneity of the studies, including that related to the use of various outcome measures. The results of the qualitative analysis led Sweetow and Palmer to conclude, albeit cautiously, that the evidence supported auditory training for adults with hearing loss, particularly from synthetic training activities. More specifically, synthetic training appeared to result in improvements in speech recognition in noise and in better use of active listening strategies. Although there was less evidence supporting the use of analytic training activities, Sweetow and Palmer noted that in addition to the methodological concerns, there was no evidence that training paradigms were optimized. Thus, they concluded that continued research was needed prior to being able to draw compelling conclusions related to individual auditory training.

Several auditory training studies have been conducted since the Sweetow and Palmer (2005) systematic review. Using EBP principals, research studies which were published subsequent to the 2005 review were identified through a literature search conducted between May and August of 2010. The inclusion criteria utilized were the same as those of Sweetow and Palmer, with one exception. Rather than include articles examining either objective or subjective outcome measures, only studies that objectively assessed speech recognition performance were included. This decision was made so that data from the studies would be similar enough to allow for a quantitative synthesis of the outcomes of a systematic review designed to determine the magnitude of the effect of auditory training in adults with acquired hearing loss, who were not cochlear implant users, on speech recognition abilities. The search terms utilized were the same as those in the Sweetow and Palmer review (i.e., "adult" and "aural rehabilitation"; "auditory training"; "hearing loss"; "hearing impaired"; "individual aural rehabilitation"; "audiological rehabilitation"; "analytic"; "top-down processing"; "listening training"). Databases searched included: PubMed, Health Reference Center Academic, MEDLINE, Cumulative Index to Nursing and Allied-Health Literature (CINAHL), and Annual Reviews. As shown in Figure 10–1, 49 articles were initially identified, with 35 eliminated after abstract review. In addition to meeting all other inclusion criteria, only studies which were at least a Level 4, cohort studies, or higher as shown in Table 1–5, were included for further review. After full article review, four studies were selected for the final analyses: two RCTs (Stecker et al., 2006; Sweetow & Sabes, 2006); and two with cohort designs, one of which utilized a control group (Humes, Burk, Strauser, & Kinney, 2009) and one that did not (Burk & Humes, 2008).

Table 10–1 provides a brief summary of the four studies identified as well as the six studies from the Sweetow and Palmer (2005) systematic review. As with the studies included in the Sweetow and Palmer systematic review, more recent research has examined both analytic (Burk & Humes, 2008; Humes et al., 2009; Stecker et al., 2006) and synthetic (Sweetow & Sabes, 2006) training paradigms. Across the ten studies speech recognition abilities were assessed using a variety of stimuli, including nonsense syllables, words, and sentences; presented stimuli in both quiet and noise conditions; and, evaluated performance via hearing alone or via

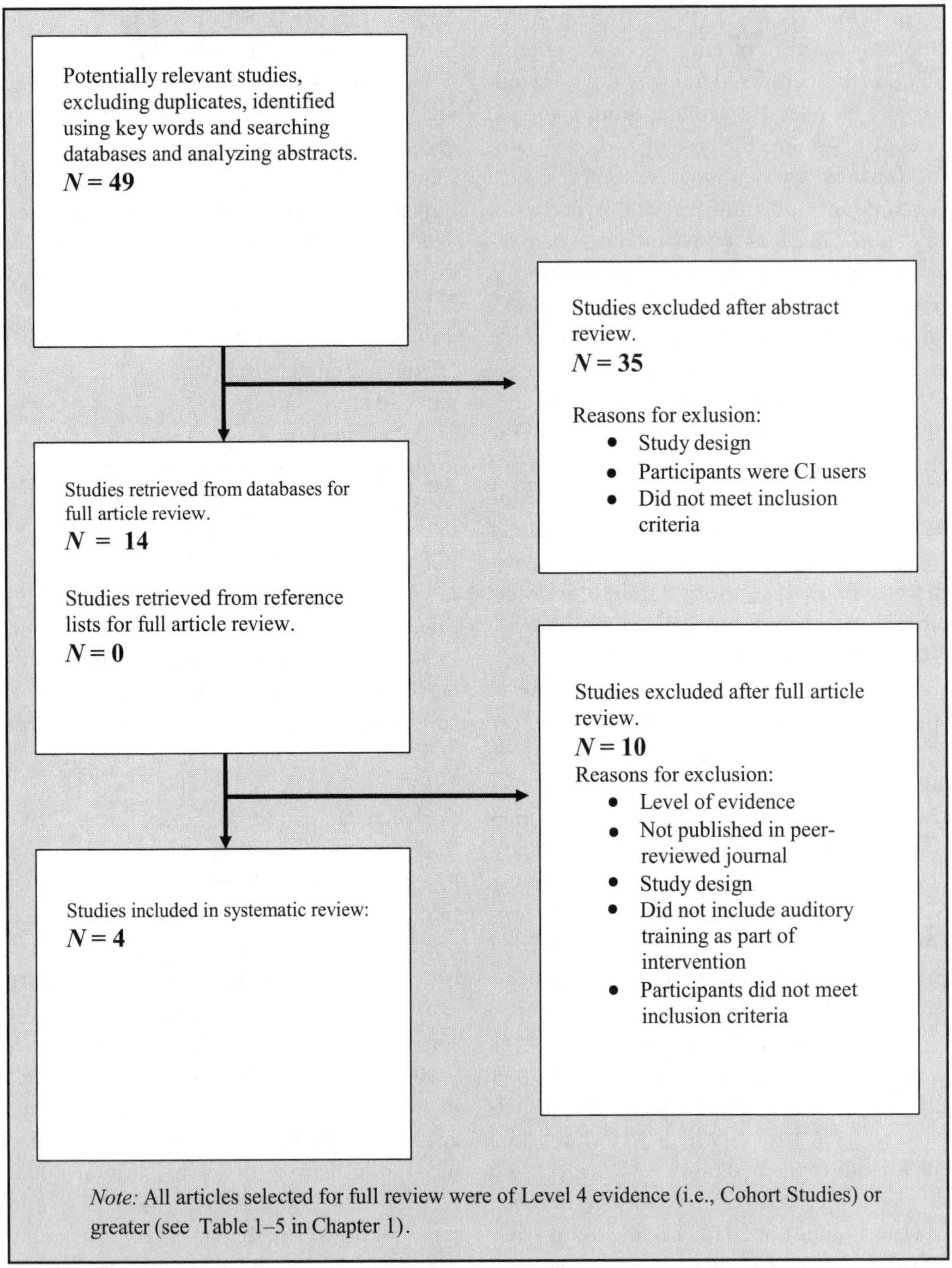

Figure 10–1. *Search flow chart for auditory training.*

hearing and speech-reading (auditory + visual) inputs. Sweetow and Palmer noted that the sample sizes were relatively small in the studies reviewed, ranging from 8 to 13 per group, for all but one study (i.e., Kricos & Holmes, 1996) which had 26 subjects per group.

Table 10–1. Summary of Auditory Training Studies Meeting Inclusion Criteria for Systematic Review

Study	*Design*	*Intervention*	*Speech Recognition Outcomes*	*Results*	*Included in Meta-Analysis?*
Bode & Oyer (1970)*	Cohort with four groups differentiated by training protocol *n* = 8 in each group 9 experienced HA users; 23 non-HA users	Analytic, word-based auditory training protocols varying by listening condition (SNR-constant vs. SNR-varied) and stimulus type (open set vs. closed set)	CID W-22 M-Rhyme test Semidiagnostic test	Significant improvements after training for W-22 and M-Rhyme test. No improvements seen for semidiagnostic test. Differences between listening conditions, stimulus types, and their interactions were not significant.	No Did not report standard deviations for posttest results
Burk & Humes (2008)	Cohort, no control group *n* = 8 HA use not reported	Combination analytic/synthetic, word- and sentence-based auditory training protocol conducted in background noise—12 weeks, 3 times per week	Open- and closed-set recognition of trained and untrained words in isolation and in phrases in sentences	Training improved for both closed-set and open-set performance for trained materials only. Training effects generalized to unfamiliar talkers. Listeners were able to retain training effects for at least 3.5 months.	No No control group and could not estimate pre/post correlation for sentence test due to adaptation to stimuli.

continues

Table 10–1. *continued*

Study	*Design*	*Intervention*	*Speech Recognition Outcomes*	*Results*	*Included in Meta-Analysis?*
Humes et al. (2009)	Cohort, with control group Four groups, two experimental older hearing impaired (OHI) and two young normal hearing (YNH) control groups. Each of the OHI and YNH groups received one of two training protocols; Young normal hearing control groups. n = 8 in each group HA use not reported	Combination analytic/synthetic, word- or sentence-based auditory training protocol conducted in ICRA background noise	Frequent words Frequent phrases VAST sentences CID sentences	Significant improvements seen for all groups for all outcomes posttraining. Improvements generalized to novel words and sentences. Effects of training not as dramatic as those seen in Burk & Humes (2008) study	Yes
Kricos et al. (1992)*	RCT, one experimental and one control group n = 13 in each group Experienced HA users	4-week, synthetic, sentence-based auditory training program	CID Everyday Sentences, auditory-visual version	Significant improvements for both the experimental and control groups.	Yes
Kricos & Holmes (1996)*	Cohort, two experimental groups and a control group n = 26 in each group Experienced HA users	Analytic training protocol vs. active listening training protocol	CST	No improvements on speech recognition scores were evident in any group.	Yes

Study	Design	Intervention	Speech Recognition Outcomes	Results	Included in Meta-Analysis?
Montgomery et al. (1984)*	RCT, two control groups, hearing impaired receiving standard treatment; and young normal hearing. n = 12 in each group. New HA users	Standard (unspecified) aural rehabilitation training (AR) alone vs. AR plus auditory + visual integration training	Auditory-Visual sentence test	Significant improvements seen for AR control group and for experimental group. Magnitude of improvement much greater for the experimental group. No improvement for the young normal-hearing control group.	Yes
Rubenstein & Boothroyd (1987)*	Cohort with two matched experimental groups, no control group n = 10 in each group	Synthetic sentence recognition training vs. analytic consonant recognition training	NST R-SPIN	Small improvement seen on high-predictability R-SPIN items only for both experimental groups. No differences seen between training protocols.	Yes
Stecker et al. (2006)	RCT, with new hearing aid user immediate treatment (IT) group, experienced hearing aid user treatment group, and delayed treatment (DT) new hearing aid user control group. n = 12 IT group n = 8 experienced hearing aid user group n = 11 DT group	Analytic, PC-based auditory training protocol completed at home	NST	NST performance significantly increased after training. Greatest training improvement seen in IT group. 8-weeks posttraining for IT and DT groups, significant improvements were maintained for up to 8-weeks posttraining and generalized to new talkers.	No Could not extrapolate variance from error bars included with figures in results section

continues

Table 10–1. *continued*

Study	*Design*	*Intervention*	*Speech Recognition Outcomes*	*Results*	*Included in Meta-Analysis?*
Sweetow & Sabes (2006)	RCT, with an immediate treatment (IT) and a delayed-treatment (DT) control group. *n* = 56 IT group *n* = 33 DT group Experienced HA users	LACE™ PC-based training completed at home. LACE contains both auditory and cognitive tasks.	QuickSIN HINT	QuickSIN improved post-LACE™ training with the exception of HINT. Both QuickSIN and HINT were used to assess generalization of training.	No[1] Did not report variance
Walden et al. (1981)*	RCT, auditory training group, lipreading training group, control standard treatment group *n* = 10 in each training group; *n* = 15 in control group New HA users	Analytic, consonant-recognition training	Auditory consonant recognition Visual consonant recognition Auditory-visual sentence recognition	All three groups showed significant improvements on the auditory-visual sentence recognition task, with the two experimental groups showing the greatest improvements. Significant improvements on the consonant recognition tasks were seen for the experimental groups only.	Yes

[1]Effect size is reported and included in Figure 10–2 stem plot. Data were not reported that allowed inclusion in meta-analytic software.

Note: Studies marked with an asterisk were identified by Sweetow and Sabes (2005), whereas the remaining studies were identified in the current literature search. CID-W22 = Central Institute for the Deaf W-22 word list (Hirsh et al., 1952) ; CID Everyday Sentence Test = Central Institute for the Deaf Everyday Sentence Test (Harris, Haines, Kelsey, & Clack, 1961); CST = Connected Speech Test (Cox, Alexander, & Gilmore, 1987); HA = Hearing aid; HINT = Hearing in Noise Test (Nilsson, Soli, & Sullivan, 1994); LACE™ = Listening & Communication Enhancement (Sweetow & Sabes, 2006); M-Rhyme Test = Modified Rhyme Test (House, Williams, Hecker, & Kryter, 1965); NST = Nonsense Syllable Test (Resnick, Dubno, Hoffnung, & Levitt, 1975); QuickSIN = Quick Speech-in-Noise (Etymotic Research, 2001); R-SPIN = Revised Speech Perception in Noise test (Bilger, Nuetzel, Rabinowitz, & Rzeczkowski, 1984); VAST = Veterans Administration Sentence Test (US Department of Veterans Affairs, 1998).

Small numbers of subjects were also noted in three of the four newly identified studies. The exception was the study by Sweetow and Sabes with 89 subjects. Participant characteristics were varied across the studies reviewed by Sweetow and Palmer, with age ranging from 19 to 85 years old. The four newly identified studies included participants with hearing loss who were primarily older with the largest age range (28 to 85 years old) in the Sweetow and Sabes investigation. Two of the studies reviewed by Sweetow and Palmer (Montgomery et al., 1984; Walden et al., 1981) and one of the newly identified studies (Stecker et al., 2006) were conducted with male veterans as participants, whereas all other studies reportedly included both male and female subjects. Sweetow and Palmer reported that, in four of the six studies, participants were hearing aid users, with two of the studies indicating that the individuals were new hearing aid users. New and experienced hearing aid users participated in the Stecker et al. and the Sweetow and Sabes studies with training occurring with the use of amplification. Hearing aid use status was not reported for the Burk and Humes or Humes et al. studies, and training occurred with stimuli presented via insert earphones. All but one of the studies reviewed (Kricos & Holmes, 1996) by Sweetow and Palmer showed statistically significant improvements in speech recognition performance as a function of training on at least one outcome measure, as did all four of the studies identified in the present literature search. Although all of the studies examined outcomes immediately postintervention, only Burk and Humes reported that there was a subsequent retention of training benefits.

In addition to considering the overall findings of the individual studies, an important step in the systematic review process is quality assessment. As recommended by Wong and Hickson in Chapter 1, the quality of the four newly identified studies, as well as those included in the Sweetow and Palmer (2005) review, was assessed utilizing Dollaghan's (2007) guidelines (see the Appendix). According to Dollaghan, it is important to determine whether or not the aims of the study were plausible and related to the clinical question, and the answer for all of the studies as indicated in Table 10–2 was "yes." All studies were prospective and analytic in nature. The results section of each study indicated that the aims were addressed although, as noted above, all but one of the studies demonstrated statistical significance with regard to objective speech recognition performance. Table 10–2 also shows that the studies differed in several of the methodological variables that are important to consider when judging both the internal and external validity of results. This finding is not surprising and is consistent with the results of the quality assessment performed by Sweetow and Palmer. Consistent with the studies examined by Sweetow and Palmer, the newly identified studies were mixed in their use of control groups, use of randomization, and discussions of group similarities. A lack of reporting of power analyses was noted by Sweetow and Palmer, and was consistently lacking in the recently identified studies. In addition, none of the studies reported the use of blinding, either of participants or experimenters, and dropout rates were presented in only one study (Sweetow & Sabes, 2006). Given the methodological concerns, the adoption of the majority of the individual study interventions was judged to be "suggestive" (i.e., different clinicians might responsibly chose to adopt or not adopt the intervention), with the interventions described in three studies judged as "equivocal" (i.e., the evidence does not support adopting the intervention). The exception was the Listening and Communication Enhancement (LACE™) at-home computer-based program examined by Sweetow and Sabes. LACE includes training focused on the perception of speech in babble,

Table 10–2. Quality Assessment of Auditory Training Studies.

Study	*Aims: Plausible and Relevant*	*Methods*	*Results: Achieve Goals and Clinically Significant*	*Control Group*	*Random-ization*	*Power*	*Groups Similar*	*Blinding*	*Dropouts <20%*	*Overall Judgment*
Bode & Oyer (1970)*	Yes	Yes	Yes	No	No	No	Yes	No	Unknown	Suggestive
Burk & Humes (2008)	Yes	Yes	Yes	No	No	No	N/A	No	None reported	Equivocal
Humes et al. (2009)	Yes	Yes	Yes	No	No	No	No	No	None reported	Suggestive
Kricos et al. (1992)*	Yes	Yes	Yes	Yes	Yes	No	Yes	No	Unknown	Suggestive
Kricos & Holmes (1996)*	Yes	Yes	Yes	Yes	Yes	No	Yes	No	Unknown	Equivocal
Montgomery et al. (1984)*	Yes	Yes	Yes	Yes	Yes	No	Yes	No	Unknown	Suggestive
Rubenstein & Boothroyd (1987)*	Yes	Yes	Yes	No	No	No	Yes	No	Unknown	Equivocal
Stecker et al. (2006)	Yes	Yes	Yes	Yes	No	No	No	No	Yes	Suggestive
Sweetow & Sabes (2006)	Yes	Yes	Yes	Yes	Yes	No	Yes	No	>30%	Suggestive
Walden et al. (1981)*	Yes	Yes	Yes	Yes	Yes	No	No	No	Unknown	Suggestive

Note: Studies included in the Sweetow and Palmer (2005) review are marked with an asterisk. "Compelling"= adoption of the intervention should be considered seriously; "Suggestive" = different clinicians might responsibly make different decision about whether to adopt the intervention; "Equivocal" = the intervention should not be adopted.

time-compressed speech, and speech in a competing speaker background, as well as a short-term memory task, the identification of missing words in sentence, and helpful hints about communication strategies. Although there were some limitations in the quality of the Sweetow and Sabes study, the use of a control group, with similarities of experimental and control groups reported, the use of randomization, the discussion of dropouts, as well as a fairly large sample size (see Table 10–1), and statistically significant off-task results (see Table 10–1), led to the conclusion that the clinicians could with some confidence, consider adopting the LACE intervention.

Although the individual studies varied in terms of training paradigms, number of subjects, methodological quality and statistically significant results, an advantage of conducting systematic reviews is the opportunity to complete a meta-analysis. By combining study results with meta-analytic techniques, even small *n* studies can make a significant contribution to knowledge. As noted, we elected to examine only outcome measures in the reviewed studies that assessed changes in speech recognition performance. Although there were differences in the type of stimuli (i.e., phonemes vs. words vs. sentences), the listening conditions (i.e., quiet or noise), and input modalities (i.e., hearing alone or hearing + vision), the construct assessed, "speech recognition" was the same across all outcome measures providing data for the meta-analysis. To conduct the analysis, the Comprehensive Meta-Analysis (version 2.0)® software package was used. Only one study (Burk & Humes, 2008) included pretest and posttest data for both short- and long-term outcomes. Thus, to maintain consistency the data utilized in the meta-analysis were those obtained immediately posttreatment. To be included, certain information had to be extractable from the studies. Thus, not all studies provided data for the meta-analysis, as reported in the last column in Table 10–1. In addition to reporting means or mean differences, measures of variability were needed. If a study reported only the *p* value, the data needed for the meta-analysis were not available. In addition, although some studies reported effect sizes as Cohen's *d*, because of software limitations, the individually reported effect sizes could not be included in the calculation of an overall average effect size unless measures of variance were also reported. In the meta-analysis, effect sizes were calculated as standardized mean differences (Cohen's *d*) for comparison across studies, and a random-effects model for variability was employed. Furthermore, individual studies were weighted for sample size, as suggested by Robey and Dalebout (1988), to ensure that the confidence interval for the average effect size was not unduly biased by studies with significant postintervention results, but a small *n*.

The results of the meta-analysis are summarized in the forest plot in Figure 10–2. A forest plot is a graphical display which illustrates the relative effect sizes from multiple quantitative scientific studies addressing the same question. As shown in Figure 10–2, the left-hand column in a forest plot lists the name of the studies, commonly in chronological order from the top down. The second column in Figure 10–2 shows the subgroup from each individual study that provided data for the meta-analysis. The specific outcome measure used in each of the studies is listed in the third column. The next three columns show the statistics for each study, including the effect size measure; Cohen's *d* in the column labeled "Std diff in means," and the upper and lower limits for the 95% confidence intervals. These data also are illustrated in the right-hand column, which is the actual plot of the effect size measures for each study, shown in the black boxes. The effect sizes are shown for a range of −1.00 to +1.00 on the x-axis in the plot. Zero on the x-axis represents "no effect" as a result of the intervention.

Study name	Subgroup within study	Outcome	Std diff in means	Lower limit	Upper limit
Kricos et al. 1992	AT (Synthetic) vs. NT	Combined	0.287	-0.487	1.060
Kricos & Holmes 1996	AT (Analytic) vs. NT	Combined	0.205	-0.340	0.750
Kricos & Holmes 1996	AT (Synthetic) vs. NT	Combined	0.033	-0.511	0.577
Montgomery et al. 1984	AT vs. HA	AV Sentences	0.654	-0.167	1.475
Rubenstein & Boothroyd 1987	AT (Analytic)	Combined	0.422	-0.193	1.037
Rubenstein & Boothroyd 1987	AT (Synthetic)	Combined	0.196	-0.399	0.792
Walden et al. 1981	AT Auditory vs. NT	AV Sentences	0.889	0.052	1.727
Walden et al. 1981	AT Visual vs. NT	AV Sentences	0.360	-0.446	1.167
Humes et al. 2009	AT vs. NT	CID Sentences	0.767	0.000	1.533
TOTAL			**0.352**	**0.128**	**0.575**
Sweetow & Sabes, 2006		HINT	0.16		
Sweetow & Sabes, 2006		QuickSIN@45dB	0.31		
Sweetow & Sabes, 2006		QuickSIN@70dB	0.23		

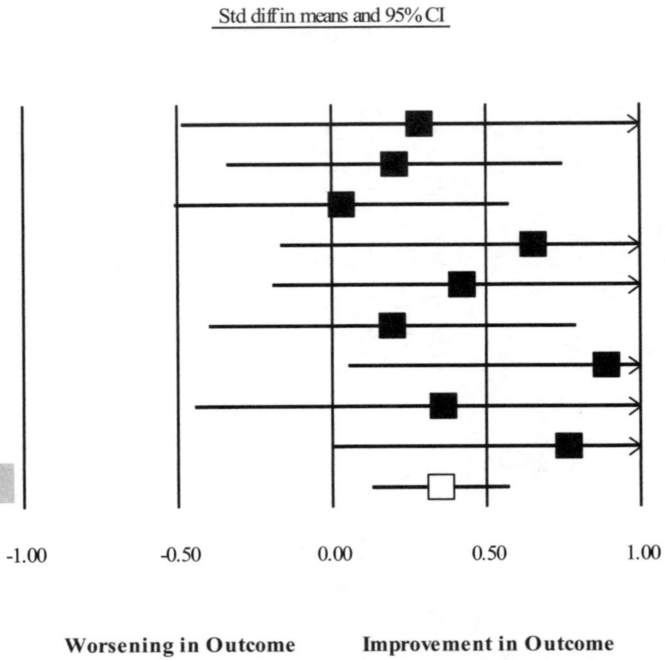

Note: AT=Auditory training; AV=Auditory+Visual; CID=Central Institute for the Deaf; HA=Hearing aid; NT=No treatment; HINT=Hearing in Noise Test; QuickSIN= Quick Speech in Noise Test

Figure 10–2. *Forest plot showing auditory training effects.*

Positive numbers indicate that speech recognition performance improved as a result of the intervention, whereas a negative number indicates that performance decreased after intervention. The horizontal lines around the effect size measures indicate the 95% confidence intervals, which provide similar information to that obtained in a test of statistical significance. If the 95% confidence interval crosses zero, the results suggest that statistically significant findings are not likely. Given the differences in the studies included in the present meta-analysis, in terms of the training paradigms and outcome measures utilized as well as the variability of methodological quality, Figure 10–2 shows that the magnitude of the effect sizes was heterogeneous across studies. Although all of the individual effect sizes were positive, indicating that speech recognition performance improved as a result of training, the reliability of this interpretation for many of the individual studies must be made with caution as the 95% confidence intervals cross the zero point. Of course, the point of the meta-analysis, and perhaps its greatest advantage, is to obtain a more reliable estimate of the effect size through the combining of the results of smaller studies. The mean effect size calculated in the present analysis, shown at the bottom of the forest plot by the open box, was .352, with the 95% confidence limits greater than zero. Thus, taken as a whole, the body of literature examining individual auditory training in adults indicates that the intervention provides a reliable, although small, effect in terms of improving speech understanding immediately postintervention. The mean effect size reported here provides a benchmark against which the results of future training studies can be compared. For example, although the data from Sweetow and Sabes (2006) shown under the total effect size line in Figure 10–2 could not be extracted for inclusion in the meta-analysis, the researchers reported effect sizes for their off-task speech recognition measures for the intervention group to be Cohen's *d* values of 0.16 for the HINT test, 0.31 for the Quick Speech-in Noise (QuickSIN) test at 45 dB HL and 0.23 for the QuickSIN test at 70 dB HL. These effect sizes fall within the 95% confidence intervals calculated for the body of literature and suggest that the magnitude of the effect of LACE training is similar to that obtained, in general, for auditory training. Certainly, auditory training paradigms must be optimized for individual patients, but the synthesis of the evidence to date indicates that individual auditory training will result in at least short-term improvements in speech understanding. Thus clinicians should have increased confidence in recommending the use of an auditory training program as a part of a comprehensive aural rehabilitation plan for adults with hearing loss, at least for improving short-term outcomes. Whether or not improvements noted immediately after intervention are maintained longer term, cannot be adequately addressed with the available research.

COUNSELING-BASED GROUP AURAL REHABILITATION PROGRAMS

A holistic approach to aural rehabilitation includes counseling as the principal mechanism for addressing deficits of participation and quality of life resulting from hearing loss (Boothroyd, 2007). Although individual counseling and instruction occur during all points in the audiological management process, issues related to participation and quality of life are also addressed through group aural rehabilitation (AR) programs, particularly after the provision of hearing aids. As with other components of aural rehabilitation, hearing aid follow-up group programs are not a new idea. In fact, the first post–hearing aid fitting follow-up group program was initiated by Raymond Carhart as a part of the post–World War II program for military personnel at the Deshon General Hospital (Bergman, 2002). As discussed by Hawkins (2005), who conducted a systematic review of the effectiveness of counseling-based group AR programs, there have been numerous publications stressing the importance of incorporating the use of communication strategies and counseling as a part of a holistic management approach for adults with hearing loss, with the most time and cost effective method for implementation being a group setting. Group settings allow participants to share their feelings, problems and solutions for dealing with communication failures. Group AR programs typically involve the use of lectures, in which information about hearing, hearing loss, speech-reading, communication strategies, and assistive devices is provided. Practice in the use of communication strategies, the use of relaxation and/or stress relaxation techniques, psychosocial discussions, and participation of significant others are also commonly employed techniques (Preminger & Yoo, 2010). In some approaches specific speech recognition practice, similar to that which is done in individual training, is implemented in the group setting (see, for example, Preminger & Ziegler, 2008).

Hawkins's (2005) systematic review was implemented to determine if participation in group AR programs by adults with hearing loss resulted in short- and/or long-term self-perceived benefits and/or satisfaction with hearing aids. To be included in the analysis, studies had to involve adults with hearing loss who participated in a group AR program emphasizing counseling, communication strategies, personal adjustment and the provision of information about hearing, hearing loss, and hearing aids. Acceptable study designs included RCTs, quasi-experimental (e.g., cohort) or nonintervention cohort designs with a sample size that was judged to be appropriate. Finally, the outcome measures utilized had to assess an aspect of personal adjustment, perceived hearing handicap, or perceived hearing aid benefit and/or satisfaction. Twelve studies were identified as meeting the criteria. The majority of the studies (Abrams, Hnath-Chisolm, Guerreiro & Ritterman, 1992; Andersson, Melin, Scott, & Lindberg, 1995a, 1995b; Benyon, Thornton, & Poole, 1997; Brewer, 2001; Brickley, Cleaver, & Bailey, 1996; Norman, George, Downie, & Milligan, 1995; Preminger, 2003; Smaldino & Smaldino, 1988) examined outcomes in terms of reductions of auditory handicap (i.e., reductions in participation restrictions). Personal adjustment and/or the use of communication strategies was assessed in four studies (Andersson et al., 1995b; Chisolm, Abrams, & McArdle, 2004; Hallberg & Barrenas, 1994; Preminger, 2003); hearing aid use, performance and adjustment in new users in two studies (Brickley et al., 1996; Norman et al., 1995); and, in one study each, relaxation issues (Andersson et al., 1995a) and generic quality of life (Abrams, Chisolm, & McArdle, 2002). In discussing the systematic review results Hawkins pointed out that the majority, but not all, of the studies demonstrated benefits of group AR in terms of reductions of participation restrictions. Although there was documentation of improved use of communication strategies, enhanced personal adjustment, and better use of hearing aids, the data were limited and had not been systematically replicated. In summarizing the body of research reviewed, Hawkins concluded that there were very few well-controlled studies and called for future studies to utilize RCT designs with adequate numbers of participants given the variability previous results. Although it is important to conduct single well-designed studies, it is also possible to further explore the evidence-base for group AR through updating the Hawkins's systematic review. In updating the Hawkins's systematic review, we focused on studies that utilized a RCT design with control groups (Level 2 evidence, as described in Table 1–5), and assessed the outcomes we believed were most related to the goals of counseling-based group aural rehabilitation programs. Specifically, this was the effect of intervention on reductions in participation restrictions and improvements in quality of life. This last criterion was implemented so that the outcome measures would be assessing a similar construct, allowing for the completion of a meta-analysis to estimate the effect size of the group aural rehabilitation intervention. In this context, participation is defined according to the World Health Organization's International Classification of Functioning, Disability and Health (WHO, 2001) as what a person "does do" in his or her everyday environment across the broad domains of learning and applying knowledge; general tasks and demands; communication; mobility; self-care; domestic life; interpersonal interactions and relationships; major life areas (e.g., employment, education, economic life); and community, social, and civic life. Participation is closely related to the construct of quality of life, which in its simplest form, can be thought of as "how good or bad you feel your life to be" (Bradley, Todd, Gorton, Symonds, Martin, & Plowright, 1999). When the impact of a disease or disorder and its treatments are considered, the outcome measures utilized assess health-related quality of life (HRQoL) of individuals (Chisolm & Abrams, 2007). Health-related quality of life can be assessed relative to a specific disease or disorder or generically.

When examining the studies identified by Hawkins (2005) it was found that seven of the studies utilized an RCT design, with six utilizing a disease-specific participation/QoL outcome measure (Abrams et al., 1992; Andersson et al., 1995a, 1995b; Benyon et al., 1997; Chisolm et al., 2004; Hallberg & Barrenas, 1994; Smaldino & Smaldino, 1988) and one utilizing a generic QoL instrument (Abrams et al., 2002). In addition to these studies, two more recent studies meeting the criteria were identified in a literature search conducted between May and August 2010 (Hickson, Worrall, & Scarinci, 2007; Preminger & Ziegler, 2008). A third study, by Preminger and Yoo (2010) was identified subsequent to the initial search and included in the present review. The search terms were the same as those used by Hawkins (2005) and included, "audiological rehabilitation," "adult aural rehabilitation," "group aural rehabilitation," and "counseling and hearing aids." The databases searched included: PubMed, Health Reference Center Academic, MEDLINE, Cumulative Index to Nursing and Allied-Health Literature (CINAHL), and Annual Reviews. Figure 10–3 shows the step-by-step results of the search and Table 10–3 provides a brief discussion of the nine studies whose results are synthesized here.

Several factors are important to consider regarding the body of literature examining the efficacy of group AR intervention. First, there were three studies with a relatively large *n*. The first, reported by Abrams et al. (2002), compared generic HRQoL outcomes from over 100 veterans who received hearing aids alone to those who received hearing aids plus participated in a 4-week post–hearing aid fitting group aural rehabilitation program. Although a statistically significant difference was not found between the groups, when disease-specific outcomes were examined for the same subjects, significant participation/QoL benefits were seen (Chisolm et al., 2004) as measured through the Communication Profile for the Hearing Impaired (Demorest & Erdman, 1987) personal adjustment factor score. The largest study to date was conducted by Hickson, Worrall, and Scarinci (2007) in which 100 individuals participated in the

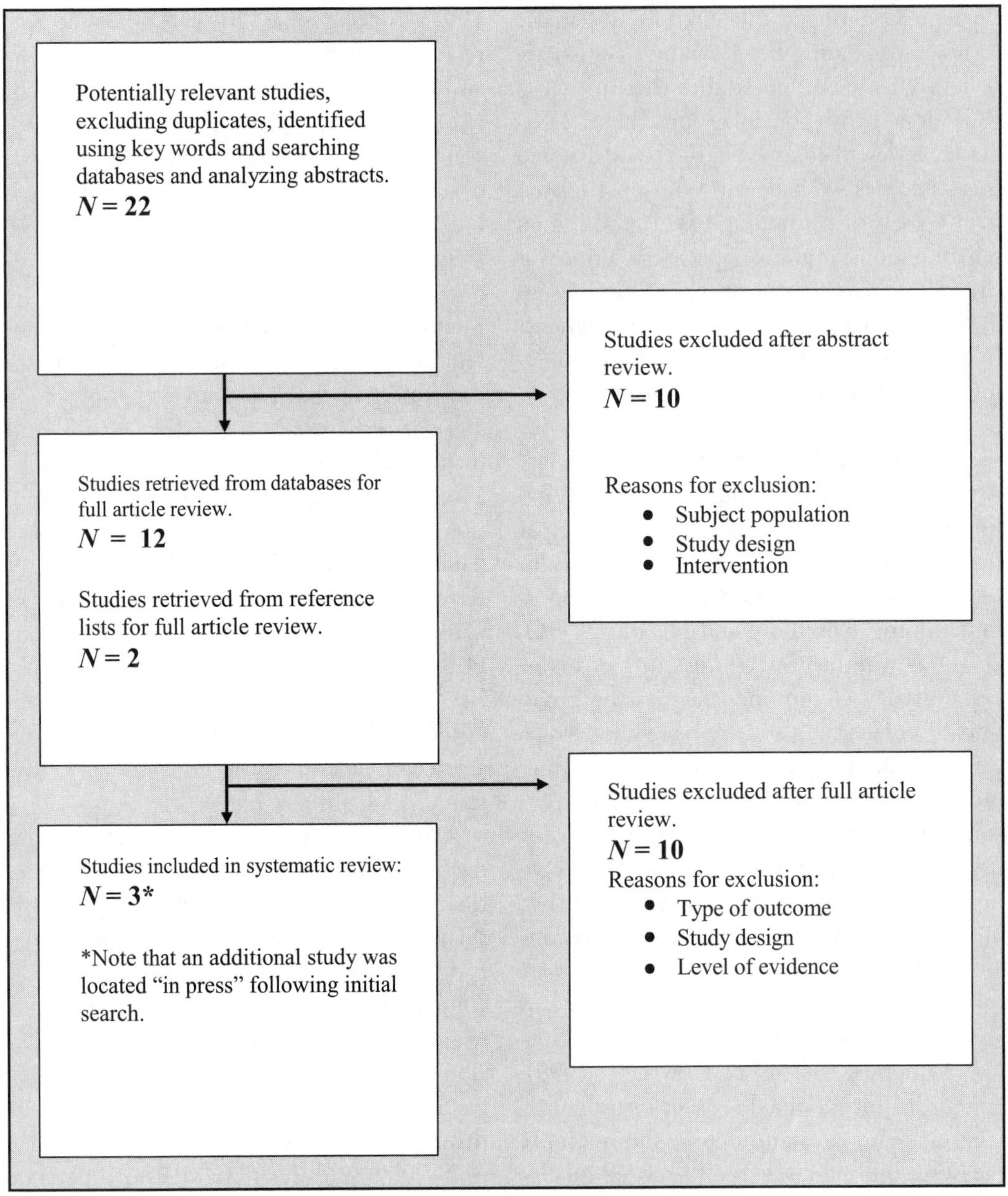

Figure 10–3. *Search flow chart for counseling-based group AR.*

experimental training, referred to as *Active Communication Education (ACE)* program and 78 older individuals participated in a placebo training condition followed by ACE. Across both groups 54% had been fitted with hearing aids, but there was no difference in the frequency of hearing aid use between the two groups. ACE consisted of a series of five, two-hour modules aimed at addressing specific, common communication difficulties encountered in daily life for individuals with hearing loss, and the placebo training condition consisted of the same amount of contact time but sessions were about general communication issues.

Table 10–3. Summary of Group Aural Rehabilitation Meeting Inclusion Criteria for Systematic Review. Studies marked with an asterisk were identified by Hawkins (2005), whereas the remaining studies were identified in the current literature search.

Study	*Design/Participants*	*Intervention*	*Participation/QoL Outcomes*	*Results*	*Included in Meta analysis?*
Abrams, Hnath-Chisolm, Guerriero, & Ritterman (1992)*	RCT; 3 groups Control Group *n* = 9 Hearing Aids Alone (HA-only) *n* = 11 HA + Group AR *n* = 11 All new HA users	AR group met 1 time per week, 1.5 hours per week for 3 weeks.	HHIE Total	HA-only and HA + AR groups showed significantly greater reduction of hearing handicap than Control group for HHIE-Total score, with greater change for the HA + AR as compared to HA-only group.	Yes Analyzed: HHIE Total postscores – HA + AR vs. Control – HA + AR vs. HA alone
Abrams, Chisolm, & McArdle (2002)*	RCT; 2 groups HA-only *n* = 52 HA + AR *n* = 53 All new HA users	AR group met 1.5 hours per week for 4 sessions	SF-36 Mental Component Scores (MCS) Physical Component Scores (PCS)	MCS scores improved more for HA + AR as compared to HA alone but difference not statistically significant. No effect seen on PCS for either group.	No Outcome measure (SF-36) generic rather than disease-specific.
Andersson, Melin, Scott, & Lindberg (1995a, 1995b)*	RCT; 2 groups Control Group *n* = 12 AR Group *n* = 12 Experienced HA users	AR group met 2 hours per week for 4 sessions	HCA	Participation in group AR did not result in a significantly different outcome (as measured by the HCA) between groups. F/U at 2 years (1995b) showed no group differences for *n* = 20.	Yes Analyzed: HCA Total postscores

continues

Table 10–3. *continued*

Study	*Design/Participants*	*Intervention*	*Participation/QoL Outcomes*	*Results*	*Included in Meta analysis?*
Benyon, Thornton, & Poole (1997)*	RCT; 2 groups HA-Only Group *n* = 26; 25 completed HA + AR Group *n* = 24; 19 completed New HA users	AR group met 4 times (number of hours and days unreported)	QDS	Greater reduction in mean QDS scores for HA + AR participants than for HA-only group.	No Data needed for effect size calculation not available in publication.
Chisolm, Abrams & McArdle (2004)[1]*	RCT; 2 groups HA-Alone *n* = 53 HA + AR *n* = 53 New HA users	AR group met 1.5 hours per week for 4 sessions	CPHI, subscale, and factor scores	Improvements in short term communication strategy usage and reaction and interaction factors seen in Group AR participants. Benefits remained stable when reassessed 1year post-AR. Benefit scores for the control group increased when measured 1year post-AR period, resulting in no differences in outcomes between groups at this time point.	Yes Analyzed: Personal Adjustment Factor Postscore from CPHI

Study	*Design/Participants*	*Intervention*	*Participation/QoL Outcomes*	*Results*	*Included in Meta analysis?*
Hallberg & Barrenas (1994)*	RCT; 2 groups Control n = 27 randomized; 12 completed Experimental n = 23 7.5% Experienced HA users 92.5% nonusers; No difference in frequency of reported HA use between groups	AR group met 3 hours per week for 4 sessions	HMS, HSS	Short-term effects, with a reduction in perceived handicap on HHS and HMS, seen in Group AR participants. No differences found posttreatment for CPHI CS subscale scores found, possibly due to an order effect (administered after video interview, possibly drawing more attention to difficulties). No differences in outcomes seen between groups when measured 4 months posttreatment.	Yes Analyzed: HMS and HSS Total postscores
Hickson, Worrall, & Scarinci (2007)	RCT; 2 groups Placebo group n = 78 Treatment Group n =100 54% experienced HA users 46% non-HA users; No difference in frequency of reported HA use between groups	(ACE) Group AR program met for 2 hours per week for 5 weeks. Social program (placebo) followed by ACE met for 2 hours per week for 10 weeks. All but 7 subjects from the social program chose to complete the ACE program in the control group following the placebo.	HHQ, QDS, SAC, Shortened Ryff Scale, SF-36	Small effect sizes measured for within-group changes following ACE and the placebo social program for all outcomes (range d = 0.09–0.36), with greater benefits seen on 4 measures for ACE program (HHQ, QDS, SAC, Ryff) than for social placebo (QDS, SF-36 Mental Component). No significant change differences were found between groups following the ACE program as compared to the placebo social program.	Yes Analyzed: HHQ, QDS, and SAC Total postscores

continues

Table 10–3. *continued*

Study	*Design/Participants*	*Intervention*	*Participation/QoL Outcomes*	*Results*	*Included in Meta analysis?*
Preminger & Yoo (2010)	RCT, 3 groups Communication Strategies (CS) Group *n* = 18 CS + Psychosocial Exercises (CS + PS) *n* = 17 Information + PS (Info + PS) *n* = 17 Experienced HA users (at least 3 mo.)	AR group met 1 time per week, 1 hour per week, for 6 weeks. All participants completed at least 5 sessions.	HHIE, WHODAS II	CS + PS and Information + PS groups demonstrated large short- and long-term (6 months) effects on the HHIE, whereas the effect size demonstrated by the CS-only Group was medium. CS and Info + PS groups demonstrated mostly small short- and long-term (6 months) effects on specific portions of the WHODAS II.	Yes Analyzed: HHIE Total postscores
Preminger & Ziegler (2008)	RCT, 3 groups Control Group *n* = 16 Auditory Training + Psychosocial Exercises (AT + PS) *n* = 16 AT-only *n* = 18 Experienced HA users (at least 3 months)	AR group met 1 time per week, 1 hour per week, for 6 weeks. All participants completed at least 5 sessions.	HHIE, WHODAS II	*F*-test revealed a significant effect on HHIE Total Scores for time between baseline and 6-wk testing as well as follow-up testing at 6 months for all 3 groups. However, follow-up analysis of the subscales on the HHIE revealed a significant decrease of perceived handicap as measured by the Emotional Subscale for the training groups only. No significant effects were found on the WHODAS II for any group.	No Variance measures not available. I-test can be used to calculate *d*, but only for studies with two or less groups (including control).

Study	*Design/Participants*	*Intervention*	*Participation/QoL Outcomes*	*Results*	*Included in Meta analysis?*
Smaldino & Smaldino (1988)*	RCT; 4 groups Control Group *n* = 10 Cognitive Style Group (Cog) *n* = 10 AR Group *n* = 10 AR + Cog Group *n* = 10 New HA users	AR Group met 4 times (number of hours and days unreported)	HPI	Participation in group AR sessions resulted in reduced self perception of hearing handicap than hearing aid use + orientation alone.	Yes Analyzed: HPI Total postscores

[1] Participants the same as in Abrams et al. (2002).

Note: Studies marked with an asterisk were identified by Hawkins (2005), whereas the remaining studies were identified in the current literature search. APHAB = Abbreviated Profile of Hearing Aid Benefit (Cox & Alexander, 1995); CSS = Communication Strategies Subscale of the CPHI = Communication Profile for the Hearing Impaired (Demorest & Erdman, 1987); CSOA = Communication Scale for Older Adults (Kaplan, Bally, Brandt, Busacco, & Pray, 1997); HCA = Hearing Coping Assessment (Andersson, Melin, Lindberg, & Scott, 1995); HHQ = Hearing Handicap Questionnaire (Gatehouse & Noble, 2004); HMS = Hearing Measurement Scale (Noble & Atherley, 1970); HPI = Hearing Performance Inventory (Giolas, Owens, Lamb, & Schubert, 1979); HSS = Hearing Handicap Support Scale (Erlandsson, Hallberg & Axelsson, 1992); QDS = Quantified Denver Scale of Communication (Alpiner, Chevrette, Glascoe, Metz, & Olsen, 1978); QOL = Quality of Life; SAC = Self-Assessment of Communication (Schow & Nerbonne, 1982); WHODAS = World Health Organization Disability Assessment Scale (World Health Organization, 2001).

Although there were within-group reductions in perceived communication participation restrictions and activity limitations following ACE for both groups, between-group differences were not statistically significant. It should be noted, however, that greater within-group benefits were seen on four outcomes for the ACE groups (Hearing Handicap Questionnaire, Gatehouse & Noble, 2004; Quantified Denver Scale of Communicative Function, Alpiner, Chevrette, Glascoe, Metz, & Olsen, 1978; Self-Assessment of Communication, Schow & Nerbonne, 1982; Ryff Psychological Well-Being Scale, Hoen, Thelander, & Worsley, 1997) as compared to within-group benefits seen for the social placebo group, which were only evident on two outcomes following intervention (Quantified Denver Scale of Communicative Function; Short Form-36 Mental Component, Ware & Sherbourne, 1992).

In general, the participants in the studies reviewed were primarily older, although a wide age-range of individuals (30 to 90 years old) participated. All but one of the studies (Abrams et al., 1992) involved both male and female participants. All studies involved at least some participants who were hearing aid users, with both new and experienced users represented across the studies. In terms of the outcome measures, the majority of studies reported the use of outcome measures specifically designed for use in adults with hearing loss (i.e., disease-specific measures), such as the Hearing Handicap Inventory for the Elderly (HHIE; Ventry & Weinstein, 1982). Four studies (Abrams et al., 2002; Hickson et al., 2007; Preminger & Yoo, 2010; Preminger & Ziegler, 2008) reported results from the use of at least one generic QoL outcome measure.

In all studies short-term significant benefits were obtained from intervention, whether intervention was through hearing aid use alone (Abrams et al., 1992; Benyon et al., 1997; Chisolm et al., 2004; Preminger & Ziegler, 2008; Smaldino & Smaldino, 1988), through hearing aid use plus group aural rehabilitation (Abrams et al., 1992; Benyon et al., 1997; Chisolm et al., 1994; Preminger & Yoo, 2010; Preminger & Ziegler, 2008) or through the use of different approaches to group intervention, whether or not individuals within the groups used hearing aids (Halberg & Barrrenas, 1994; Hickson et al., 2007). Although the magnitude of pre- to postintervention differences were typically larger for those receiving the experimental forms of group aural rehabilitation, statistical significance in support of group aural rehabilitation was not always observed, and depended on the analyses conducted. For example, Abrams et al. (1992) demonstrated that treatment by hearing aids in combination with group aural rehabilitation participation resulted in a significantly greater reduction in the self-perception of hearing handicap than occurred for those who did not receive any intervention. The difference between hearing aid use alone and hearing aid use combined with group aural rehabilitation was statistically significant only when a 1-tailed *t*-test was utilized. In another study Chisolm et al. (2004) found a statistically significant interaction between test-time and treatment group (i.e., hearing aids alone vs. hearing aids plus group aural rehabilitation), with the results of post hoc analyses demonstrating a significant difference between the two intervention groups at the immediate, postintervention assessment. More recently, Preminger and Zeigler (2008) found significant improvements on the emotional subscale of the HHIE (Ventry & Weinstein, 1982) for hearing aid users who received group psychosocial and speech perception training and a treatment group that received speech perception training alone, but not for those who used hearing aids alone. There was no significant difference in outcome, however, between the groups that received treatment in addition to using hearing aids. Thus, as a whole the research provides support, albeit at times relatively weak, that led Hawkins (2005) to conclude that there were short-term benefits from participation in group aural rehabilitation.

As reported by Hawkins (2005), Hallberg and Barrenas (1994) found that their initial differential benefits of group AR participation were not maintained at 4 months postintervention. In contrast, the participants in the Chisolm et al. (2004) study maintained the differential benefits at 6 months. The maintenance of treatment benefits at 6-months postintervention was noted in the more recent studies by Hickson et al. (2007) and Preminger and Yoo (2010). Only two studies examined benefits at longer than 6 months postintervention, with Chisolm et al. showing no differential benefit of group AR participation after 1 year and Andersson et al. (1995b) showing no differential benefit of group AR participation after 2 years. Finally, there is minimal evidence that participation in a group AR program significantly impacts on generic measure of health-related QoL, either short- or long-term (Abrams et al., 2002; Hickson et al., 2007; Preminger & Yoo, 2010; Preminger & Ziegler, 2008).

In assessing the quality of the studies utilizing Dollaghan's (2007) guidelines (see the Appendix), it was determined that the aim of each of the studies was plausible and addressed the clinical question of whether or not participation in a group AR program positively impacted participation/QoL in adults with hearing loss (Table 10–4). All of the studies were analytic and prospective in nature, with the results section demonstrating that the aims of the study had been achieved and had clinical relevance. Although there was great similarity of the studies in factors that impact on both internal and external validity, there were several notable differences, which are summarized in Table 10–4. The primary differences between studies had to do with reporting of power analysis, blinding, and dropout rates. One outcome of EBP is increased attention to the adequacy of the sample size, and as reflected in Table 10–4, more recent studies have addressed sample size through reporting of power analyses. The study by Hickson and colleagues (2007) is the only one to report blinding of experimenters and participants. Although blinding participants may be difficult in studies examining the effects of aural rehabilitation (Boothroyd, 2007), the blinding of experimenters is not only feasible as demonstrated by Hickson and colleagues, but the lack of blinding can result in an inflation of the effect size (Cox, 2005). Finally, dropout rates varied across the studies with all but the study by Hallberg and Barrenas (1994) indicating a dropout rate of greater than 20%. Based on the quality assessment criteria utilized, the results of most studies were considered to be *suggestive;* that is different clinicians might responsibly make a different decision with regard to adopting the treatment. However, the three most recent studies were judged to provide *compelling* evidence for the inclusion of group aural rehabilitation (Chisolm et al., 2004; Hickson et al., 2007; Preminger & Yoo, 2010).

The lack of robust findings from individual studies highlights the need to further examine the research assessing the effect of participation in counseling-based group aural rehabilitation through conducting a meta-analysis. The same procedures as those described above for individual auditory training studies were utilized. To maintain consistency, data for meta-analysis was extracted from disease-specific outcomes immediately following treatment. Effect sizes were reported as standardized mean differences (*d*) for comparison across studies, a random-effects model for variability was employed, and individual studies were weighted for sample size. For counseling-based group aural rehabilitation, a standardized mean difference of −0.352 was found (Figure 10–4), with the 95% confidence intervals not crossing the zero point, suggesting the effect is statistically significant, despite the large amount of variability in the data among the individual studies analyzed.

Table 10–4. Quality Assessment of Group Aural Rehabilitation Studies

Study	*Aims: Plausible and Relevant*	*Methods*	*Results: Achieve Goals and Clinically Significant*	*Control Group*	*Random-ization*	*Power*	*Groups Similar*	*Blinding*	*Dropouts <20%*	*Overall Judgment*
Abrams et al. (1992)*	Yes	Prospective, Analytic	Yes	Yes	Yes	No	Yes	No	Yes	Suggestive
Abrams et al. (2002*)	Yes	Prospective, Analytic	Yes	Yes	Yes	Yes	Yes	No	Yes	Suggestive
Andersson et al. (1995a, 1995b)*	Yes	Prospective, Analytic	Yes	Yes	Yes	No	Yes	No	Yes	Suggestive
Benyon et al. (1997)*	Yes	Prospective, Analytic	Yes	Yes	Yes	No	Yes	No	Yes	Suggestive
Chisolm et al. (2004)*	Yes	Prospective, Analytic	Yes	Yes	Yes	Yes	Yes	No	Yes	Compelling
Hallberg & Barrenas (1994)*	Yes	Prospective, Analytic	Yes	Yes	Yes	No	Yes	No	No	Suggestive
Hickson et al. (2007)	Yes	Prospective, Analytic	Yes	Yes	Yes	Yes	Yes	Yes	Yes	Compelling
Preminger & Ziegler (2008)	Yes	Prospective, Analytic	Yes	Yes	Yes	Yes	Yes	No	Yes	Compelling
Preminger & Yoo (2010)	Yes	Prospective, Analytic	Yes	No	Yes	Yes	Yes	No	Yes	Compelling
Smaldino & Smaldino (1988)*	Yes	Prospective, Analytic	Yes	Yes	Yes	No	Yes	No	Yes	Equivocal

Note: Studies included in the Hawkins (2005) review are marked with an asterisk. “Compelling” = adoption of the intervention should be considered seriously; “Suggestive” = different clinicians might responsibly make different decision about whether to adopt the intervention; “Equivocal” = the intervention should not be adopted.

Study name	Subgroup within study	Outcome	Statistics for each study: Std diff in means	Lower limit	Upper limit
Abrams et al. 1992	HA+AR vs. HA	HHIE Total	-0.623	-1.479	0.233
Abrams et al. 1992	HA+AR vs. NT	HHIE Total	-1.757	-2.792	-0.721
Andersson et al. 1995a	HA+AR vs. HA	HCA	-0.230	-1.033	0.573
Chisolm et al. 2004	HA+AR vs. HA	CPHI ADJ	-0.333	-0.716	0.050
Hallberg & Barrenas 1994	AR vs. NT	Combined	-0.299	-0.996	0.398
Smaldino & Smaldino 1988	HA+AR1 vs. HA	HPI	-0.435	-1.322	0.452
Smaldino & Smaldino 1988	HA+AR2 vs. HA	HPI	-0.172	-1.050	0.706
Smaldino & Smaldino 1988	HA+AR3 vs. HA	HPI	-1.171	-2.119	-0.222
Hickson et al. 2007	AR vs. Placebo	Combined	-0.303	-0.454	-0.153
Preminger & Yoo 2010	HA+AR1 vs. HA	HHIE Total	-0.445	-45.328	44.438
Preminger & Yoo 2010	HA+AR2 vs. HA	HHIE Total	-0.787	-35.674	34.100
Preminger & Yoo 2010	HA+AR3 vs. HA	HHIE Total	-0.775	-40.758	39.208
TOTAL			**-0.352**	**-0.483**	**-0.221**

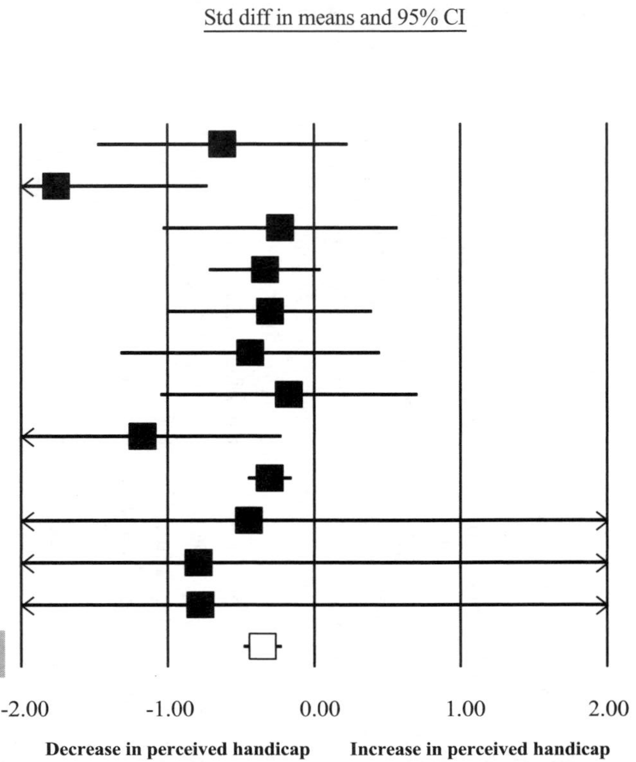

Std diff in means and 95% CI
-2.00
-1.00
0.00
1.00
2.00
Decrease in perceived handicap
Increase in perceived handicap

Note: AR=Aural rehabilitation; CPHI ADJ=Communication Profile for the Hearing Impaired Adjustment Factor; HA=Hearing aid; HCA=Hearing Coping Assessment; HHIE=Hearing Handicap Inventory for the Elderly; HPI=Hearing Performance Inventory; Info=Informational counseling; NT=No treatment

Figure 10–4. *Forest plot showing group AR effects.*

In Figure 10–4, negative effect sizes indicate a reduction in the self-perception of hearing handicap, which is the desired treatment outcome. As with individual auditory training, participation in group aural rehabilitation programs provides a small, yet reliable effect. In addition to providing a benchmark to which the results of future studies can be compared, the effect size found here suggests that clinicians can recommend participation in a group aural rehabilitation program with increased confidence. Furthermore, at least in the short term, there are benefits of adult AR groups with regard to improving outcomes related to self-perceived participation restrictions due to a hearing loss.

CLINICAL IMPLICATIONS AND RESEARCH NEEDS

As evidence-based practitioners, it is important that we seek to guide adult aural rehabilitation through the highest quality of research evidence available. Current approaches to adult aural rehabilitation often include individual auditory perceptual training and participation in group aural rehabilitation programs. As EBP gained momentum in the last decades, two systematic reviews were published addressing these two key components of adult aural rehabilitation. The systematic reviews of by Sweetow and Palmer (2005) and Hawkins (2005) provided evidence that clinical services including individual perceptual training and/or participation in a group AR program was at least minimally supported through the research literature. In both reviews, however, the need for completion of continued, high quality research studies was noted. In the present chapter, we have updated the Sweetow and Palmer and Hawkins systematic reviews, and conducted meta-analyses to provide estimates of effect sizes. These updated reviews indicated that both individual auditory-perceptual training and counseling-based group aural rehabilitation programs have a small, but reliable positive effect on outcomes related to the activities of speech recognition and participation restriction, respectively. These findings suggest that, for the average patient, clinicians should be fairly confident that auditory-perceptual and/or counseling-based group aural rehabilitation will likely lead to positive outcomes, at least in the short-term. As discussed by Chisolm et al. (2004), short-term outcomes may be particularly important for the new hearing aid user, as it is during the initial trial period that the decision of whether or not to continue use of amplification occurs. If outcomes can be improved, this may lead to greater satisfaction, lower return rates, and ultimately better outcomes for individual patients.

A critical issue for clinicians, and thus for future research, relates to the identification of which individual clients will benefit most from which aspects of aural rehabilitation. A key tenet of EBP is that it starts with the individual client and ends with the individual client. Perceptual training and group AR have a reliable effect, but the effects are not large. This may be due to differences in individual need. For example, Sweetow and Sabes (2006) demonstrated that individuals with poorer baseline performance on LACE™ tasks ultimately ended up showing greater improvement gains following computerized auditory training, given essentially similar hearing losses, as those who performed significantly better on baseline measures. It is also possible that certain individuals may be more responsive to certain types of intervention. For example, it has been shown that personality type is associated with self-reported hearing aid outcomes (Cox, Alexander, & Gray, 2007).

Of course, expanding services can increase the costs of intervention, which is another reason that individual need for and responsiveness to various components of adult aural rehabilitation needs to be further explored. Despite the need for further research, the addition of many components to adult aural rehabilitation does not have to be financially prohibitive. With the advent of computer-based approaches to perceptual training, the cost benefit ratio is likely to be highly favorable. Furthermore, group treatment can be very cost effective. For example, Abrams et al. (2002) demonstrated that cost-effectiveness of group AR participation, in conjunction with hearing aid fitting, was actually less expensive in terms of costs per quality-adjusted life-year gained (QALY) than was hearing aid intervention alone. It will be important in future studies to measure cost benefits as well as clinical outcomes in order to increase the evidence-base for adult aural rehabilitation. Absolute costs may increase as a result of holistic aural rehabilitation as opposed to simple hearing aid dispensing, but the costs do not have to be enormous and can be justified when we demonstrate improved outcomes.

REFERENCES

Abrams, H. B., Chisolm, T., & McArdle, M. S. (2002). A cost-utility analysis of adult group audiologic rehabilitation: Are the benefits worth the cost? *Journal of Rehabilitation Research and Development, 39*(5), 549–558.

Abrams, H. B., Hnath-Chisolm, T., Guerreiro, S. M., & Ritterman, S. I. (1992). The effects of intervention strategy on self-perception of hearing handicap. *Ear and Hearing, 13*(5), 371–377.

Alpiner, J. G., Chevrette, W., Glascoe, G., Metz, M., & Olsen, B. (1978). The Denver scale of communication function. In J. Alpiner (Ed.), *Adult rehabilitative audiology* (pp. 53–56). Baltimore, MD: Williams & Wilkins.

American Psychological Association. (1994). *Publication manual of the American Psychological Association* (5th ed.). Washington, DC: Author.

Andersson, G., Melin, L., Lindberg, P., & Scott, B. (1995). Development of a short scale for self-assessment of experiences of hearing loss: The hearing coping assessment. *Scandinavian Audiology, 24*(3), 147–154.

Andersson, G., Melin, L., Scott, B., & Lindberg, P. (1995a). An evaluation of a behavioral treatment approach to hearing impairment. *Behavioral Research and Therapy, 33*(3), 283–292.

Andersson, G., Melin, L., Scott, B., & Lindberg, P. (1995b). A two-year follow-up examination of a behavioural treatment approach to hearing tactics. *British Journal of Audiology, 29*, 347–354.

Benyon, G., Thornton, F., & Poole, C. (1997). A randomized, controlled trial of the efficacy of a communication course for first time hearing aid users. *British Journal of Audiology, 31*(5), 345–351.

Bergman, M. (2002). On the origins of Audiology: American wartime military audiology. *Audiology Today, Monograph 1.*

Bilger, R. C., Nuetzel, J. M., Rabinowitz, W. M., & Rzeczkowski, C. (1984). Standardization of a test of speech perception in noise. *Journal of Speech and Hearing Research, 27*, 32–48.

Bode, D. L., & Oyer, H. J. (1970). Auditory training and speech discrimination. *Journal of Speech and Hearing Research, 13*(4), 839–855.

Boothroyd, A. (2007). Adult aural rehabilitation: What is it and does it work? *Trends in Amplification, 11*(2), 63–71.

Borenstein, M., Hedges, L.V., Higgins, J. P. T., & Rothstein, H. R. (2009). *Introduction to meta-analysis.* Hoboken, NJ: John Wiley & Sons.

Bradley, C., Todd, C., Gorton, T., Symonds, E., Martin, A., & Plowright, R. (1999). The development of an individualized questionnaire measure of perceived impact of diabetes on quality of life: The ADDQoL. *Quality of Life Research, 8*, 79–91.

Brewer, D. (2001). Considerations in measuring effectiveness of group audiologic rehabilitation classes. *Journal of the Academy of Rehabilitative Audiology, 34*, 53–60.

Brickley, G., Cleaver, V., & Bailey, S. (1996). An evaluation of a group follow-up scheme for new NHS hearing aid users. *British Journal of Audiology, 30*, 307–312.

Burk, M. H., & Humes, L. E. (2008). Effects of long-term training on aided speech-recognition performance in noise in older adults. *Journal of Speech, Language, and Hearing Research, 51*, 759–771.

Chisolm, T., Abrams, H., & McArdle, R. (2004). Short and long-term outcomes of adult audiologic rehabilitation. *Ear and Hearing, 25*(5), 464–477.

Chisolm, T. H., & Abrams, H. (2007). Measuring the effects of audiology treatment on health-related quality of life. *Perspectives on Aural Rehabilitation and its Instrumentation, ASHA Special Interest Division 7, 14*(1), 2–6.

Cox, R. M. (2005). Evidence-based practice in provision of amplification. *Journal of the American Academy of Audiology, 16*, 419–438.

Cox, R. M., & Alexander, G. C. (1995). The abbreviated profile of hearing aid benefit. *Ear and Hearing, 16*(2), 176–186.

Cox, R. M., Alexander, G. C., & Gilmore, C. (1987). Development of the Connected Speech Test (CST). *Ear and Hearing, 8*(Suppl.), 119S–126S.

Cox, R. M., Alexander, G. A., & Gray, G. A. (2007). Personality, hearing problems, and amplification characteristics: Contributions to self-report hearing aid outcomes. *Ear and Hearing, 28*, 141–162.

Dalton, D. S., Cruickshanks, K. J., Klein, B. E., Klein, R., Wiley, T. L., & Nondahl, D. M. (2003). The impact of hearing loss on quality of life in older adults. *Gerontologist, 4*, 661–668.

Demorest, M. E., & Erdman, S. A. (1987). Development of the communication profile for the hearing impaired. *Journal of Speech and Hearing Disorders, 52*(2), 129–143.

Dollaghan, C. (2007). *Handbook for evidence based practice in communication disorders.* Baltimore, MD: Paul H. Brookes.

Erlandsson, S. I., Hallberg, L. M., & Axelsson, A. (1992). Psychological and audiological correlates of perceived tinnitus severity. *Audiology, 31*, 168–179.

Gatehouse, S., & Noble, W. (2004). The Speech, Spatial, and Qualities of Hearing scale (SSQ). *International Journal of Audiology, 43(2)*, 85–99.

Giolas, T. G., Owens, E., Lamb, S. H., & Schubert, E. D. (1979). Hearing performance inventory. *Journal of Speech and Hearing Disorders, 44*(2), 169–195.

Hallberg, L., & Barrenas, M. (1994). Group rehabilitation of middle-aged males with noise induced hearing loss and their spouses: Evaluation of short- and long-term effects. *British Journal of Audiology, 28*, 71–79.

Harris, J., Haines, H., Kelsey, P., & Clark, T. (1961). The relation between speech intelligibility and electroacoustic characteristics of low fidelity circuitry. *Journal of Audiological Research, 1*, 357–381.

Hawkins, D. B. (2005). Effectiveness of counseling-based adult group aural rehabilitation programs: A systematic review of the evidence. *Journal of the American Academy of Audiology, 16*, 485–493.

Hickson, L., Worrall, L., & Scarinci, N. (2007). A randomized controlled trial evaluating the active communication education program for older people with hearing impairment. *Ear and Hearing, 28*(2), 212–230.

Hirsch, I. J., Davis, H., Silverman, S. R., Reynolds, E. G., Eldert, E., & Benson, R.W. (1952). Development of materials for speech audiometry. *Journal of Speech and Hearing Disorders, 17*, 321–337.

Hoen, B., Thelander, M., & Worsley, J. (1997). Improvement in psychological well-being of people with aphasia and their families: Evaluation of a community-based programme. *Aphasiology, 11*(7), 681–691.

House, A., Williams, C., Hecker, M., & Kryter, K. (1965). Articulation testing methods: Consonantal differentiation with a closed response set. *Journal of the Acoustical Society of America, 37*, 158–166.

Humes, L. E., Burk, M. H., Strauser, L. E., & Kinney, D. L. (2009). Development and efficacy of a frequent-word auditory training protocol for older adults with impaired hearing. *Ear and Hearing, 30*(5), 613–627.

Kaplan, H., Bally, S., Brandt, F., Busacco, D., & Pray, J. (1997). Communication scale for older adults (CSOA). *Journal of the American Academy of Audiology, 8*(3), 203–217.

Kricos, P., Holmes, A., & Doyle, D. (1992). Efficacy of a communication training program for hearing impaired elderly adults. *Journal of the Academy of Rehabilitative Audiology, 25*, 69–80.

Kricos, P., & Holmes, A. (1996). Efficacy of audiologic rehabilitation for older adults. *Journal of the American Academy of Audiology, 7*, 219–229.

Kricos, P. B., & McCarthy, P. (2007). From ear to there: Historical perspective on auditory training. *Seminars in Hearing, 26*, 89–99.

Montgomery, A., Walden, B., Schwartz, D., & Prosek, R. (1984). Training auditory-visual speech recognition in adults with moderate sensorineural hearing loss. *Ear and Hearing, 5*(1), 30–36.

Mulrow, C. D., Aguilar, C., Endicott, J. E., Velez, R., Tuley, M. R., Charlip, W. S., & Hill, J. A. (1990). Association between hearing impairment and the quality of life of elderly individuals. *Journal of the American Geriatric Society, 38*, 45–50.

Nilsson, M., Soli, S. D., & Sullivan, J. A. (1994). Development of the hearing in noise test for the measurement of speech reception thresholds in quiet and in noise. *Journal of the Acoustical Society of America, 95*, 1085–1099.

Noble, W. G., & Atherley, G. R. C. (1970). The Hearing Measure Scale: A questionnaire for the assessment of auditory disability. *Journal of Auditory Research, 10*, 229–250.

Norman, M., George, C., Downie, A., & Milligan, J. (1995). Evaluation of a communication course for new hearing aid users. *Scandiavian Audiology, 24*, 63–69.

Pratt, S. (2005). Adult audiologic rehabilitation. *Access Audiology, 4*(2). Retrieved December 27, 2010, from http://www.asha.org/aud/articles/adultaudrehab.htm

Preminger, J. (2003). Should significant others be encouraged to join adult group aural rehabilitation classes? *Journal of the American Academy of Audiology, 14*(10), 545–555.

Preminger, J. E. (2007). Issues associated with the measurement of psychosocial benefits of group audiological rehabilitation programs. *Trends in Amplification, 11*(2), 113–123.

Preminger, J. E., & Yoo, J. K. (2010). Do group audiologic rehabilitation activities influence psychosocial outcomes? *American Journal of Audiology, 19*(2), 109–125.

Preminger, J. E., & Ziegler, C. H. (2008). Can auditory and visual speech perception be trained within a group setting? *American Journal of Audiology, 17*, 80–97.

Resnick, S., Dubno, J. R., Hoffnung, S., & Levitt, H. (1975). Phoneme errors on a nonsense syllable test. *Journal of the Acoustical Society of America, 58*(Suppl.), 114.

Rubenstein, A., & Boothroyd, A. (1987). Effect of two approaches to auditory training on speech recognition by hearing impaired adults. *Journal of Speech and Hearing Research, 30*(2), 153–160.

Schow, R. L., & Nerbonne, M. A. (1982). Communication screening profile: Use with elderly clients. *Ear and Hearing, 3*, 134–147.

Smaldino, S., & Smaldino, J. (1988). The influence of aural rehabilitation and cognitive style disclosure on the perception of hearing handicap. *Journal of the Academy of Rehabilitative Audiology, 21*, 57–64.

Stecker, G., Bowman, G. A., Yund, E. W., Herron, T. J., Roup, C. M., & Woods, D. L. (2006). Perceptual training improves syllable identification in new and experienced hearing aid users. *Journal of Rehabilitation Research and Development, 43*(4), 537–552.

Sweetow, R., & Palmer, C. V. (2005). Efficacy of individual auditory training in adults: A systematic review of the evidence. *Journal of the American Academy of Audiology, 16*, 494–504.

Sweetow, R. W., & Sabes, J. H. (2006). The need for and development of an Adaptive Listening and Communication Enhancement (LACE) program. *Journal of the American Academy of Audiology, 17*, 538–558.

Taylor, B., & Shrive, A. (2008). The economics of computer-based auditory training. *Audiology Online.* Retrieved December 27, 2010, from http://www.audiologyonline.com/articles/article_detail.asp?article_id=2060

Thalheimer, W., & Cook, S. (2002). *How to calculate effect sizes from published research: A simplified methodology.* Retrieved September 15, 2010, from http://work-learning.com/effect_sizes.htm

United States Department of Veteran Affairs. (1998). *Veterans Administration Sentence Test (VAST).* Mountain Home, TN: VA Medical Center.

Ventry, I. M., & Weinstein, B. E. (1982). The hearing handicap inventory for the elderly: A new tool. *Ear and Hearing, 3(3)*, 128–134.

Walden, B., Erdman, S., Montgomery, A., Schwartz, D., & Prosek, R. (1981). Some effects of training on speech recognition by hearing-impaired adults. *Journal of Speech and Hearing Research, 24*(2), 207–216.

Ware, J. E., & Sherbourne, C. D. (1992). The MOS 36-item short-form health survey (SF-36). I. Conceptual framework and item selection. *Medical Care, 30*(6), 473–483.

World Health Organization. (2001). *International Classification of Functioning, Disability, and Health (ICF).* Geneva, Switzerland: Author.

World Health Organization. (2006). *Primary ear and hearing care training resource: Advanced.* Geneva, Switzerland: Author.

CHAPTER 11

Evidence About the Effectiveness of Treatments Related to Tinnitus

William Noble

TINNITUS EFFECTS AND THEIR ASSESSMENT

In a recent study (Noble, Naylor, Bhullar, & Akeroyd, 2012), respondents were asked to answer "yes" or "no" to the question, "Do you have difficulty with your hearing?" They were also asked to rate their ability on six items from the Speech, Spatial and Qualities of Hearing scale (SSQ: Gatehouse & Noble, 2004). Two groups from the general population, aged 50 to 80 years, each of about 100 people, were constructed, comprising: (1) Those who said yes they did have hearing difficulty and gave low ratings of their abilities; and (2) those who said no they did not have hearing difficulty and gave high ratings of their abilities. Both of these response patterns were consistent with what would be expected. But it was also possible to construct similarly-sized and otherwise matched groups who gave inconsistent answers, in particular, one group comprising those who said they *did* have hearing difficulty yet gave high ability ratings.

It turned out that the group with self-reported hearing difficulty but high ability ratings had a significantly greater incidence of tinnitus than the group who said they did not have hearing difficulty and also gave high ability ratings. This suggests that the factor of tinnitus can provoke a "yes" response to a general question about "hearing difficulty," even among people who otherwise rate their hearing ability as high. Such an outcome reinforces the point that tinnitus interferes with hearing function, a finding observed by Tyler and Baker (1983), where respondents noted decrements in, for example, speech signal discrimination and spatial localization, as direct effects of tinnitus on hearing. This feature of tinnitus can get overlooked among the more common reports about the sheer persistence and distressfulness of this auditory phenomenon (e.g., McKenna, 2004).

It is, nonetheless, the emotional response to tinnitus that seems to have attracted the greater amount of clinical and research attention. Most people who report persistent tinnitus are not unduly or continually distressed by it. Somewhere between 10 to 20% of the adult population reports persistent tinnitus (Preece, Tyler, & Noble, 2003): these estimates probably vary with different definitions of chronicity. But a significant minority, about one-tenth of people with persistent tinnitus, are very much distressed by it (Axelsson & Ringdahl, 1989). Many fear they are being driven insane by the uncontrollable and unwanted noise internal to their ears/head (Henry & Wilson, 2001). The strength of such emotional distress, long-term, can be predicted by initial reactions of anxiety, and anxiety-related behaviors, such as sleeplessness (Langenbach, Olderog, Michel, Albus, & Kohle, 2005). Fear about the implications of tinnitus, well-founded or not, along with its sheer persistence, drive overattention to and continuing distress about the experience. These reactions sit alongside the sheer interference with hearing mentioned above.

Clinicians thus are confronted by people who are often "at the end of their tether" emotionally because of chronic tinnitus. And in company of researchers and practitioners with pharmaceutical, neurophysiological, or biomedical/bioengineering backgrounds and interests, they strive to identify interventions that will simply remove or at least moderate the tinnitus sound, and hence their patients' distress. There are a number of clinical questions that may arise in the quest to engage in Evidence-Based Practice (EBP) in this context. For example, the clinician and the client could formulate the following question using the PICO format described in Chapter 1: For tinnitus (P = Problem), is hearing aid fitting (I = Intervention) superior to Cognitive Behavior Therapy (C = Comparison) for reducing distress (O = Outcome) associated with the tinnitus? There are many similar questions in this field that could be posed. In a recent issue of the Tinnitus Research Initiative Newsletter there was a short piece titled: "We must cure tinnitus, we can cure tinnitus, and we will cure tinnitus" (Langguth, Elgoyhen, De Ridder, & Staudinger, 2010). Such a heroic stand raises strong expectations that the tools of medical science, so effectively applied in many other areas of clinical intervention and management, will indeed be made to work in this area too.

How confident can we be that an effective treatment for tinnitus is identifiable? A significant feature in seeking to answer such a question is methodical literature reviewing. A high standard of reviewing is represented in the Cochrane Database of Systematic Reviews, a library of reviews and, where feasible, meta-analyses, resulting from selection of reports according to criteria described in the *Cochrane Handbook for Systematic Reviews of Interventions* (Higgins & Green, 2009). This reviewing system relies on independent investigators working critically with each other on bodies of literature. The reviews are updated from time to time to check the currency of earlier conclusions. Wherever possible in the present chapter, use has been made of any such review or meta-analysis.

A further key feature in identifying effective treatment is represented by the measures used to assess tinnitus. The Tinnitus Effects Questionnaire (Hallam, Jakes, & Hinchcliffe, 1988) and the Tinnitus Handicap Questionnaire (Kuk, Tyler, Russell, & Jordan, 1990) are referred to at several points in the ensuing review as recognized standard measures of tinnitus disabilities and handicaps.[1] The Tinnitus Effects Questionnaire is also in a German version, known as the Tinnitus Questionnaire (Hiller & Goebel, 1992). The Tinnitus Reaction Questionnaire (Wilson, Henry, Bowen, & Haralambous, 1991) is focused more on emotional and social handicaps; it has also achieved general recognition. The psychometric properties of these scales are robust and

[1] *Handicap* is defined here as nonauditory consequences of hearing disorder, for example, emotional distress and depression due to tinnitus (World Health Organization, 1980); the term contrasts with *disability*, which refers to auditory consequences of disorder: for example, the problems of discrimination and spatial localization mentioned at the start of the chapter.

have been independently verified (see Noble, 2001, for a review). Newman, Jacobson, and Spitzer (1996) developed the Tinnitus Handicap Inventory; the claimed three-factor structure of this scale has not been independently verified. Baguley, Andersson, Moffat, Humphriss, and Moffat (2002) reported a single-factor structure; Zachariae et al. (2000) applied a Danish version of the Tinnitus Handicap Inventory, and their results also suggested a single-factor structure. The Tinnitus Handicap Inventory otherwise has good psychometric performance. It is widely used, reflecting its origin in the US Veterans Administration. As noted, some researchers have used other measurement devices, including custom-designed questionnaires and visual analogue scales.

The next two sections of the following review address, respectively, evidence about the effectiveness of a range of pharmaceutical and physical procedures that have been offered as possible cures for tinnitus. None of these provides a reliable or lasting remedy. Some, such as electrical stimulation, show considerable promise; one, acoustic amplification, offers a useful palliative. The subsequent section gives a review of evidence about the effectiveness of psychological and biobehavioral treatment approaches to the tinnitus sufferer's reaction to the tinnitus. The latter approaches have the aim, not of addressing the tinnitus as such, but of modifying distressed reactions to it. It emerges that cognitive behavior therapy (CBT) is the most effective of such interventions (Hesser, Weise, Westin, & Andersson, 2011; Martinez-Devesa, Perera, Theodoulou, & Waddell, 2010). A recent development links application of CBT with biofeedback training (Heinecke, Weise, & Rief, 2009; Weise, Heinecke, & Rief, 2008), and looks like a worthwhile and effective combination treatment. Finally, a case is set out for the management of tinnitus that combines the skills of clinical audiology with clinical psychology.

TYPES OF TREATMENT ADDRESSED DIRECTLY TO TINNITUS

Pharmacological Treatments

Topical application of pharmacological agents such as local anaesthetics and anticonvulsants are known to have immediate suppressive effects on certain kinds of tinnitus (e.g., Baguley, Jones, Wilkins, Axon, & Moffat, 2005; Kallio et al., 2008; Nam, Handzel, & Levine, 2010). But there are no lasting effects from treatment using such substances. That patients seek possible remedies of this sort for their tinnitus is an indication of the desperate situation many people confront.

Less dramatically, a wide range of proprietary compounds and herbal products variously used to address depression, anxiety, or as dietary supplements have been proposed as candidates for the direct treatment of tinnitus. In the case of some of these agents, a plausible or hypothetical mechanism can be argued for (e.g., Fornaro & Martino, 2010). In other cases, it is hard to see what logic informs the case for using the substance. For example, ginkgo biloba is often advocated for, but there is no obvious reason why, and there is no good evidence of its effectiveness (Hilton & Stuart, 2004). On a more general note, reviews by Dobie (1999, 2004) and Langguth, Salvi, and Belen Elgoyhen, (2009) indicate no lasting direct effect on tinnitus presence or severity for any of the substantial set of pharmacological preparations that have been tried to date.

A recently updated Cochrane review (Baldo, Doree, Lazzarini, Molin, & McFerran, 2009) addressed specifically to the use of antidepressants for tinnitus relief identified six studies that met threshold inclusion criteria, namely, "randomized controlled clinical studies of antidepressant drugs versus placebo in patients with tinnitus" (p. 1). The studies were by Bayar, Boke, Turan, and Belgin (2001), Dib, Casse, Alives de Andrade, Testa, and Cruz (2007), Mihail et al. (1988), Podoshin, Ben-David, Fradis, Malatskey, and Hafner (1995), Robinson et al. (2005), and Sullivan, Katon, Russo, Dobie, and Sakai (1993). Of those six, only the trial by Robinson et al. (2005) achieved top rating for overall methodological quality. Across the six trials there was heterogeneity of populations (e.g., depressed/nondepressed), of drugs used, and level of standardization of the measures of tinnitus severity. There were also variable standards for ensuring participants and researchers were blind to the treatment versus placebo condition, and there was little attention paid to long-term follow-up.

A consequence of these shortcomings was that the reviewers could come to no firm conclusion about the effectiveness of the class of the more traditional tricyclic antidepressants in tinnitus reduction. The study by Robinson et al. (2005) involved use of the more recently developed type of antidepressant (selective serotonin reuptake inhibitor—SSRI), claimed to be more specific as an agent. The theory behind antidepressant action is that altering serotonin levels in the nervous system affects auditory action potentials, and this may directly reduce the spontaneous neural activity understood to be one possible generator of the tinnitus experience. Additionally, reducing signs of anxiety and depression may indirectly improve the person's capacity to cope with tinnitus. As it happens, Robinson et al. (2005) had only one case of diagnosable depression, so there was little headroom for measures on that dimension to show any change. The main outcome, however, was no difference between the SSRI paroxetine and placebo control groups on various measures of tinnitus loudness and severity (sensation level; Tinnitus Handicap Questionnaire [Kuk et al., 1990]). An exception was response to one informal inquiry about the extent to which tinnitus was aggravating. The difference here was as much due to an increase in the placebo group's ratings on this dimension as it was to a decrease in the treatment group.

A subgroup of participants in the Robinson et al. (2005) study reached the highest dosage of the active drug and did show significant reduction in tinnitus self-ratings and sensation level compared to the placebo group. In their own review of studies of antidepressant treatments for tinnitus, Robinson, Viirre, and Stein (2004) concluded that the effect of SSRI is to make tinnitus less annoying. Baldo et al. (2009) note that reported dropout rates were high in the studies they reviewed, and Robinson et al. (2005) observed a substantial occurrence of adverse side effects in the treatment condition. Given that the participants in their study did not show signs of depression, it may be concluded that use of antidepressants as an approach to tinnitus unaccompanied by other relevant pathology is somewhat heroic.

Physical Treatments

Hearing Aids

Hearing aids have long been used in this area with Vernon (e.g., 1977) a consistent advocate of the benefit of amplification as a means of relieving tinnitus. Early evidence came from Surr, Montgomery, and Mueller (1985) who reported that fitting of hearing aids in a sample of Veterans had beneficial effects in about 50% of 200 new cases, as assessed with a custom questionnaire 1 to 2 months after fitting.

Trotter and Donaldson (2008) reported the results of a long-running program of hearing aid fitting that formed part of the protocol in their tinnitus clinic. Over a 25-year period, a total of 2,153 patients were fitted either with one or with two hearing aids, depending on presentation and amplification needs. As this was not an experimental design there was no control group, and so the "subjective symptomatic improvement" in tinnitus perception (reflected in scores on a visual analogue scale), following hearing aid provision, cannot be compared with what may have happened in the absence of such provision. But a feature of these data is a change from analogue to digital devices in the last 5 years of the reporting period. The degree of "symptomatic improvement" showed a distinct increase following introduction of the digital device. The authors attribute this upturn to the broader bandwidth offered by the more recent hearing aid models, providing improved tinnitus masking at higher frequencies. It should be noted that use of amplification only acts as a partial tinnitus masker, and appears to have little or no influence on the tinnitus signal itself (Moffat et al., 2009).

The case where patients do not opt to use a hearing aid, or a personally worn noise masker, is illustrated in a study by Folmer and Carroll (2006). They followed up on 50 patients who adopted the recommendation to use hearing aids, 50 who opted for noise maskers and 50 who opted for neither. Among measures used in this study was a custom 12-item self-report scale inquiring about personal, social and emotional handicaps due to tinnitus. The custom self-report scale used by Folmer and Carroll (2006) was administered at pre-treatment and, on average, 18 months following that treatment. The three groups (hearing aid, masker, neither) all showed statistically significant reduction in handicap scores, but the hearing aid group's score went from 38.2 (out of maximum 56) to 29.6, whereas the no-device group went from 38.1 to 33.8. The masker group had an intermediate change in score. It is important to note that there were also differences between the groups in terms of average hearing threshold levels in the 0.5 to 4 kHz range: the hearing aid group had the poorest hearing (i.e., 40 dB average), the no device group had an average of about 26 dB and the masker group had the best hearing with an average of 15 dB. The contrast in hearing level between people opting to use a hearing aid versus a masking device features again in the next section of this review.

Searchfield, Kaur, and Martin (2010) compared pretreatment with 12-months posttreatment responses on the Tinnitus Handicap Questionnaire (Kuk et al., 1990) in a group of 29 tinnitus patients opting to use hearing aids, compared with 29 patients opting for a brief counseling session. The groups were matched for age, duration of tinnitus, and pretreatment THQ scores. The aided group's hearing threshold levels were about 10 to 15 dB higher than those of the brief counseling group at 4 and 6kHz. The hearing aid group showed a substantial, statistically significant reduction in THQ score (from 59% to 37%), in contrast to the counseling group (51% to 44%). It is mentioned in Searchfield's report that open earmould fittings were often selected by those opting to use hearing aids. Del Bo and colleagues (2006) assessed the results of use of such fittings in a group of 22 tinnitus patients with hearing threshold levels similar to those in the Searchfield et al. (2010) sample. Del Bo et al. used the Tinnitus Handicap Inventory (Newman, Jacobson, & Spitzer, 1996) and observed 50% reduction in tinnitus severity using that measure at 7 months follow-up.

Some earlier reports (e.g. Melin, Scott, Lindberg, & Lyttkens, 1987) have concluded that hearing aids do not seem to offer moderation of experienced tinnitus severity. But improvements in device design and signal delivery have occurred in the last two decades, and these seem to address tinnitus masking more effectively, as shown in the Trotter and Donaldson (2008) study. Thus, where otherwise indicated (and this would surely be for a large proportion of tinnitus sufferers), broadband acoustic amplification and open-earmold coupling could be of benefit. Certainly, the studies reviewed here strongly suggest that systematic investigation of different hearing aid profiles and frequency responses in relation to tinnitus experience is a worthy research topic and would make a substantial contribution to EBP in this field.

Masker

As shown from the Folmer and Carroll (2006) report, referred to in the previous section, masking devices are more favored by people whose tinnitus is not paired with reduced hearing ability. This was also observed by Stephens and Corcoran (1985). Such findings make intuitive sense; in the comparative absence of hearing loss, low-level masking may be tolerable as a form of distraction from the tinnitus, but could become aversive as masking level has to be increased to match increasing hearing threshold levels, causing further interference with the already challenging task of detecting/discriminating wanted external signals. There is not enough known about factors influencing the use and acceptance of masking devices; this is an area that might repay further investigation.

Laser

A recent report (Teggi, Bellini, Piccioni, Palonta, & Bussi, 2009) confirms an earlier one (Mirz et al., 1999) that exposure of the cochlea via the ear canal to low-level laser energy (a highly coherent form of light) has no influence on tinnitus severity. The evidence for the lack of an effect here is strong with both studies using a double-blind, placebo-controlled design, with random assignment of cases to the laser or inactive treatment. The findings are not surprising as there is little or no theoretical ground on which to expect an outcome using this kind of intervention. Claims are made for the effectiveness of this treatment in the case of chronic pain; by analogy, tinnitus may be conceptualized as a form of "pain response," especially if it is induced by repeated exposure to painfully loud noise.

Magnetic and Electrical Stimulation

Supracranial. There has been increasing attention to repetitive transcranial magnetic stimulation based on an argument that this may reduce the amount of overactivity observed in the auditory cortex, taken as a sign of tinnitus (De Ridder et al., 2004). Anders et al. (2010) observed a persistent, small difference between real and sham treatment groups on the Tinnitus Handicap Inventory (Newman et al., 1996) and the Tinnitus Questionnaire (Hiller & Goebel, 1992). The data indicated that the difference persisted for at least 14 weeks.

Attention has also been given to the related procedure of applying direct, low-level electrical stimulation to cranial surfaces: more radically, subcranial electrical stimulation has become a topic of clinical research investigation. It should be noted in this context that significant reduction in rated tinnitus loudness (visual analog scale) and significant reduction in self-rated tinnitus distress (Tinnitus Questionnaire [Hiller & Goebel, 1992]) have been observed following the activation of a cochlear implant (Van de Heyning et al., 2008): there are also, more rarely, cases of distinct worsening of tinnitus following this form of direct electrical stimulation of the auditory nerve (Summerfield et al., 2006).

As regards surface electrical stimulation, Vanneste, Plazier, Van de Heyning, and De Ridder (2010) applied the technique of direct electrical stimulation of the dorsolateral prefrontal region of the auditory cortex in cases of what they termed somatic tinnitus. This is a relatively common form of tinnitus that involves interaction between the auditory and somatosensory systems. The tinnitus can be modified by a variety of motor manipulations of and about the head, neck, eyes, and so forth, indicating a role for upper cervical nerves in tinnitus maintenance. Stimulation was applied to those nerves, and modest to substantial, statistically significant, temporary reduction of tinnitus experience (visual analog scale) was observed in about 18% of the 240 patients in the study. This is an experimental procedure; results for a modest proportion of participants are encouraging, but how readily it might be applied clinically is uncertain.

Subcranial. Friedland, Gaggl, Runge-Samuelson, Ulmer, and Kopell (2007) recruited eight tinnitus sufferers presenting a specific profile, that is, tinnitus that was unilateral, narrowband, continuous and of greater than 1 year duration. They reported on outcomes from the first 12 weeks of a year-long treatment program. The average tinnitus duration of the eight patients was 15.8 years (SD = 13.7), two outliers had durations of 3 and 48 yr; the average duration of the other six cases was 12.5 years (SD = 2.9). The substantial duration and continuous nature of tinnitus in this sample is a feature that can be argued to play an important explanatory role in the results obtained by Friedland et al. (2007). For this and other reasons, it is instructive to consider outcomes of this report in some detail.

Friedland and colleagues (2007) used brain-scanning observations to locate the auditory cortical area, in each of the eight cases, that showed maximal excitation, hence assumed as the site of tinnitus activity, with implant location determined accordingly. In seven of the eight cases, at initial induction using the implanted neurostimulator, there were experiences reported of temporary tinnitus suppression. In the study proper, there was an initial 2 × 2-week single-blind cross-over design (stimulation versus no stimulation); no consistent effects were observed in this period in terms of ongoing ratings of tinnitus loudness or device effectiveness. Self-assessments were reported as being obtained using the Tinnitus Handicap Questionnaire (Kuk et al., 1990) and the Tinnitus Reaction Questionnaire (Wilson et al., 1991), although the citation details given here were not listed in the Friedland et al. (2007) paper. Consistent improvements on both of these self-assessment measures were observed for two of the eight patients in the four-week cross-over phase.

Following the crossover phase, all patients were exposed for 8 weeks to an "open label" treatment, that is, non-blinded continuous electrical stimulation. Six of the eight patients reported episodes of complete tinnitus suppression during this period (in two cases this was subsequent to the open-label phase). The Friedland et al. (2007) study included an extensive program of psychophysical measurements: hearing threshold and speech recognition tests, tinnitus loudness matching, minimum masking level, and tinnitus frequency matching. There were no consistent changes in any of these measures from baseline to completion of the four-week cross-over plus 8-week open-label phase. The Tinnitus Handicap Questionnaire (Kuk et al., 1990) and Tinnitus Reaction Questionnaire (Wilson et al., 1991) were readministered at the end of the open-label phase. All patients showed improvement on one or both self-assessment measures; in several cases this was substantial. Self-assessed change was unrelated to change, if any, in the psychophysical measurements. A measure of depression was also applied (Beck, Steer, Ball, & Ranieri, 1996), citation details not listed by Friedland et al. (2007), and generally showing improvement on this factor.

It is evident that there was much high-level technical investment in this project and all the researchers had specialist technical backgrounds (otology, radiology, neurosurgery). The only positive outcomes from the project were in the realm of self-assessed reduction in tinnitus-related disabilities and handicaps (and self-rated depression). It is clear the authors were expecting that a complex and carefully devised neurophysiological intervention should have beneficial consequences at least at a psychophysical level. In discussing their results the authors see themselves as faced with a problem about how to interpret the contrast between the absence of signs of meaningful change in the psychophysics accompanied by stronger signs of change on the basis of self-assessment. They suggest placebo effect/s may account for such subjective changes unrelated to the more objective ones.

In appraising their results, Friedland and colleagues (2007) seem to have overlooked the history and experiences of their participants. As these authors state (p. 1010), "All subjects noted that [tinnitus suppression] had never occurred previously," and (p. 1011), "almost all participants had distinct episodes of total tinnitus suppression despite reporting that cessation of tinnitus had never occurred in the past." Among these eight participants the shortest history of continuous tinnitus was three years (average 15.8 yr). Thus, for the first time in many years these patients had an experience, even if transient, of relief from this constant noise, and resulting from application of a direct physical mechanism they knew was underpinning that relief. The intervention may have had no impact on the character of the tinnitus, once it recurred, but it surely had the powerful effect of offering hope to these people. They now were confronting a future holding the prospect of recurring episodes of suppression, as against one of relentless experience of their tinnitus. The direct experience of tinnitus suppression due to an identifiable treatment would allow them to rate their response to tinnitus, and the level of depression associated with its ongoing presence, as less distressed and severe.

There is nothing in the result observed by Friedland et al. (2007) that demonstrates a cure for tinnitus. Rather, the significance of their findings is in showing the potential for use of implants of one or another kind to suppress tinnitus in certain cases. The data also offer confirmation, if this was needed, of the substantial impact on quality of life that would accrue in the event that a direct remedy for tinnitus can be found.

Other reports (e.g., Cheung & Larson, 2010; De Ridder et al., 2006; Seidman et al., 2008) confirm that stimulation of different regions of auditory cortex, and in brain regions outside the cortex, yet implicated in distribution of auditory inputs, can moderate tinnitus loudness, sometimes substantially. Outcomes are not consistently beneficial, but do show a sufficient proportion of evidently positive results as to make it clear this direction of clinical research should continue to be actively pursued and refined.

PSYCHOLOGICAL/ BIOBEHAVIORAL TREATMENTS

Biofeedback, Hypnosis, Relaxation Training

There have been somewhat inconsistent outcomes from the three treatment approaches listed in this subsection. In previous reviews (Dobie, 1999; Noble, 1998), biofeedback and relaxation training were both reported as having borderline beneficial effects, mixed effects, or no effect. In the case of hypnosis, Dobie (1999) reported that studies to that date had been characterized by a conjunction of hypnosis procedures with one or more form of psychotherapy; hence, it was difficult to unpack whatever might be attributable to hypnosis as such. This problem remains. In a large-scale recent study (Ross, Lange, Unterrainer, & Laszig, 2007), hypnosis was administered over a 28-day period to 393 inpatients, along with education about tinnitus, relaxation training, and music therapy. Substantial and long-term reduction was observed in tinnitus distress (using the Tinnitus Questionnaire [Hiller & Goebel, 1992]), but it is not possible to identify if the hypnosis component was the driver of this change.

In a later section of this chapter (headed CBT plus biofeedback), a recent tinnitus treatment program is described that combines cognitive behavior therapy and biofeedback. This offers a promising direction for psychological/biobehavioral clinical research, and, in addition, helps to illustrate the complexity of the response to tinnitus.

Neuromonics

This procedure is based on a combination of counselling and masking/partial masking using filtered music plus broadband noise. It has been reported on by its original authors (e.g., Davis, Paki, & Hanley, 2007) and there appears to be one small-scale independent study (Goddard, Berliner, Luxford, 2009) applying the approach. In that study there were as many people who discontinued the treatment (n = 15) as completed it (n = 14). Of those completing, there was a significant reduction in Tinnitus Reaction Questionnaire (Wilson et al., 1991) scores after 8 months of treatment. It remains unclear whether the counselling component or the masking component of this procedure provides whatever benefit may be observed. Some illumination on this point can be derived from studies of the next approach to be reviewed here, Tinnitus Retraining Therapy.

Tinnitus Retraining Therapy (TRT)

In their Cochrane Review, Phillips and McFerran (2010) could identify only one study (Henry et al., 2006) of TRT that represented a trial of this procedure based on its original formulation (Jastreboff & Hazell, 2004). That formula comprises a combination of partial masking of the tinnitus sound and what its authors call "directive counselling"—a procedure largely designed to offer an explanation of how tinnitus arises as a neural phenomenon. Henry et al. (2006) parsed the components of TRT and compared the original protocol with partial masking alone, in two independent groups of veterans. They observed that partial masking alone had statistically significant beneficial effect at 3 months after initial treatment allocation, but tended not to show much further improvement at 6, 12, and 18 months after entering this treatment arm, at least as reflected in Tinnitus Handicap Questionnaire (Kuk et al., 1990) scores. By contrast, the full TRT protocol continued to show improving effects through the life of the trial, and had broadly a 3:1 improvement rate over partial masking. A confound in this study is due to the choice to use hearing aids by about one-quarter of participants. Given the evidence reviewed here, indicating that amplification can be beneficial in relieving tinnitus distress, analysis should have involved separate scrutiny of data provided by hearing aid users versus those using noise maskers.

The outcome from the Henry et al. (2006) study accords with that observed by Hiller and Haerkötter (2005). These investigators used a standard CBT protocol instead of the TRT directive counselling procedure. (Standard CBT procedure typically involves about 8 to 12 weekly 1- to 2-hour sessions designed to train people in relaxation techniques, strategies for reducing stress, and cognitive re-framing so as to acquire more accepting evaluation of tinnitus; the "directive counselling" component of TRT involves about three 1- to 2-hour sessions spaced widely over an 18-month period and focused on explanation of the tinnitus mechanism.) Hiller and Haerkötter (2005) found that groups using only a partial masking device showed improvement in tinnitus-related distress over an 18-month observation period, as assessed using the Tinnitus Questionnaire (Hiller & Goebel, 1992), but not to the extent of improvement observed in the CBT group. Furthermore, there was no incremental effect over CBT alone observable in a group treated with the combination of CBT and partial masking. It thus looks as though the counseling component of TRT is what delivers whatever beneficial effect it may offer.

The absence of control groups compromises the above conclusion because it remains unknown what would be the natural time-course of adaptation to tinnitus in the case of no intervention. The study by Folmer and Carroll (2006), described in the Hearing Aid section of this chapter, enables comparison of device use versus nonuse. A recent meta-analysis (Hesser, Weise, Rief & Andersson, 2011) reports small but statistically significant reductions in measures of tinnitus distress of between 3% and 8% in wait-list control groups.

A conclusion regarding the relative ineffectiveness of masking procedures does not gainsay the reports of individuals who find masking devices of one or other kind beneficial in self-management of tinnitus. Here, though, the earlier point (in the section on Maskers) should be noted about interaction between increasing degree of any accompanying hearing loss and declining preference for use of masking.

Cognitive Behavior Therapy (CBT)

As noted at the start of this chapter, most people with chronic tinnitus are not distressed by it: they have habituated to the noise/s (Hallam, Rachman, & Hinchcliffe, 1984). Finding ways to enable the distressed patient to attain such habituation is the aim of CBT. This therapy has emerged as a standard form of treatment for a range of chronic conditions (e.g., pain, depression, anxiety), and rests on a set of procedures aimed at re-orienting a person's thoughts, emotions and coping strategies, in relation to the condition in question. CBT is not expected to influence the condition as such.

Cochrane Review

Martinez-Devesa et al. (2010), in an updated Cochrane review, identified eight studies (Andersson, Porsaeus, Wiklund, Kaldo, & Larsen, 2005; Henry & Wilson, 1996; Kaldo, Cars, Rahnert, Larsen, & Andersson, 2007; Kröner-Herwig et al., 1995; Kröner-Herwig, Frenzel, Fritsche, Schilkowsky, & Esser, 2003; Rief, Weise, Kley, & Martin, 2005; Weise et al., 2008; Zachriat & Kröner-Herwig, 2004) as meeting the inclusion criterion of a randomized controlled trial, and with sufficient similarity of procedures and outcome measures to enable meta-analyses (total $N = 468$). This systematic review is Level 1 evidence (see Table 1–5). The primary outcome measure chosen by Martinez-Devesa et al. (2010) was subjective tinnitus loudness, assessed using visual analog scales: not unexpectedly, this showed no signs of difference between treatment and (wait-list) control conditions. The secondary measures identified by these reviewers were self-assessments of depression and of quality of life, the latter reflected in response to one or other standard measure of tinnitus severity (typically, the Tinnitus Questionnaire [Hiller

& Goebel, 1992] or the Tinnitus Handicap Questionnaire [Kuk et al., 1990]). In the case of depression, the data from six of the eight included studies were able to be pooled and a significant difference in favour of the treatment condition was observable between that and the control condition. Significant differences in favour of the treatment group were also observed on measures of tinnitus severity. Thus, these reviewers concluded that CBT is reliably observed to have a positive influence on the coping strategies of those with distressing tinnitus; they noted, though, a lack of long-term follow-up data in the research literature they reviewed. That conclusion is confirmed by Hesser, Weise, Westin, and Andersson (2011).

CBT Plus Biofeedback

Weise et al. (2008) argued that a combination of biofeedback training with CBT ought to capture a larger proportion of chronic tinnitus sufferers, on the ground that some people are unconvinced by purely psychotherapeutic (e.g., CBT) procedures, holding the understandable view that tinnitus is a somatic complaint, requiring a somatically-directed intervention. One purpose of the CBT approach is to draw each person's attention to their "thinking as usual" and to challenge ways of responding (in this case to the tinnitus) that generate distressing thoughts, feelings, and behaviors. The biofeedback procedure used electromyography to allow participants to achieve progressive muscle relaxation; the CBT regime was a standard procedure developed with specific focus on tinnitus. Measures included the Tinnitus Questionnaire (Hiller & Goebel, 1992), the Beck Depression Inventory (Beck et al., 1996), diary entries, self-efficacy, and general well-being. A total of 125 people were entered at random into one or other arm of the trial: CBT/biofeedback intervention; wait-list control. Findings showed substantial and persistent improvements in tinnitus annoyance, and (unusually) rated tinnitus loudness. Findings also indicated improved self-efficacy and general well-being. Finally, patients reported high levels of satisfaction with the treatment, and drop-out rates were minor, bearing out the initial argument.

In a subsequent analysis, Heinecke et al. (2009) examined the changes in muscle control due to biofeedback, which were significant, and the equally significant changes in the psychological measures (Tinnitus Questionnaire [Hiller & Goebel, 1992], Beck Depression Inventory [Beck et al., 1996], etc.). There were virtually no signs of correlation between the two domains; the two sets of changes were independent of each other. The authors hypothesized that the biofeedback procedure may well have acted positively for patients with a strongly somatic orientation to their tinnitus, enabling them to be more responsive to the psychological component of treatment. This is an intriguing possibility; overall, the combined procedure offers quite a promising direction for a biobehavioral approach to tinnitus management.

TREATMENT COALITIONS

Tinnitus too often has been prey to treatment offers that have no evidentiary basis. Because it is essentially subjective, the risk of exposure to such offers is increased. As has been argued elsewhere (Noble & Tyler, 2007, p. 573) people who experience chronic tinnitus can be understood as "curious, concerned or distressed." In the first two sorts of case, and after care has been taken to rule out the rare instance of tinnitus as a sign of something more sinister, an evidence-based explanation of its origin may be sufficient to enable the person to reduce their curiosity/concern and habituate to the noise. The person who is distressed, however, may need more careful management, and this calls upon skills that are likely beyond the scope of someone trained in clinical audiology. An obvious collaboration is between clinical audiology and clinical psychology.

In the case where implant technology of one or other kind is indicated as likely to be beneficial, it is of course necessary to engage the skills of neurosurgery and related specialties. But as the study by Friedland and colleagues (2007) illustrates (described in the section on Subcranial Stimulation), absence of an appropriate psychosocial appreciation of tinnitus experience can lead to incomplete understanding of the reality of tinnitus for the person suffering with it. Thus, clinical psychology can also serve a useful function in the context of such technical intervention.

CONCLUSIONS

On the basis of the evidence reviewed here it is feasible to identify two potentially effective approaches to successful tinnitus treatment: (1) physical and (2) psychological/biobehavioral. A physical approach seeks to remove, or at least moderate the tinnitus as a signal, and a promising treatment involves electromagnetic stimulation over a range of sites in the nervous system. It is not clear if all instances of tinnitus could be addressed or addressed effectively by such an approach, but results in individual instances are impressive. A psychological/biobehavioral approach can be understood as having two forms or two components: (1) effective acoustic amplification to achieve optimal masking in the (quite common) case of tinnitus as accompaniment to hearing loss; and (2) cognitive-behavior therapy, especially if enhanced with biofeedback training.

The evidence indicates that there do not seem to be any currently viable pharmacological approaches to tinnitus management; and physical intervention, such as use of a noise masker, seems limited to the uncommon case of tinnitus in the absence, or relative absence, of hearing loss. Given the complex nature of tinnitus suffering, that is, tinnitus experience resistant to adaptation, it seems vital, in such a case, to engage a coalition of skills drawn from clinical audiology and clinical psychology.

REFERENCES

Anders, M., Dvorakova, J., Rathova, L., Havrankova, P., Pelcova, P., Vaneckova, M., . . . Raboch, J. (2010). Efficacy of repetitive transcranial magnetic stimulation for the treatment of refractory chronic tinnitus: A randomized, placebo-controlled study. *Neuroendocrinology Letters*, *31*(2), 238–249.

Andersson, G., Porsaeus, D., Wiklund, M., Kaldo, V., & Larsen, H. C. (2005). Treatment of tinnitus in the elderly: A controlled trial of cognitive behavior therapy. *International Journal of Audiology*, *44*(11), 671–675.

Axelsson, A., & Ringdahl, A. (1989). Tinnitus—a study of its prevalence and characteristics. *British Journal of Audiology*, *23*(1), 53–62.

Baguley, D. M., Andersson, G., Moffat, M., Humphriss, R. L., & Moffat, D. A. (2002). *Factor analysis of the tinnitus handicap inventory*. Paper presented at the VIIth International Tinnitus Seminar, Perth, Australia.

Baguley, D. M., Jones, S., Wilkins, I., Axon, P. R., & Moffat, D. A. (2005). The inhibitory effect of intravenous lidocaine infusion on tinnitus after translabyrinthine removal of vestibular schwannoma: A double-blind, placebo-controlled, crossover study. *Otology and Neurotology*, *26*(2), 169–176.

Baldo, P., Doree, C., Lazzarini, R., Molin, P., & McFerran, D. (2009). Antidepressants for patients with tinnitus. *Cochrane Database of Systematic Reviews*, Issue 4. doi: 10.1002/14651858.CD003853.pub2

Bayar, N., Boke, B., Turan, E., & Belgin, E. (2001). Efficacy of amitriptyline in the treatment of subjective tinnitus. *Journal of Otolaryngology, 30*(5), 300–303.

Beck, A. T., Steer, R. A., Ball, R., & Ranieri, W. F. (1996). Comparison of Beck Depression Inventories-IA and -II in psychiatric outpatients. *Journal of Personality Assessment, 67*(3), 588–597.

Cheung, S. W., & Larson, P. S. (2010). Tinnitus modulation by deep brain stimulaiton in locus of caudate neurons. *Neuroscience, 169*(4), 1768–1778.

Davis, P. B., Paki, B., & Hanley, P. J. (2007). Neuromonics tinnitus treatment: Third clinical trial. *Ear and Hearing, 28*(2), 242–259.

De Ridder, D., De Mulder, G., Verstraeten, E., Van der Kelen, K., Sunaert, S., Smits, M., . . . Moller, A. R.(2006). Primary and secondary auditory cortex stimulation for intractable tinnitus. *Journal of Oto-Rhino-Laryngology and its Related Specialties, 68*, 48–55. doi: 10.1159/000090491.

De Ridder, D., De Mulder, G., Walsh, V., Muggleton, N., Sunaert, S., & Moller, A. (2004). Magnetic and electrical stimulation of the auditory cortex for intractable tinnitus—Case report. *Journal of Neurosurgery, 100*(3), 560–564.

Del Bo, L., Ambrosetti, U., Bettinelli, M., Domenichetti, E., Fagnani, E., & Scotti, A. (2006). Using open-ear hearing aids in tinnitus therapy. *Hearing Review, 13*(9), 30–33.

Dib, G. C., Casse, C. A., Alives de Andrade, T., Testa, J. R. G., & Cruz, O. L. M. (2007). Tinnitus treatment with trazodone. *Brazilian Journal of Otorhinolaryngology, 73*(3), 390–397.

Dobie, R. A. (1999). A review of randomized clinical trials in tinnitus. *Laryngoscope, 109*(8), 1202–1211.

Dobie, R. A. (2004). Clinical trials and drug therapy for tinnitus. In J. B. Snow (Ed.), *Tinnitus: Theory and management* (pp. 266–277). Hamilton, ON: BC Decker.

Folmer, R. L., & Carroll, J. R. (2006). Long-term effectiveness of ear-level devices for tinnitus. *Otolaryngology—Head and Neck Surgery, 134*(1), 132–137.

Fornaro, M., & Martino, M. (2010). Tinnitus psychopharmacology: A comprehensive review of its pathomechanisms and management. *Neuropsychiatric Disease and Treatment, 6*, 209–218.

Friedland, D. R., Gaggl, W., Runge-Samuelson, C., Ulmer, J. L., & Kopell, B. H. (2007). Feasibility of auditory cortical stimulation for the treatment of tinnitus. *Otology and Neurotology, 28*, 1005–1012.

Gatehouse, S., & Noble, W. (2004). The Speech, Spatial and Qualities of Hearing Scale (SSQ). *International Journal of Audiology, 43*(1), 85–99.

Goddard, J. C., Berliner, K., & Luxford, W. M. (2009). Recent experience with the neuromonics tinnitus treatment. *International Tinnitus Journal, 15*(2), 168-173.

Hallam, R. S., Jakes, S. C., & Hinchcliffe, R. (1988). Cognitive variables in tinnitus annoyance. *British Journal of Clinical Psychology, 27*, 213–222.

Hallam, R. S., Rachman, S., & Hinchcliffe, R. (1984). Psychological aspects of tinnitus. In S. Rachman (Ed.), *Contributions to medical psychology* (Vol. 3, pp. 31–53). Oxford, UK: Pergamon.

Hayes, S. C., Strosahl, K. D., & Wilson, K. G. (1999). *Acceptance and commitment therapy: An experiential approach to behavior change.* New York, NY: Guilford Press.

Heinecke, K., Weise, C., & Rief, W. (2009). Psychophysiological effects of biofeedback treatment in tinnitus sufferers. *British Journal of Clinical Psychology, 48*, 223–239.

Henry, J. A., Schechter, M. A., Zaugg, T. L., Griest, S., Jastreboff, P. J., Vernon, J. A., . . . Stewart, B. J. (2006). Outcomes of clinical trial: tinnitius masking versus tinnitus retraining therapy. *Journal of the American Academy of Audiology, 17*(2), 104–132.

Henry, J. L., & Wilson, P. H. (1996). The psychological management of tinnitus: Comparison of a combined cognitive educational program, education alone and a waiting-list control. *International Tinnitus Journal, 2*, 1–12.

Henry, J. L., & Wilson, P. H. (2001). *The psychological management of chronic tinnitus: A cognitive-behavioral approach.* Boston, MA: Allyn & Bacon.

Hesser, H., Weise, C., Rief, W., & Andersson, G. (2011). The effect of waiting: A meta-analysis of wait-list control groups in trials for tinnitus distress. *Journal of Psychosomatic Research, 70,* 378–384.

Hesser, H., Weise, C., Westin, V. Z., & Andersson, G. (2011). A systematic review and meta-analysis of randomized controlled trials of cognitive-behavioral therapy for tinnitus dstress. *Clinical Psychology Review, 31,* 545–553.

Higgins, J. P. T., & Green, S. (Eds.). (2009). *Cochrane handbook for systematic reviews of interventions Version 5.0.2: The Cochrane Collaboration.*

Hiller, W., & Goebel, G. (1992). A psychometric study of complaints in chronic tinnitus. *Journal of Psychosomatic Research, 36*(4), 337–348.

Hiller, W., & Haerkötter, C. (2005). Does sound stimulation have additive effects on cognitive-behavioral treatment of chronic tinnitus? *Behaviour Research and Therapy, 43,* 595–612.

Hilton, M. P., & Stuart, E. L. (2004). Ginkgo biloba for tinnitus. *Cochrane Database of Systematic Reviews,* Issue 2. doi: 10.1002/14651858.CD003852.pub2

Holgers, K. M., Axelsson, A., & Pringle, I. (1994). Ginkgo biloba extract for the treatment of tinnitus. *Audiology, 33*(2):85–92.

Jastreboff, P. J., & Hazell, J. W. P. (2004). *Tinnitus retraining therapy.* Cambridge, UK: Cambridge University Press.

Kaldo, V., Cars, S., Rahnert, M., Larsen, H. C., & Andersson, G. (2007). Use of a self-help book with weekly therapist contact to reduce tinnitus distress: A randomized controlled trial. *Journal of Psychosomatic Research, 63,* 195–202.

Kallio, H., Niskanen, M. L., Havia, M., Neuvonen, P. J., Rosenberg, P. H., & Kentala, E. (2008). I.V. ropivacaine compared with lidocaine for the treatment of tinnitus. *British Journal of Anaesthesia, 101*(2), 261–265.

Kröner-Herwig, B., Frenzel, A., Fritsche, G., Schilkowsky, G., & Esser, G. (2003). The management of chronic tinnitus—Comparison of an outpatient cognitive-behavioral group training to minimal-contact interventions. *Journal of Psychosomatic Research, 54*(4), 381–389.

Kröner-Herwig, B., Hebing, G., Van Rijn-Kalkman, U., Frenzel, A., Schilkowsky, G., & Esser, G. (1995). The management of chronic tinnitus—comparison of a cognitive-behavioural group training with yoga. *Journal of Psychosomatic Research, 39*(2), 153–165.

Kuk, F. K., Tyler, R. S., Russell, D., & Jordan, H. (1990). The psychometric properties of a tinnitus handicap questionnaire. *Ear and Hearing, 11*(6), 434–445.

Langenbach, M., Olderog, M., Michel, O., Albus, C., & Kohle, K. (2005). Psychosocial and personality predictors of tinnitus-related distress. *General Hospital Psychiatry, 27,* 73–77.

Langguth, B., Elgoyhen, A. B., de Ridder, D., & Staudinger, S. (2010). We must cure tinnitus, we can cure tinnitus, and we will cure tinnitus. *TRI Newsletter, 13,* 1.

Langguth, B., Salvi, R., & Belen Elgoyhen, A. (2009). Emerging pharmacotherapy of tinnitus. *Expert Opinion on Emerging Drugs, 14*(4), 687–702.

Martinez-Devesa, P., Perera, R., Theodoulou, M., & Waddell, A. (2010). Cognitive behavioural therapy for tinnitus. *Cochrane Database of Systematic Reviews,* Issue 9. doi: 10.1002/14651858.CD005233.pub3

McKenna, L. (2004). Models of tinnitus suffering and treatment compared and contrasted. *Audiological Medicine, 2,* 1–14.

Melin, L., Scott, B., Lindberg, P., & Lyttkens, L. (1987). Hearing aids and tinnitus—an experimental group study. *British Journal of Audiology, 21,* 91–97.

Mihail, R. C., Crowley, J. M., Walden, B. E., Fishburne, J. F., Reinwall, J. E., & Zajtchuk, J. T. (1988). The tricyclic trimipramine in the treatment of subjetive tinnitus. *Annals of Otology Rhinology and Laryngology, 97*(2), 120–123.

Mirz, F., Zachariae, R., Andersen, S. E., Nielsen, A. G., Johansen, L. G., Bjerring, P., & Pedersen, C. B. (1999). The low-power laser in the treatment of tinnitus. *Clinical Otolaryngology, 24*(4), 346–354.

Moffat, G., Adjout, K., Gallego, S., Thai-Van, H., Collet, L., & Norena, A. J. (2009). Effects of hearing aid fitting on the perceptual characteristics of tinnitus. *Hearing Research, 254,* 82–91.

Nam, E. C., Handzel, O., & Levine, R. A. (2010). Carbamazepine responsive typewriter tinnitus from basilar invagination. *Journal of Neurology, Neurosurgery and Psychiatry, 81*(4), 456–458.

Newman, C. W., Jacobson, G. P., & Spitzer, J. B. (1996). Development of the tinnitus handicap inventory. *Archives of Otolaryngology—Head and Neck Surgery, 122*, 143–148.

Noble, W. (1998). *Self-assessment of hearing and related functions.* London, UK: Whurr.

Noble, W. (2001). Tinnitus self-assessment scales: Domains of coverage and psychometric properties. *Hearing Journal, 54*(11), 20–25.

Noble, W., Naylor, G., Bhullar, N., & Akeroyd, M. (2012). Self-assessed hearing abilities in middle- and older-age adults: A stratified sampling approach. *International Journal of Audiology, 51*(3), 174–180.

Noble, W., & Tyler, R. S. (2007). Physiology and phenomenology of tinnitus: Implications for treatment. *International Journal of Audiology, 46*(10), 569–574.

Phillips, J. S., & McFerran, D. (2010). Tinnitus retraining therapy (TRT) for tinntus. *Cochrane Database of Systematic Reviews*, Issue 3. doi: 10.1002/14651858.CD007330pub2

Podoshin, L., Ben-David, Y., Fradis, M., Malatskey, S., & Hafner, H. (1995). Idiopathic subjective tinnitus treated by amitriptyline hydrochloride/biofeedback. *International Tinnitus Journal, 1*(1), 54–60.

Preece, J. P., Tyler, R. S., & Noble, W. (2003). The management of tinnitus. *Geriatrics and Aging, 6*(6), 22–28.

Rief, W., Weise, C., Kley, N., & Martin, A. (2005). Psychophysiologic treatment of chronic tinnitus: a randomized clinical trial. *Psychosomatic Medicine, 67*, 833–838.

Robinson, S. K., Viirre, E. S., Bailey, K. A., Gerke, M. A., Harris, J. P., & Stein, M. B. (2005). Randomized placebo-controlled trial of a selective serotonin reuptake inhibitor in the treatment of nondepressed tinnitus subjects. *Psychosomatic Medicine, 67*(6), 981–988.

Robinson, S. K., Viirre, E. S., & Stein, M. B. (2004). Antidepressant therapy for tinnitus. In J. B. Snow (Ed.), *Tinnitus: Theory and management* (pp. 278–293). Hamilton, ON: BC Decker.

Ross, U. H., Lange, O., Unterrainer, J., & Laszig, R. (2007). Ericksonian hypnosis in tinnitus therapy: effects of a 28-day inpatient multimodal treatment concept measured by Tinnitus-Questionnaire and Health Survey SF-36. *European Archives of Oto-Rhino-Laryngology, 264*, 483–488.

Searchfield, G. D., Kaur, M., & Martin, W. H. (2010). Hearing aids as an adjunct to counselling: Tinnitus patients who choose amplification do better than those that don't. *International Journal of Audiology, 49*, 574–579.

Seidman, M. D., De Ridder, D., Elisevich, K., Bowyer, S. M., Darrat, I., Dria, J., . . . Zhang, J. (2008). Direct electrical stimulation of Heschl's gyrus for tinnitus treatment. *Laryngoscope, 118*, 491–500.

Stephens, S. D. G., & Corcoran, A. L. (1985). A controlled study of tinnitus masking. *British Journal of Audiology, 19*, 159–167.

Sullivan, M., Katon, W., Russo, J., Dobie, R., & Sakai, C. (1993). A randomized trial of nortriptyline for severe chronic tinnitus—effects on depression, disability, and tinnitus symptoms. *Archives of Internal Medicine, 153*(19), 251–259.

Summerfield, A. Q., Barton, G. R., Toner, J., McAnallen, C., Proops, D., Harries, C., . . . Pringle, M.. (2006). Self-reported benefits from successive bilateral cochlear implantation in postlingually deafened adults: Randomised controlled trial. *International Journal of Audiology, 45* (Suppl. 1), S99–S107.

Surr, R. K., Kolb, J. A., Cord, M. T., & Garrus, N. P. (1999). Tinnitus Handicap Inventory (THI) as a hearing aid outcome measure. *Journal of the American Academy of Audiology, 10*, 489–495.

Surr, R. K., Montgomery, A. A., & Mueller, H. G. (1985). Effect of amplification on tinnitus among new hearing aid users. *Ear and Hearing, 6*(2), 71–75.

Teggi, R., Bellini, C., Piccioni, L. O., Palonta, F., & Bussi, M. (2009). Transmeatal low-level laser therapy for chronic tinnitus with cochlear dysfunction. *Audiology and Neurotology, 14*(2), 115–120.

Trotter, M. I., & Donaldson, I. (2008). Hearing aids and tinnitus therapy: A 25-year experience. *Journal of Laryngology and Otology, 122*, 1052–1056.

Tyler, R. S., & Baker, L. J. (1983). Difficulties experienced by tinnitus sufferers. *Journal of Speech and Hearing Disorders, 48*, 150–154.

Van de Heyning, P., Vermeire, K., Diebl, M., Nopp, P., Anderson, I., & De Ridder, D. (2008). Incapacitating unilateral tinnitus in single-sided deafness treated by cochlear implantation. *Annals of Otology, Rhinology, and Laryngology, 117*(9), 645–652.

Vanneste, S., Plazier, M., Ost, J., van der Loo, E., Van de Heyning, P. H., & De Ridder, D. (2010). Bilateral dorsolateral prefrontal cortex modulation for tinnitus by transcranial direct current stimulation: A preliminary clinical study. *Experimental Brain Research, 202*, 779–785.

Vanneste, S., Plazier, M., Van de Heyning, P. H., & De Ridder, D. (2010). Transcutaneous electrical nerve stimulation (TENS) of upper cervical nerve (C2) for the treatment of somatic tinnitus. *Experimental Brain Research, 204*, 283–287.

Vernon, J. (1977). A tinnitus clinic. *Ear, Nose, and Throat Journal, 56*, 58–71.

Weise, C., Heinecke, K., & Rief, W. (2008). Biofeedback-based behavioral treatment for chronic tinnitus: Results of a randomized controlled trial. *Journal of Consulting and Clinical Psychology, 76*(6), 1046–1057.

Wilson, P. H., Henry, J., Bowen, M., & Haralambous, G. (1991). Tinnitus reaction questionnaire: Psychometric properties of a measure of distress associated with tinnitus. *Journal of Speech and Hearing Research, 34*, 197–201.

World Health Organization. (1980). *International Classification of Impairments, Disabilities, and Handicaps*. Geneva, Switzerland: Author.

Zachariae, R., Mirz, F., Johansen, L. V., Andersen, S. E., Bjerring, P., & Pedersen, C. B. (2000). Reliability and validity of a Danish adaptation of the Tinnitus Handicap Inventory. *Scandinavian Audiology, 29*, 37–43.

Zachriat, C., & Kröner-Herwig, B. (2004). Treating chronic tinnitus: Comparison of cognitive-behavioural and habituation-based treatments. *Cognitive Behaviour Therapy, 33*(4), 187–198.

CHAPTER 12

Evidence of the Effectiveness of Interventions for Auditory Processing Disorder

Wayne J. Wilson and Wendy Arnott

INTRODUCTION

Reviewing the evidence about the effectiveness of interventions for auditory processing disorder (APD) is a complex task. It is tempting to rush straight to an analysis of the interventions themselves, but this would ignore the fundamental controversies engulfing APD. We therefore begin this chapter by addressing the question: what is APD and how is it diagnosed? We continue by attempting to answer the following clinical questions, formed using the PICO format of Needleman (2003) discussed in Chapter 1:

1. For school-age children with APD with or without spoken language, reading, or learning difficulties (Patient/Problem), does auditory intervention (Intervention) improve auditory processing (AP) (Outcome), compared to no treatment or placebo treatments (Comparison)?
2. For school-age children with spoken language or reading disorders, with or without APD (Patient/Problem), does auditory intervention (Intervention) improve spoken language, reading, spelling and phonological awareness skills (Outcome), compared to no treatment or placebo treatments (Comparison)?

We then briefly consider the role of phonological interventions in APD. Finally, we end the chapter by considering the future of AP intervention and offering our final conclusions.

WHAT IS APD AND HOW IS IT DIAGNOSED?

Despite several decades of investigation, we still lack "gold standards" for defining and diagnosing APD. There remains much debate (Cacace & McFarland, 2005; Cowan, Rosen & Moore, 2009; Dawes & Bishop, 2009; Dillon, Cameron, Glyde, Wilson & Tomlin, in press; Jerger, 2009; McFarland & Cacace, 2009; Moore, 2006; Wilson, Heine, & Harvey, 2004) about:

- Which individual process or processes comprise the nondisordered process, AP.
- The relationship between AP, language and cognition.

- The roles of bottom-up versus top-down processing, active versus passive processing, and general auditory versus speech specific processing.
- The roles of the peripheral versus the central auditory system, and the central auditory system versus nonauditory nervous systems.
- Whether APD is a unimodal disorder or part of a multimodal disorder.
- Which individual deficit or deficits comprise APD, and in turn, whether APD consists of a primary deficit or a series of subprofiles.
- The roles of the three historical approaches to APD: the audiological approach, which is based on the study of brain injured adults and its application to children; the psychoeducational approach, which is based on the concept of discrete auditory perceptual abilities; and a third approach, based on the possible impact of APD on language acquisition and learning.
- Whether APD is a disorder (a clinically significant and discrete syndrome or pattern of disturbance of function and/or structure, resulting from failure in development or from exogenous factors) or an impairment (a loss or abnormality of body structure or of physiological or psychological function). It should be noted that established nosological systems (e.g., APA, 1995; WHO, 1980) favor an impairment-based theory of APD.
- Which tests should be used to assess APD and which skills do these tests really assess.

This led Jerger (2009, p. 10) to conclude that "APD means different things to different people," and Dawes and Bishop (2009, p. 440) to state that "APD, as currently diagnosed, is not a coherent category" but "rather than abandoning the construct, we need to develop improved methods for assessment and diagnosis, with a focus on interdisciplinary evaluation."

Rather than be paralyzed by the above debates, we emphasize two sets of APD definitions and diagnostic criteria (Table 12–1) in this chapter: those of the widely cited American Speech-Language-Hearing Association (ASHA) Working Group on Auditory Processing Disorders (ASHA, 2005; an update on ASHA, 1996), and those more recently offered by the British Society of Audiology (BSA, 2011a; an update on BSA, 2007). We note that although these definitions and diagnostic criteria are widely cited, they are not necessarily widely accepted (e.g., Katz et al., 2002; McFarland & Cacace, 2002). We purposely avoided more pragmatic definitions such as "AP is what we do with what we hear" (Katz, Stecker & Henderson, 1992, pp. 5–6), and "APD is when something goes wrong with what we do with what we hear" (Wilson et al., 2004, p. 84), because they lack the precision needed for systematic, evidence-based review and they fail to differentiate APD from other disorders such as those involving receptive language or cognition.

Although the ASHA (2005) and BSA (2011a) positions on APD share several common features, two particular differences are apparent. The first is BSA's (2011a) explicit statement that APD is characterized by poor perception of *both* speech *and* nonspeech sounds. This addresses the widespread use of both types of sounds in most APD test batteries (e.g., ASHA, 1996, 2005; Bellis & Ferre, 1999; BSA, 2007; Domitz & Schow, 2000; Jerger & Musiek, 2000; Katz et al., 1992; Musiek & Chermak, 1994; Musiek, Geurkink, & Kietel, 1982; Neijenhuis, Stollman, Snik, & van der Broek, 2001; Willeford, 1977), with examples of speech tests being time-compressed speech (Beasley, Schwimmer, & Rintelmann, 1972) and dichotic digits (Musiek, 1983), and examples of non-

Table 12–1. Definitions and Diagnostic Criteria for APD According to ASHA (2005) and BSA (2011)

ASHA (2005)	*BSA (2011a)*
Definition	**Definition**
APD refers to difficulties in the perceptual processing of auditory information in the central nervous system, as demonstrated by poor performance in one or more of the following skills: • sound localization and lateralization • auditory discrimination • auditory pattern recognition • temporal aspects of audition, including temporal integration, temporal discrimination (e.g., temporal gap detection) • temporal ordering and temporal masking • auditory performance in competing acoustic signals (including dichotic listening), and • auditory performance with degraded acoustic signals.	APD is characterized by poor perception of both speech and nonspeech sounds. APD has its origins in impaired neural function. APD impacts on everyday life primarily through a reduced ability to listen, and so respond appropriately to sounds. APD does not result from a failure to understand simple instructions. APD is a collection of symptoms (although the specific symptoms are not explicitly stated) that usually co-occurs with other neurodevelopmental disorders.
Although APD may coexist with, lead to, or be associated with disorders of higher order language, cognition or related factors, it is not the result of such disorders.	Cognitive factors such as attention, rather than being a potential confound, may make a significant contribution to APD.
Diagnostic Criteria	**Diagnostic Criteria**
Demonstration of a deficit in the neural processing of auditory stimuli that is not due to higher order language, cognitive, or related factors. Performance deficits at least two standard deviations (SDs) below the mean on two or more tests, or at least three SDs below the mean on one test, in an APD test battery conducted by the audiologist to assess the AP skills listed above. Inconsistencies (although this is not explicitly defined) across tests can indicate the presence of nonauditory confounds such as deficits in attention. Whether the test battery should involve specific combinations of speech and/or nonspeech stimuli, or assess lexical and/or sublexical processing is not explicitly stated.	Not explicitly stated. The above definition implies the need for performance deficits on at least two tests, one involving nonspeech sounds and one involving speech sounds.

speech test being the Pitch Pattern Sequence Test (Pinhiero, 1977) and the Random Gap Detection Test (Keith, 2000b). In considering the role of speech versus nonspeech testing, several authors favor nonspeech tests for their APD test batteries to avoid the confounding influence of language (Bamiou, Campbell, & Sirimanna, 2006; Moore, 2006; Moore, Ferguson, Edmondson-Jones, Ratib, & Riley, 2010). Others adopt a more psycholinguistic approach, suggesting that the influence of top-down language processing be monitored by distinguishing between stimuli processed at a lexical (e.g., words & sentences) versus a sublexical (e.g., nonspeech sounds, simple speech sounds, and nonsense letter strings) level (Dawes & Bishop, 2009; Findlen & Roup, 2011; McArthur, 2009).

The second particular point of difference between the ASHA (2005) and BSA (2011a) positions on APD is the manner in which they differentiate APD from other associated disorders. Both ASHA (2005) and BSA (2011a) have a discrepancy component where the diagnosis of APD requires a discrepancy between a child's test performance and that of an age-matched normal population. In this regard, ASHA (2005) requires a discrepancy of at least two SDs on two or more tests or at least three SDs on one test involving nonspeech *and/or* speech sounds; BSA (2011a) requires a discrepancy (of unstated quantity) on at least one test involving nonspeech sounds (which may exclude some language confounds) *and* at least one test involving speech sounds. Only ASHA (2005) also has exclusionary criteria requiring demonstration that the discrepancy is not due to higher order language, cognitive or related factors (although they do not explicitly quantify the age-appropriate language or cognitive performance required to exclude these factors). BSA (2011a), on the other hand, argues that the cognitive factor of attention is a key element of AP and that poor attention may contribute significantly to APD.

Conclusion

There are no universally accepted "gold standards" for defining and diagnosing APD, with the widely cited (but not necessarily widely accepted) positions of ASHA (1996, 2005) and BSA (2007, 2011a) differing essentially on the manner in which they account for the potential confounds of higher order language and cognitive processing. To this end, ASHA (2005) allows for deficient processing of nonspeech and/or speech sounds but suggests any deficit should not be the result of higher order processing problems, whereas BSA (2011a) requires deficient processing of nonspeech and speech sounds and suggests higher order processing contributes significantly to APD.

ARE AUDITORY INTERVENTIONS EFFECTIVE TREATMENTS FOR APD?

In recent years, there have been a number of systematic reviews (level 1, see Table 1–5) conducted into AP interventions (Fey et al., 2011; Lemos et al., 2009; Loo, Bamiou, Campbell, & Luxon, 2010; McArthur, 2009). In this section of the chapter, we attempt to synthesize the findings of these reviews and of other published research in the light of the PICO clinical question outlined in the introduction. In doing so, we consider the AP outcomes following both indirect and direct APD interventions in school-age children with APD, with or without associated spoken language and/or reading disorders. Although favoring studies involving subjects diagnosed with an APD, we also consider studies lacking such diagnoses if APD interventions had been used and AP outcomes had been measured. We took this decision in an attempt to mitigate some of the controversies surrounding the definitions and diagnosis of APD discussed in the first section of this chapter. Finally, we used Valente et al's (2006) levels of evidence to rate each study (Table 1–5) and Cox (2005) and Valente et al's (2006) grade of recommendation of research quality (Table 1–6) to draw overall conclusions.

Before beginning this review, it is worth noting that just as we lack consensus on how to differentiate APD from language disorders, so too do we lack consensus on what distinguishes auditory interventions from spoken language interventions (Fey et al., 2011). One approach, similar to that used in the assessment of AP, has been to distinguish the two interventions based on the stimuli used. In this regard, auditory intervention is defined by its use of nonspeech stimuli (such as pure tones) and language intervention by its use of speech stimuli (such as phonemes or words). This approach breaks down, however, when the intervention includes nonspeech and speech stimuli, or nonspeech modifications of speech stimuli. To deal with this problem, other authors have defined auditory intervention by its manipulation of the auditory features of nonspeech and speech stimuli, such as rate, interstimulus interval, frequency, intensity, and presence of background noise; and language intervention by its manipulation of linguistic features of speech stimuli such as language form (syntax, morphology, phonology), content (semantics, vocabulary), and use (pragmatics) (Fey et al., 2011).

Indirect Auditory Interventions

Indirect interventions such as frequency modulation (FM) systems, and similar technologies such as infra red (IR) systems, are proposed as a prima facie solution for improving the signal-to-noise ratio for the listener. FM systems typically consist of a microphone and transmitter worn by the speaker, and a receiver worn with earphones by the listener (personal FM) or a receiver strategically placed with loudspeakers in the room (sound field amplification [SFA] or distribution [SFD]). The microphone and transmitter detects and transmits the speaker's voice via radio (FM) or light (IR) waves to the receiver, which converts the signal back to sound for the listener. The research regarding the effectiveness of personal FM and SFA systems is reviewed in turn below.

In 2009, Lemos et al. (2009) systematically reviewed the evidence regarding the effectiveness of personal FM systems in the treatment of APD. They searched seven electronic databases, as well as Google Academico (Google Scholar), using various combinations of the terms auditory, processing, personal, FM, technolog*, system*, frequency modula*, auditory diseases, and central, as well as the reference sections in the articles they found. They only considered studies that attempted randomized, controlled clinical trials of FM systems to treat APD; studies that mentioned APD intervention in the title and the use of FM systems in any part of the text; and studies of subjects with normal peripheral hearing. Lemos et al. (2009) also appear to have accepted whatever diagnostic criteria for APD individual studies had employed, although ASHA (1996, 2005) or ASHA-like criteria were dominant.

Lemos et al.'s (2009) initial search revealed 1,589 citations, only 20 of which met their inclusionary criteria of randomized, controlled clinical attempts (but not randomized controlled trials) which could evidence the use of FM systems in the treatment of APD; the inclusion of interventions for APD in the title of the study and of FM systems anywhere in the text; and the use of subjects with normal peripheral hearing. Of the 20 studies reviewed, most represented low levels of evidence with Lemos et al. rating no studies at levels 1, 2, or 3, three at level 4, three at level 5, and 14 at level 6 (see Table 1–5).

The three studies receiving the highest rating (level 4) from Lemos and colleagues (2009) all reported descriptive findings only. Young, McPherson, Hickson, and Lawson (1997) found teacher reports of more on-task behavior and independent learning (not statistically tested) in seven subjects (aged 8 to 13 years) with APD who had been wearing FM systems for at least 2 months. Although the diagnosis of APD had been confirmed by poor results on at least one of the Goldman-Fristoe-Woodcock Auditory Skills Battery (Brown, 1987), Synthetic Sentence Identification (Jerger, Speaks, & Trammell, 1968) or Staggered Spondaic Words (Katz, Basil, & Smith, 1963) tests, the study also lacked a control group and its outcome measures (subjective teacher reports) had been anecdotal. Another study that did employ an age matched control group and objective outcome measures (Phonak, 2006) investigated 10 children with APD who were aged 7 to 14 years and had used a personal FM system for one year. Phonak found that 70% to 94% of parents whose children had used the FM systems reported improved classroom behaviors on parental questionnaires. They also found that, relative to control children, children who used the FM systems showed improved psychoacoustic performances on frequency discrimination and temporal ordering tasks, and improved auditory evoked potentials on auditory late latency response and auditory P300 testing. This study was limited, however, by its lack of statistical procedures and inability to determine whether reported improvements were significantly better for the treatment group, and its use of personal histories to diagnose APD. The study was also conducted by the manufacturer of the FM systems and was published in the manufacturer's unrefereed newsletter. Finally, Kreisman and Crandell (2002) reported significantly improved (p value not provided) speech recognition scores in 20 subjects aged 18 to 29 years in an aided condition (wearing an FM system, of which two types were trialed) versus an unaided condition (not wearing an FM system), but this was a single group study of adult subjects with no self-report of APD (or any other impairments). Accordingly, whether results can be generalized to children with APD is unclear.

More recently, BSA (2011b) manually searched Medline and identified a further two FM studies, both providing statistically tested level 4 evidence. In the first study, Johnston, John, Kreisman, Hall, and Crandell (2009) compared the performance of 10 children aged 8 to 15 years who had been diagnosed with APD according to ASHA (2005) and had used an FM system in the classroom for a period of at least 5 months, versus 13 matched control children. Prior to using the FM systems, the children with APD showed significantly ($p < 0.05$) poorer scores on some measures of classroom performance and on the Hearing in Noise (HINT) test (Nilsson, Soli, & Sullivan, 1994) in both aided and unaided conditions, compared to the children in the control group. After using the FM systems, the children with APD showed fewer examples of significantly ($p < 0.05$) poorer scores compared to the control group prior to the FM fitting (i.e., the control group had been only assessed once, prior to the FM fitting), and some examples of significantly ($p < 0.05$) improved performance compared to their own prefitting performances. This study was limited by its assessment of the control group in the pre-treatment phase only, which meant the effects of practice and maturation on the APD group could not be determined. It was also limited by its use of sentence stimuli in the measurement of treatment outcomes, which meant the contribution of language expertise and exposure could not be determined. This study was funded by the manufacturer of the FM systems used in the study.

In the second study (published in German), Hanschmann, Wiehe, Müller-Mazzotta, and Berger (2010) reported significantly ($p < 0.001$) improved performance on a sentence-in-noise test in aided (wearing the FM system) versus unaided (not wearing the FM system) conditions in 66 children aged 6 to 11 years. These improvements appeared to be independent of APD as they were observed in the children regardless of whether they had passed the sentence test initially and finally (described as the control group), failed initially and passed finally (described as APD group 1), and failed initially and finally (described as APD group 2). Furthermore, that the sentence-in-noise test was used both as the sole diagnostic criterion for APD and the sole outcome measure suggests that the results may reflect generalized improvements in listening rather than improved AP.

To our knowledge, there have been no studies on the use of soundfield amplification systems (SFA) conducted specifically on children with APD. There have, however, been many studies conducted on the more general use of SFA systems in the classroom. These studies are often limited by their use of subjective measurements that are susceptible to response bias (e.g., behavioral questionnaires completed by nonblinded classroom teachers), and their lack of rigorous peer review. Some exceptions are noted, with Rosenberg (2002, a level 3 study with total $n = 2054$) showing greater improvement in listening and learning behaviors and skills, and Heeney (2007, a level 3 study with total $n = 626$) reporting significantly greater improvements in listening comprehension, reading comprehension and reading vocabulary (with a smaller effect for mathematics), for children in classrooms with SFA systems ($p < 0.0001$ to $p < 0.05$) than for children in classrooms without SFA systems ($p < 0.0001$ to not significant). Importantly, however, neither study compared the absolute performances of children in the two classroom conditions. Similar evidence from smaller studies is also noted (Arnold & Canning, 1999; Crandell, 1996; Massie & Dillon, 2006a, 2006b; Massie, Theodoros, Byrne, McPherson, & Smaldino, 1999; Massie, Theodoros, McPherson, & Smaldino, 2004; McSporran, Butterworth, & Rowson, 1997). These findings are mitigated by Wilson, Marinac, Pitty, and Burrows (2011), who conducted a level 3 study with a total of 147 student participants in four classrooms with SFA and four matched classrooms without SFA. Overall, Wilson et al. (2011) found small but significantly ($p < 0.01$ to $p < 0.05$) larger improvements in students' listening and auditory analysis skills in classrooms with SFA systems compared to classrooms without SFA systems. On closer inspection, it was identified that the significant improvements had only occurred in one SFA classroom, with its lower background noise levels and reverberation times potentially contributing to the effectiveness of its SFA system.

Conclusions

Despite prima facie evidence that personal FM systems (Intervention) can improve the signal-to-noise ratio for the listener, the evidence is equivocal (see the Appendix) regarding their ability to improve AP (Outcome) in school-age children with APD with or without spoken language, reading, or learning difficulties (Patient/Problem), compared to no treatment or placebo treatments (Comparison). In general, this evidence came mostly from level 5 and 6 studies, with the smaller number of level 3 and 4 studies often showing adequate external validity but limited internal validity and impact (mostly due to a lack of diagnostic confirmation of APD, a lack of specific AP outcome measures, biases in outcome measures, and a lack of control groups and statistical procedures). The overall grade of recommendation was considered to be a C or D (see Table 1–6).

Direct Auditory Interventions

In 2011, Fey et al. (2011) published a systematic review of the peer-reviewed literature on the efficacy of direct auditory interventions for school-age children with APD. They considered all treatment studies involving school-age children diagnosed with spoken language disorders and/or APD as defined by the individual studies themselves. They defined auditory intervention by its manipulation of auditory features and language intervention by its manipulation of linguistic features, as described above in the introduction to this part of the chapter. As a result, Fey et al. classified Earobics as a language intervention arguing that it predominantly manipulates linguistic rather than acoustic features of speech.

Fey et al. (2011) systematically searched 28 electronic databases for studies published from 1978 to 2008 using key words related to central auditory processing or AP interventions. They only considered studies written in English in peer-reviewed journals that contained original data pertaining to their review; that assessed school-age children (6 to 12 years old) diagnosed with APD and/or primary spoken language disorders; and that used active, direct treatment designed to influence children's ability to process speech and language. They excluded studies where the participants had a primary diagnosis of reading or learning disability without an accompanying APD or spoken language disorder; where the participants had autism or autism spectrum disorder, hearing loss, or cognitive disability; that used passive treatment approaches designed to compensate for children's APD (such as preferential seating and FM systems); or that used mixed treatment regimes, vestibular interventions, or pharmacological interventions. Each eligible study was classified by level of evidence according to ASHA (2004; see also Table 1–5), and the methods were rated on seven quality indicators: (1) study protocol, (2) blinding, (3) sampling/allocation, (4) treatment fidelity, (5) statistical significance, (6) precision, and (7) intention to treat.

Fey et al.'s (2011) search identified 192 citations, from which 23 studies met the selection criteria. Only six studies, involving a total of 121 participants, reported the outcomes of auditory interventions for children who had been diagnosed with APD (with or without co-morbid spoken language disorders). The diagnoses of APD had been based mostly on teacher concern for listening and related academic abilities, or low overall performance on one or more tests, including the Staggered Spondaic Word test (SSW; Katz et al., 1963), the SCAN-C Test for Auditory Processing Disorders in Children — Revised (Keith, 1999), and tests of speech in noise. None of the six studies satisfied more than four of the seven quality indicators, with the most common problems relating to blinding, random group assignment, and treatment fidelity.

Two of the six auditory intervention studies in Fey et al. (2011) were level 3 nonrandomized studies with control groups. The first study (Jirsa, 1992; total $n = 40$) evaluated a traditional auditory training approach involving intensive listening in competing noise. It demonstrated significant ($p < 0.05$) changes in auditory evoked potentials (tone-evoked auditory late latency response and auditory P300) and behavioral tasks in the treatment group. Unfortunately, this study received a quality score of only 2 out of 7 points most notably due to a failure to adequately describe the study design and to blind examiners to participants' groups. Although not included in the Fey et al. review, similar results have since been obtained by a level 3 study (Schochat, Musiek, Alonso, & Ogata, 2010; total $n = 52$) that evaluated an auditory training approach involving frequency, intensity, temporal and dichotic listening training as well as informal home training. It demonstrated significant ($p < 0.05$ to 0.001) treatment-related changes in the amplitude of middle latency evoked potentials in the APD group (as well as significant [$p < 0.001$] improvements in this group on the behavioral APD tests).

The second level 3 study reviewed by Fey et al. (2011) involved 36 participants who completed a 10 hour, modified Auditory Integration Therapy (AIT) program (Yencer, 1998). AIT uses filtered music to stimulate the auditory system in an attempt to enhance listening skills. This study failed to find positive treatment effects on any of the 26 behavioral and physiological outcome measures employed.

The other four auditory intervention studies reviewed by Fey et al. (2011) were level 4 studies (Valente et al., 2006) that included smaller sample sizes, no control groups, and speech-dependent outcome measures (e.g., speech recognition). Three of these studies evaluated traditional auditory training approaches such as degraded and dichotic listening treatments, with significant ($p < 0.05$) gains reported by Miller et al. (2005; $n = 2$) and Putter-Katz et al. (2002; $n = 20$) but not by English, Martonik, and Moir (2003; $n = 10$). Two of these studies (Miller, et al., 2005; $n = 3$ and Deppeler, Taranto, & Bench, 2004; $n = 8$) evaluated Fast ForWord (Scientific Learning Corporation, 1998), which uses computer games to deliver acoustically modified nonspeech, simple speech, and more complex speech sounds such as syllables, words, and sentences in an attempt to improve spoken language processing. Most children (9 out of 11) in these two studies showed significant ($p < 0.05$) gains on at least one measure of either the SSW (Katz et al., 1963) or AB words (Boothroyd, 1968) in noise. Maintenance of these gains, however, was poor. One study (Miller et al., 2005) also evaluated Earobics (Cognitive Concepts, 1997), which uses computer-delivered games designed to improve listening, memory, and phonological awareness skills. Although this component of the Miller et al. (2005) study involved only two children with APD, both showed improved AP as measured by the SSW (Katz et al., 1963) or SCAN-C (Keith, 2000a).

Another recent systematic review of auditory training was conducted by McArthur (2009). Based on an earlier review (McArthur & Bishop, 2001) that had identified 75 studies showing children with specific reading disability (SRD) and specific language impairment (SLI) perform poorly on nonspeech auditory tests and a smaller number of studies showing similar findings for children with autism, McArthur's overall aim was to determine if children's developmental disorders can be treated by training AP skills. Within this, she also considered whether APD can be treated by training AP skills. McArthur operationally defined auditory training as involving nonspeech or simple speech sounds and APD as poor performance on a test that requires the detection, identification, discrimination, ordering, grouping, or localization of sounds with the cutoff for "poor" performance being as defined by the individual studies. She also stated that, although an APD may impact upon the processing of both nonspeech and speech sounds, the best tests for APD use nonspeech sounds to avoid language confounds.

McArthur (2009) identified six studies published between 2007 and 2008 that used auditory training programs with school-age children (6 to 15 years old) diagnosed with SRD, SLI and/or autism. These studies represented level 3 and 4 evidence. McArthur categorized their interventions based on the types of sound stimuli used: (1) nonspeech interventions, which presented nonspeech sounds differing in frequency, (2) simple speech interventions, which presented vowels and consonant-vowels (CVs), (3) Fast ForWord-Language (FFW-L; Scientific Learning Corporation, Inc., Berkeley, California, USA), which presented nonspeech, simple speech, and complex speech (syllables, words, and sentences) sounds, and (4) Tomatis therapy, which presented frequency filtered music and speech. Like Fey et al. (2011), McArthur critically evaluated the quality of each study by considering whether: (1) the trainees had an APD prior to training, (2) the trainees had significantly better AP after training, (3) the trainees had symptoms of SLI, SRD, Attention Deficit Hyperactivity Disorder, and autism before training, (4) the trainees' symptoms were significantly better after training, (5) the study included a second group of children who did no training, to gauge the effects of repeated testing and maturation on the measures, and (6) the study included a third group of children who did an unrelated type of training (e.g., math training), to detect placebo effects. One of the studies reviewed by McArthur (2009), the only study involving Tomatis, neglected to test participants for AP before and after therapy. Accordingly, no conclusions can be drawn regarding the impact of Tomatis on APD and so this study is omitted from the following review.

One level 3 study that met five of McArthur's (2009) six quality measures examined the impact of computer-based nonspeech and simple speech training on children with confirmed APD and SRD and/or SLI (McArthur, Ellis, Atkinson, & Coltheart, 2008). There were three groups, an experimental training group, a control training or placebo group, and an untrained group, with the children in the experimental training group receiving nonspeech (frequency discrimination and/or rapid auditory processing) and/or simple speech (vowel discrimination and/or consonant-vowel discrimination) training that specifically targeted their particular AP deficit. Group comparisons revealed significant ($p < 0.05$) improvements in the experimental group's nonspeech and simple speech test scores that were not due to repeated testing or maturation.

The other four studies reviewed by McArthur (2009) evaluated Fast ForWord-Language in children with SRD and/or SLI, but only three of the studies (Gaab, Gabrieli, Deutsch, Tallal, & Temple, 2007; Gillam et al., 2008; Stevens, Fanning, Coch, Sanders, & Neuille, 2008) measured AP outcomes. Furthermore, only one of these (Gaab et al., 2007) also confirmed that subjects had an APD prior to commencing the study. Gillam et al. (2008), a level 2 study with total $n = 216$ and meeting three of McArthur's six quality measures and Stevens et al. (2008) a level 3 study with total $n = 33$ and meeting four of McArthur's six quality measures, both identified significant ($p < 0.05$) improvements in auditory evoked potentials and auditory masking tests after training. However, neither study had confirmed the presence of APD prior to training. Furthermore, Gillam et al.'s (2008) study lacked an untrained control group that could have ruled out retest or maturation effects. In contrast, Gaab et al. (2007), a level 3 study with total $n = 22$ and meeting five of McArthur's six quality measures, established that trainees had an APD prior to training, and included a control group but found that Fast ForWord-Language had no effect on their APD.

Like Fey et al. (2011) and McArthur (2009), Loo et al. (2010) reviewed the research regarding auditory interventions, however, their focus was solely on computer-based auditory training. Accordingly, some of the studies included in Loo et al.'s review are examined also by Fey et al. and McArthur. In particular, Loo et al. wished to examine the effectiveness of computer-based auditory training for children with language- and reading-related learning difficulties due to the close relationship between APD and language, learning, and reading difficulties (Sharma, Purdy, & Kelly, 2009). Loo et al. did not define their criteria for diagnosing APD, possibly because only two of the studies in their review (Gaab et al., 2007; McArthur et al., 2008) had confirmed that their subjects had an APD (defined as a failure on a nonspeech or simple speech test of APD). They also claimed that a review of the existing evidence for computer-based auditory training in children with language learning and reading difficulties could guide the use of this approach as an intervention for APD.

Loo et al. (2010) systematically searched three electronic databases (MED-LINE, Pubmed, and Web of Science) for studies published between 2000 and 2008, as well as references from several textbooks on APD, using key words related to AP. They only considered studies written in English where the participants were school-age children between 6 and 15 years of age and where the intervention had contained nonspeech and/or simple speech sound training. Unlike Fey et al. (2011) and McArthur (2009), however, Loo et al. accepted both Earobics and Fast ForWord into the auditory intervention category. Using these criteria, Loo et al. reviewed 21 Level 2 to 4 studies. The 13 studies that measured AP outcomes, eight relating to commercially available programs (Earobics and Fast ForWord) and five to other programs, are discussed below.

Three studies reviewed by Loo et al. (2010) evaluated the Earobics program in school-age children. These were level 3 studies, all conducted by the same group of researchers and involving total participant numbers ranging from 19 to 49 (Hayes, Warrier, Nicol, Zecker, & Kraus, 2003; Russo, Nicol, Zecker, Hayes, & Kraus, 2005; Warrier, Johnson, Hayes, Nicol, & Kraus, 2004). All studies showed significantly ($p < 0.05$) improved speech evoked auditory brainstem and cortical responses in noise postintervention. In addition, Warrier et al. (2004) demonstrated a correlation between these electrophysiological changes and behavioral auditory perceptual changes (such as improved speech discrimination abilities).

The commercially available program, Fast ForWord, was evaluated by six studies reviewed by Loo et al. Three of these studies (Gaab et al., 2007; Gillam et al., 2008; Stevens et al., 2008) are also reviewed by McArthur (2009) and are outlined above. The remaining three studies, all level 4, reported significant ($p < 0.05$) improvements in temporal processing tasks but did not include untrained comparison groups and generally included small subject numbers (Agnew, Dorn, & Eden, 2004, with $n = 7$; Valentine, Hedrick, & Swanson, 2006, with $n = 26$; and Marler, Champlin, & Gillam, 2001, with total $n = 7$). Accordingly, it is unclear whether reported improvements are the result of the treatment or due to other factors such as repeated testing or maturation.

Other noncommercially available nonspeech (e.g., tone) and simple speech (e.g., phonemes or consonant-vowel syllables) sound training programs were the subject of a further five studies reviewed by Loo et al. (2010). In addition to the McArthur et al.(2008) level 3 study mentioned above, Loo et al. reviewed four more level 3 studies that had included both treatment and control groups: Kujala et al. (2001, $n = 48$), Schaffler, Sonntag, Hartnegg, and Fischer (2004, $n = 182$), Strehlow et al. (2006, $n = 44$); and Veuillet, Magnan, Ecalle, Thai-Van, & Collet (2007, $n = 18$). All of these studies showed significant ($p < 0.05$) treatment-related gains on measures ranging from frequency, intensity and temporal discrimination to auditory evoked potentials.

Conclusions

The evidence that direct auditory interventions (Intervention) improve AP (Outcome) in school-age children with APD with or without spoken language, reading, or learning difficulties (Patient/Problem), compared to no treatment or placebo treatments (Comparison), is:

- suggestive-to-compelling (see the Appendix) for interventions involving nonspeech and/or simple speech stimuli (noncomputer or computer-based),
- suggestive for Earobics, and
- equivocal for Fast ForWord.

The evidence that AIT has no effect on AP is suggestive.

In general, this evidence contained mostly level 3 and 4 studies with adequate internal validity and impact but often limited external validity (mostly due to the use of stimuli not easily obtained in general clinical environments). As a result, the overall grade of recommendation was considered to be a B or C (see Table 1–6).

Are Auditory Interventions Effective Treatments for Spoken Language and Reading Disorders?

Intervention for APD often extends beyond APD itself. This is driven by widespread reports that APD coexists with other disorders of language, attention, and/or cognition. For example, in a clinical sample of 68 children, Sharma et al. (2009) diagnosed three children (4%) as having APD only, and 46 children (67%) as having APD and a spoken language and/or reading disorder. Adding to this is the vigorous and ongoing debate over whether APD causes disorders in language, literacy or cognition, or whether children with primary disorders of language and cognition are being incorrectly diagnosed with APD due to the confounds present in some APD tests (ASHA, 2005; Bailey & Snowling, 2002; Dawes & Bishop, 2009). With these factors in mind, this section briefly reviews the evidence for direct auditory interventions in the treatment of language, reading, and spelling disorders in school-age children, as presented by Fey et al. (2011), McArthur (2009) and Loo et al. (2010). It must be noted that these reviews included many of the same studies considered in the previous section of this chapter, and many of the studies were included in more than one of these reviews. A further meta-analysis of the Fast ForWord program only (Strong, Torgerson, Torgerson, & Hulme, 2011) is also included.

Fey et al. (2011) considered auditory interventions used to treat spoken language disorders in school-age children who had not been identified as having APD (although this was sometimes due to the child not receiving an AP assessment rather than the confirmation of normal AP skills). Their search yielded 17 articles involving 19 separate studies. One study, however, was a case study from which no firm conclusions could be drawn (Crosbie & Dodd, 2001). Eleven studies examined the effect of Fast ForWord on language, with the three largest and most rigorous studies (levels 2 to 3) showing either no improvements in language (Pokorni, Worthington, & Jamison, 2004), or improvements similar to other, equally intensive language interventions or control conditions involving no auditory or language manipulations (Cohen et al., 2005; Gillam et al., 2008). One level 3 and two level 4 studies (Agnew et al., 2004; Loeb, Stoke, & Fey, 2001; Pokorni et al., 2004) examined the effect of Fast ForWord on reading, with no firm conclusions drawn due to inconsistent results. Finally, two level 3 studies examined the effect of language-based interventions (that incorporated graded acoustic modifications similar to those employed in Fast ForWord) on sentence comprehension (Bishop et al., 2006) and phonological awareness (Segers & Verhoeven, 2004), with both studies showing similar gains for the treatment and control groups.

McArthur (2009) reviewed six intervention studies that used auditory training programs to treat school-age children with APD and SRD and/or SLI. One level 3 study (McArthur et al., 2008) involving nonspeech and simple speech training failed to demonstrate treatment-related improvements in the language, reading, spelling or attention skills of participants with APD and SRD and/or SLI, beyond those seen in the control group. Four level 2 to 3 studies (Gaab et al., 2007; Gillam et al., 2008; Given, Wasserman, Chari, Beattie, & Eden, 2008; Stevens et al., 2008) examined Fast ForWord intervention, from which McArthur (2009) concluded that the program had no effect on expressive language and phoneme awareness, inconsistent (at best) effects on reading and receptive language, and possible effects on some forms of rapid naming or the retrieval of information from phonological memory. One level 3 study (Corbett, Shickman, & Ferrer, 2008) examined the effect of Tomatis therapy on the language abilities of children with autism and found no effects on receptive and expressive vocabulary beyond those seen in the control training (placebo) group.

Loo et al.'s (2010) review of 21 studies examined the efficacy of computer-based training programs (Fast ForWord, Earobics, and other programs) in treating language and cognitive disorders in school-age children with SRD or SLI. Nine studies (levels 2 to 4) examined Fast ForWord, and although the majority reported treatment-related improvements in language (Agnew et al., 2004; Cohen et al., 2005; Gillam et al., 2008; Given et al., 2008; Hook, Macaruso, & Jones, 2001; Rouse & Krueger, 2004; Valentine et al., 2006), only two level 3 studies could show these improvements were not the result of test-retest or maturational effects (Stevens et al., 2008; Troia & Whitney, 2003). Inconsistent results were also noted with Stevens et al. (2008) reporting significant ($p < 0.05$) gains in receptive (but not expressive) language, Troia and Whitney (2003) reporting significant ($p < 0.05$) gains in phonological skills and expressive (but not receptive) language, but Pokorni et al. (2004) reporting no change in receptive or expressive language, phonological skills or reading. Loo et al. (2010) concluded that Fast ForWord may help to improve some aspects of phonological awareness (such as rhyming and blending), but is not effective in remediating reading and spelling.

Three level 3 studies reviewed by Loo et al. examined the efficacy of the Earobics program (Hayes et al., 2003; Russo et al., 2005; Warrier et al., 2004). Although all three showed significant ($p < 0.05$) improvements in phonological awareness skills, none measured the impact on language, reading or spelling.

Finally, five level 3 studies in Loo et al. (2010) examined nonspeech (e.g. tone) and simple speech (e.g., phonemes or consonant-vowel syllables) training. These showed significantly ($p < 0.05$) improved reading in children if the training was delivered using audiovisual methods (Kujala et al., 2001; Veuillet et al., 2007) rather than auditory alone (McArthur et al., 2008; Strehlow et al., 2006). Three of these studies showed no significant training effect for spelling (Kujala et al., 2001; McArthur et al., 2008; Strehlow et al., 2006), and two showed no evidence of treatment-related change in language or phonological awareness (McArthur et al., 2008; Schaffler et al., 2004).

Loo et al. (2010) concluded that the current literature provides some evidence that computer-based auditory training may enhance phonological awareness, but no clear evidence that this approach improves reading and spoken language in school-age children with language, reading, and learning deficits.

Strong et al. (2011) searched eight electronic databases for level 2 or 3 studies that included a matched control group to examine the impact of the Fast ForWord program on standardized tests of oral language or reading. Studies had to have been published in peer-reviewed journals but their participants could be of any age and learner characteristics. After numerous screenings, an initial 79 studies was reduced to six studies with a total of 795 participants with reading and spoken language impairments. Of the six studies, five have been outlined above (Cohen et al., 2005; Gillam et al., 2008; Given et al., 2008; Pokorni et al., 2004; Rouse & Krueger, 2004). A further level 2 study (Borman, Benson, & Overman, 2009) compared the effects of "pull-out" Fast ForWord intervention and other nonliteracy instruction for children with below average reading skills in the school setting. A meta-analysis conducted on two reading measures, single word and passage reading, and two spoken language measures, receptive and expressive vocabulary, compared results for Fast ForWord intervention to control training groups and control groups who did not receive any training. The resultant 8 pooled effect sizes (range = −.10 to .17) indicated no reliable difference from zero or no group differences with negative effect sizes suggesting worse performance for some children receiving the Fast ForWord program.

Conclusions

The evidence is suggestive to compelling (see the Appendix) that direct auditory interventions including computer-based interventions involving nonspeech and/or simple speech training and Fast ForWord (Intervention) do not improve spoken language and/or reading skills (Outcome) in school-age children with spoken language and/or reading disorders with or without APD (Patient/Problem), compared to no treatment or placebo treatments (Comparison). The evidence is suggestive that Earobics improves phonological awareness skills in this patient population. In general, this evidence contained level 1 to 3 studies with adequate internal validity and impact but often limited external validity (mostly due to the use of stimuli not easily obtained in general clinical environments). The overall grade of recommendation was considered to be an A or B (except for the conclusions regarding Earobics, which was considered to be a grade C).

In considering the conclusion above, it is important to note that developmental disorders such as SLI may have several underlying impairments (Dawes & Bishop, 2009; McArthur et al., 2008). This makes it unrealistic to expect that remediating one deficit (such as APD) should automatically lead to the remediation of all surface symptoms (McArthur et al., 2008).

ARE PHONOLOGICAL INTERVENTIONS EFFECTIVE TREATMENTS FOR APD?

Phonological awareness training is widely used to treat children with reading difficulties with a phonological basis (the "phonological dyslexias") and is also considered an important component of early intervention for children at risk for later literacy problems. According to the National Reading Panel (National Institute of Child Health and Human Development, 2000), phonemic awareness instruction, a specific area of phonological awareness instruction that encompasses the ability to reflect upon and manipulate individual sounds as opposed to larger segments such as syllables, is highly effective in improving reading. The reader is referred to the National Institute of Child Health and Human Development (2000), Al Otaiba, Puranik, Ziolkowski, and Montgomery (2009) and Schuele and Boudreau (2008) for more detailed reviews of phonological awareness interventions for children with reading and spelling deficits.

Although the linguistic basis of phonological awareness training aligns it more closely to language intervention than to auditory intervention, its manipulation of sound could be considered by some to be an auditory intervention under broader definitions of auditory training. It is perhaps for this reason that phonological awareness intervention is sometimes recommended for children with APD (BSA, 2011b). It is important to note, however, that the efficacy of traditional phonological awareness training on the auditory, language, reading, and spelling skills of children with APD, remains largely unexplored.

FUTURE RESEARCH INTO APD INTERVENTION

In addition to the obvious need for universally accepted definitions of APD and its various interventions, and the general need for more Level 1 and 2 research (McArthur, 2007; McArthur et al., 2008; Moore, 2006), we propose that future research into APD and APD intervention should address at least six main issues, which we discuss below.

Problems with Current Tests of AP

The many problems with current tests of AP are well recognized but poorly addressed (Dawes & Bishop, 2009). These include the widespread lack of normative and reliability data, and ongoing concerns about test validity. The latter is of particular concern considering many AP tests use linguistic stimuli and require a spoken response, and the relative contribution of language and cognition to test outcomes is often unknown. Greater efforts to address these problems are beginning to emerge. Authors such as Moore, Cowan, Riley, Edmondson-Jones, and Ferguson (2011) have provided developmental standards on a variety of temporal, spectral, and binaural AP (psychoacoustic) tests in typically developing school-age children. Other authors such as Findlen and Roup (2011) have begun to address the effects of varied lexical content (with constant phonetic content) on commonly used tests of APD. More work is needed, however, before a reliable and valid suite of APD tests can be claimed for clinical or research use.

The Relative Contribution of AP to Language and General Listening Behaviors

The fact that language development and general listening ability can be severely compromised by hearing loss has been offered as prima facie evidence that AP contributes significantly to language and listening. Although such a contribution is difficult to deny, its relative size needs to be determined particularly as the effects of APD are more subtle than those of hearing loss (Bailey & Snowling, 2002; McArthur et al., 2008).

The relative contribution of AP to language has long been debated (e.g., Rees, 1973) with recent reviews suggesting this contribution may not be as significant as previously thought, at least in the school-age child. This is highlighted by McArthur et al. (2008; included in the review by McArthur, 2009). These authors hypothesize that improving AP (nonspeech and simple speech) may not immediately improve language and reading in children with SLI and SRD because improving AP may simply ready the auditory system for learning. To improve language and reading skills, further intervention that specifically targets language and reading may be required. In this regard, McArthur et al. (2008) stress a distinction between being ready to learn language and reading versus learning language and reading. They also stress the need for longitudinal studies to further elucidate the contribution of AP to this potential progression.

The relative contribution of AP to general listening behaviors has been the topic of more recent debate with growing evidence that this contribution may also be limited, at least in the school-age child (Dawes, Bishop, Sirimanna, & Bamiou, 2008; Wilson et al., 2011). This was considered in detail by Moore et al. (2010) who studied 1469 randomly chosen, normally hearing school children (aged 6 to 11 years). A computer-based suite of tests was used to assess AP (backward masking, simultaneous masking and frequency discrimination), speech-in-noise performance, cognition (IQ, memory, language, and literacy), and attention (auditory and visual) (Barry, Ferguson, & Moore, 2010; Margolis, Glasberg, Creeke, & Moore, 2010), as well as questionnaires to measure listening and communicative performance in the classroom. These authors also used their AP test results to derive separate measures of the sensory component of AP ("pure" AP, separated from cognition and attention). Their results showed that, whereas the AP scores improved with age and correlated with poor speech-in-noise, cognitive and communicative performance, the "pure" AP scores did not. Their results also showed that whereas response variability in AP scores (thought to be a measure of attention and cognition) predicted overall listening, communication, and speech-in-noise skills, the "pure" AP scores did not. In other words, auditory sensory processing ("pure" AP) was largely unrelated to the presenting symptoms of APD (poor communication and listening). Instead, these symptoms were better predicted by auditory attention (as measured by response variability and cognitive performance). Moore et al. concluded that the clinical diagnosis and management of APD, as well as its further research, be based on the premise that APD is primarily a problem of auditory attention (potentially reigniting arguments that APD is an auditory manifestation of attention deficit disorder). This not only affects the future of APD, but also its past. It is possible that many of the inconsistencies seen in previous APD interventions could be explained (at least in part) by unmeasured fluctuations in attention.

AP and the Greater Complexity of Sensory/Perceptual Learning

AP is but one contributor to the greater concept of sensory/perceptual learning. Goldstone (1998) states that sensory/perceptual learning refers to performance changes that are brought about through practice or experience and lead to improvements in an organism's ability to respond to its environment (as distinct from procedural learning, which results from learning the response demands of the task). Moore and Amitay (2007) build on this to define auditory training as being any experience that leads to auditory learning, and auditory learning as "any measurable improvement in performance of a listening task that is produced by a period of stimulation" (Moore, Halliday, & Amitay, 2009, p. 409). This approach highlights the possibility that APD intervention need not be auditory or deliberate, as long as it resolves the APD.

Before the principles of sensory/perceptual learning can be fully applied to APD intervention, its complexities need further elucidation. This is highlighted by Wright and Zhang (2009) who note that many auditory perceptual skills improve with practice (e.g., frequency-discrimination, intensity-discrimination, temporal-judgment, spatial-hearing, and signal-detection); that some improvements generalize to untrained stimuli, to untrained tasks, to untrained testing procedures, and to other sensory modalities; but this generalization can be limited, varied, and difficult to predict. Moore et al. (2009) further suggested that the best auditory training tasks are relevant, challenging, and engaging, that significant auditory learning can occur during relatively brief periods of training, and that improvements can generalize to some untrained listening and language skills. Moore et al. contend that attention plays a fundamental role in learning and that simply performing an engaging, though apparently unrelated, task can induce learning. They also warn that, although the field of sensory/perceptual learning holds much promise for APD intervention, it is not a panacea, with realistic outlooks needed when considering its place in larger contexts of listening and education.

The Role of AP in the Development of the Younger Child

The findings of most of the studies reviewed in this chapter apply only to the school-age child. The relative contribution of AP to language and cognitive development in the younger child could differ dramatically. Assessing AP in the younger child presents many challenges however, with many behavioral tests of AP limited to children aged 7 years or older due to the highly variable performances seen in younger children. If, as outlined by McArthur et al. (2008), normal AP can be trained and lead to optimal conditions for learning language and cognitive skills, early diagnosis and remediation of APD should be a priority. Evoked potentials and neural imaging could be useful in this regard, although these measures can also be hindered by high variability in younger children.

The Potential Contribution of Evoked Potentials and Neural Imaging

Evoked potentials and neural imaging have long held significant promise as tools for investigating APD and its intervention, particularly as they allow for greater control over variables such as language and cognition. Despite the inclusion of some auditory evoked potential studies in reviews of APD intervention (e.g., Gillam et al., 2008; Jirsa, 1992; Phonak, 2006; Stevens et al., 2008), the bulk of auditory evoked potential and imaging studies have yet to be fully integrated into current models of APD (e.g., Abrams, Nicol, Zecker, & Kraus, 2010; Dick et al., 2007; Gaillard, Balsamo, Xu, Grandin, & Braniecki, 2001; Johnson, Nicol, & Kraus, 2005; Kraus & Banai, 2007; Krizman, Skoe, & Kraus, 2010; Musacchia, Sams, Skoe, & Kraus, 2007; Patterson & Johnsrude, 2008). Although some of this research has been reviewed (e.g., Eisner & Scott, 2009), a systematic review of how this work guides APD intervention is needed.

The Application of Research to Clinic and Vice Versa

Researchers often investigate single APD interventions in an attempt to control for multiple variables. In contrast, clinicians often apply multiple APD interventions (as well as linguistic, metalinguistic, cognitive, and metacognitive interventions) in the hope that at least one will have a positive effect (e.g., Bellis, 2003; Geffner, Ross-Swain, Geffner, & Ross-Swain, 2007; Katz et al., 1992; Masters, Stecker, & Katz, 1998).

To mitigate this apparent mismatch, clinicians should consider abandoning the simultaneous use of multiple interventions in favor of a staged rollout of individual interventions (or small, related groups of interventions). This could allow for a more confident determination of which interventions are providing the greater benefit for an individual child. Clinicians should also use a structured evidence-based decision-making process to regularly reconsider their choice of interventions. Authors such as Gillam and Gillam (2006) provide excellent advice for making such decisions in practical settings, and although their article addresses evidence-based decision making for child language intervention in schools, its principles remain directly applicable to APD intervention.

In return, researchers should reconsider how they disseminate their findings to clinicians, particularly with regards to distinguishing level 1 to 4 evidence from level 5 and 6 (case reports and expert opinion) evidence (see Table 1–5). In cases where benefits are gained by combining interventions (e.g., Kujala et al., 2001; Veuillet et al., 2007), then researchers must be careful to clearly report the details of these combinations.

CONCLUSIONS

When the criteria in the Appendix are used to evaluate the evidence presented here, we conclude:

1. The evidence that auditory interventions (Intervention) improve AP (Outcome) in school-age children with APD with or without spoken language, reading, or learning difficulties (Patient/Problem), compared to no treatment or placebo treatments (Comparison), is:
   - equivocal for personal FM systems,
   - suggestive to compelling for interventions involving nonspeech and/or simple speech stimuli (noncomputer or computer-based),
   - suggestive for Earobics, and
   - equivocal for Fast ForWord.

   With respect to AIT, the evidence is suggestive that it has no effect on AP.
2. The evidence is suggestive to compelling that direct auditory interventions including computer-based interventions involving nonspeech and/or simple speech training and Fast ForWord (Intervention) do not improve spoken language and/or reading skills (Outcome) in school-age children with spoken language and/or reading disorders with or without APD (Patient/Problem), compared to no treatment or placebo treatments (Comparison). With respect to Earobics, the evidence is suggestive that it improves phonological awareness skills in this patient population.

Our ability to make these conclusions was confounded by the lack of universally accepted "gold standards" for defining and diagnosing APD. Although the substantial efforts of groups such as ASHA (2005) and BSA (2011a) are acknowledged, the role of potential confounds such as language and cognition remain as particular points of confusion. Finally, our conclusions are limited to the school-age child, and the need for higher level evidence remains strong in all areas of APD intervention.

REFERENCES

Abrams, D. A., Nicol, T., Zecker, S., & Kraus, N. (2010). Rapid acoustic processing in the auditory brainstem is not related to cortical asymmetry for the syllable rate of speech. *Clinical Neurophysiology, 121*(8), 1343–1350.

Agnew, J. A., Dorn, C., & Eden, G. F. (2004). Effect of intensive training on auditory processing and reading skills. *Brain and Language, 88*(1), 21–25.

Al Otaiba, S., Puranik, C. S., Ziolkowski, R. A., & Montgomery, T. M. (2009). Effectiveness of early phonological awareness interventions for students with speech or language impairments. *Journal of Special Education, 43*(2), 107–128.

American Psychiatric Association. (1995). *Diagnostic and statistical manual of mental disorders: DSM-IV* (4th ed.). Washington, DC: Author.

Arnold, P., & Canning, D. (1999). Does classroom amplification aid comprehension? *British Journal of Audiology, 33*(3), 171–178.

American Speech-Language-Hearing Association. (1996). Central auditory processing: Current status of research and implications for clinical practice. *American Journal of Audiology, 5*(2), 41–54.

American Speech-Language-Hearing Association. (2004). *Evidence-based practice in communication disorders: An introduction* (Technical report). Retrieved from http://www.asha.org/docs/pdf/PS2005-00221.pdf

American Speech-Language-Hearing Association. (2005). *(Central) auditory processing disorders* (Technical report). Retrieved from http://www.asha.org/docs/pdf/TR2005-00043.pdf

Bailey, P. J., & Snowling, M. J. (2002). Auditory processing and the development of language and literacy. *British Medical Bulletin, 63*, 135–146.

Bamiou, D. E., Campbell, N., & Sirimanna, T. (2006). Management of auditory processing disorders. *Audiological Medicine, 4*, 46–56.

Barry, J. G., Ferguson, M. A., & Moore, D. R. (2010). Making sense of listening: The IMAP test battery. *Journal of Visualized Experiments, 44*, e2139. doi: 10.3791/2139

Beasley, D. S., Schwimmer, S., & Rintelmann, W. F. (1972). Intelligibility of time-compressed CNC monosyllables. *Journal of Speech and Hearing Research, 15*, 340–350.

Bellis, T. J. (2003). *Assessment and management of central auditory processing disorders in the educational setting: From science to practice* (2nd ed.). San Diego, CA: Singular Publishing Group.

Bellis, T. J., & Ferre, M. F. (1999). Multidimensional approach to the differential diagnosis of central auditory processing disorders in children. *Journal of the American Academy of Audiology, 10*(3), 319–328.

Bishop, D. V. M., Adams, C. V., & Rosen, S. (2006). Resistance of grammatical impairment to computerized comprehension training in children with specific and non-specific language impairments. *International Journal of Language & Communication Disorders, 41*(1), 19–40.

Boothroyd, A. (1968). Developments in speech audiometry. *Sound, 2*, 3-10.

Borman, G. D., Benson, J. G., & Overman, L. (2009). A randomized field trial of the Fast ForWord language computer-based training program. *Educational Evaluation and Policy Analysis, 31*, 82–106.

Brown, J. R. (1987). Assessing assessment: The Goldman-Fristoe-Woodcock auditory skills battery. *Ear and Hearing, 8*(5), 262–269.

British Society of Audiology. (2007). *Interim position statement on APD.* Retrieved from http://www.thebsa.org.uk/apd/BSA_APD_Position_statement_Final_Draft_Feb_2007.pdf

British Society of Audiology. (2011a). *Position statement: Auditory processing disorder (APD).* Retrieved from http://www.thebsa.org.uk/images/stories/docs/BSA_APD_PositionPaper_31March11_FINAL.pdf

British Society of Audiology. (2011b). *Practice guidance: An overview of current management of auditory processing disorder (APD).* Draft document to Council for approval to press ahead with consultation. Retrieved from http://www.thebsa.org.uk/images/stories/docs/BSA_APD Mgmt_31March2011_Consultation.pdf

Cacace, A. T., & McFarland, D. J. (2005). The importance of modality specificity in diagnosing central auditory processing disorder. *American Journal of Audiology, 14*, 112–123.

Cognitive Concepts. (1997). *Earobics: Auditory development and phonics program* [Computer software]. Cambridge, MA: Author.

Cohen, W., Hodson, A., O'Hara, A., Boyle, J., Durram, T., McCartney, E., . . . Watson, J. (2005). Effects of computer-based intervention through acoustically modified speech (Fast ForWord) in severe mixed receptive-expressive language impairment: Outcomes from a randomized controlled trial. *Journal of Speech, Language, and Hearing Research, 48*(3), 715–729.

Corbett, B. A., Shickman, K., & Ferrer, E. (2008). Brief report: The effects of Tomatis sound therapy on language in children with autism. *Journal of Autism and Developmental Disorders, 38*, 562–566.

Cowan, J., Rosen, S., & Moore, D. R. (2009). Putting the auditory processing back into auditory processing disorder in children. In A. T. Cacace & D. J. McFarland (Eds.), *Controversies in central auditory processing disorder* (pp. 187–198). San Diego, CA: Plural Publishing.

Cox, R. M. (2005). Evidence-based practice in provision of amplification. *Journal of the American Academy of Audiology, 16*(7), 419–438.

Crandell, C. (1996). Effects of sound field FM amplification on the speech perception of ESL children. *Educational Audiology Monograph, 4*, 1–5.

Crosbie, S., & Dodd, B. (2001). Training auditory discrimination: A single case study. *Child Language Teaching and Therapy, 17*(3), 173–194.

Dawes, P., & Bishop, D. (2009). Auditory processing disorder in relation to developmental disorders of language, communication and attention: A review and critique. *International Journal of Language and Communication Disorders, 44*(4), 440–465.

Dawes, P., Bishop, D. V. M., Sirimanna, T., & Bamiou, D. E. (2008). Profile and aetiology of children diagnosed with auditory processing disorder (APD). *International Journal of Pediatric Otorhinolaryngology, 72*(4), 483–489.

Deppeler, J. M., Taranto, A. M., & Bench, J. (2004). Language and auditory processing changes following Fast ForWord. *Australian and New Zealand Journal of Audiology, 26*(2), 94–109.

Dick, F., Saygin, A. P., Galati, G., Pitzalis, S., Bentrovato, S., D'Amico, S., . . . Pizzamiglio, L. (2007). What is involved and what is necessary for complex linguistic and nonlinguistic auditory processing: Evidence from functional magnetic resonance imaging and lesion data. *Journal of Cognitive Neuroscience, 19*(5), 799–816.

Dillon, H., Cameron, S., Glyde, H., Wilson, W., & Tomlin, D (in press). An opinion on the assessment of people who may have an auditory processing disorder. *Journal of the American Academy of Audiology.*

Domitz, D. M., & Schow, R. L. (2000). A new CAPD battery - Multiple auditory processing assessment (MAPA): Factor analysis and comparisons with SCAN. *American Journal of Audiology, 9*, 101–111.

Eisner, F., & Scott, S. K. (2009). Speech and auditory processing in the cortex: Evidence from functional neuroimaging. In A. T. Cacace & D. J. McFarland (Eds.), *Controversies in central auditory processing disorder* (pp. 47–60). San Diego, CA: Plural Publishing.

English, K., Martonik, J., & Moir, L. (2003). An auditory training technique to improve dichotic listening. *Hearing Journal, 56*(1), 34.

Fey, M. E., Richard, G. J., Geffner, D., Kamhi, A. G., Medwetsky, L., Paul, D., . . . Schooling, T. (2011). Auditory processing disorders and auditory/language interventions: An evidence-based systematic review. *Language Speech and Hearing Services in Schools*, 42, 246–264.

Findlen, U. M., & Roup, C. M. (2011). Dichotic speech recognition using CVC words and nonsense CVC syllable stimuli. *Journal of the American Academy of Audiology, 22*(1), 13–22.

Frattali, C. M., & Colper, L. A. (Eds.). (2007). *Evidence-based pratice and outcome oriented approaches in speech-langauge pathology* (2nd ed.). New York, NY: Thieme.

Gaab, N., Gabrieli, J. D., Deutsch, G. K., Tallal, P., & Temple, E. (2007). Neural correlates of rapid auditory processing are disrupted in children with developmental dyslexia and ameliorated with training: An fMRI study. *Restorative Neurology and Neuroscience, 25*(3–4), 295–310.

Gaillard, W. D., Balsamo, L., Xu, B., Grandin, C. B., & Braniecki, S. H. (2001). Language neural networks of auditory processing in young children identified with functional magnetic resonance imaging. *Annals of Neurology, 50*(3), S94–S95.

Geffner, D., Ross-Swain, D., Geffner, D., & Ross-Swain, D. (2007). *Auditory processing disorders: Assessment, management and treatment.* San Diego, CA: Plural Publishing.

Gillam, R. B., Loeb, D. F., Hoffman, L. M., Bohman, T., Champlin, C. A., Thibodeau, L., . . . Friel-Patti, S. (2008). The efficacy of Fast ForWord Language intervention in school-age children with language impairment: A randomized controlled trial. *Journal of Speech, Language, and Hearing Research, 51*(1), 97–119.

Gillam, S. L., & Gillam, R. B. (2006). Making evidence-based decisions about child language intervention in schools. *Language Speech and Hearing Services in Schools, 37*(4), 304–315.

Given, B. K., Wasserman, J. D., Chari, S. A., Beattie, K., & Eden, G. F. (2008). A randomized, controlled study of computer-based intervention in middle school struggling readers. *Brain and Language, 106*(2), 83–97.

Goldstone, R. L. (1998). Perceptual learning. *Annual Review of Psychology, 49*, 585–612.

Hanschmann, H., Wiehe, S., Müller-Mazzotta, J., & Berger, R. (2010). Speech perception in noise with and without FM technology. *HNO, 58*(7), 674–679.

Hayes, E. A., Warrier, C. M., Nicol, T. G., Zecker, S. G., & Kraus, N. (2003). Neural plasticity following auditory training in children with learning problems. *Clinical Neurophysiology, 114*, 673–684.

Heeney, M. F. (2007). *Classroom sound field amplification, listening and learning.* PhD Thesis, University of Newcastle, NSW, Australia, Newcastle.

Hook, P. E., Macaruso, P., & Jones, S. (2001). Efficacy of Fast ForWord training on facilitating acquisition of reading skills by children with reading difficulties—A longitudinal study. *Annals of Dyslexia, 51*, 75–96.

Jerger, J. (2009). The concept of auditory processing disorder: A brief history. In A. T. Cacace & D. J. McFarland (Eds.), *Controversies in central auditory processing disorder* (pp. 1–14). San Diego, CA: Plural Publishing.

Jerger, J., & Musiek, F. (2000). Report of the consensus conference on the diagnosis of auditory processing disorders in school-aged children. *Journal of the American Academy of Audiology, 11*(9), 467–474.

Jerger, J., Speaks, C., & Trammell, J. A. (1968). A new approach to speech audiometry. *Journal of Speech and Hearing Disorders, 33*, 318–328.

Jirsa, R. E. (1992). The clinical utility of the P3 AERP in children with auditory processing disorders. *Journal of Speech and Hearing Research, 35*, 903–912.

Johnson, K. L., Nicol, T. G., & Kraus, N. (2005). Brain stem response to speech: A biological marker of auditory processing. *Ear and Hearing, 26*(5), 424–434.

Johnston, K. N., John, A. B., Kreisman, N. V., Hall, J. W., & Crandell, C. C. (2009). Multiple benefits of personal FM system use by children with auditory processing disorder (APD). *International Journal of Audiology, 48*(6), 371–383.

Katz, J. (1992). Classification of auditory processing disorders. In J. Katz, N. Stacker, & D. Henderson (Eds.), *Central auditory processing: A transdisciplinary view* (pp. 81–91). St Louis, MO: Mosby Year Book.

Katz, J., Basil, R. A., & Smith, J. M. (1963). A staggered spondaic word test for detecting central auditory lesions. *Annals of Otology Rhinology and Laryngology, 72*(4), 908–918.

Katz, J., Johnson, C. D., Tillery, K. L., Bradham, T., Brandner, S., Delagrange, T. N., . . . Stecker, N.A. (2002). Clinical and research concerns regarding Jerger and Musiek (2000) APD recommendations. *Audiology Today, 14*(2), 14–17.

Katz, J., Stecker, N. A., & Henderson, D. (1992). Introduction to central auditory processing. In J. Katz, N. A. Stecker, & D. Henderson (Eds.), *Central auditory processing: A transdisciplinary view* (pp. 3–8). St. Louis, MO: Mosby Year Book.

Keith, R. W. (1999). Clinical issues in central auditory processing disorders. *Language, Speech, and Hearing Services in Schools, 30*, 339–344.

Keith, R. W. (2000a). Development and standardization of SCAN-C test for auditory processing disorders in children. *Journal of the American Academy of Audiology, 11*, 438–445.

Keith, R. W. (2000b). *Random Gap Detection Test.* St Louis, MO: AUDiTEC.

Kraus, N., & Banai, K. (2007). Auditory-processing malleability—Focus on language and music. *Current Directions in Psychological Science, 16*(2), 105–110.

Kreisman, B. M., & Crandell, C. C. (2002). Frequency modulation (FM) systems for children with normal hearing. Retrieved from http://www.audiologyonline.com/articles/pf_article_detail.asp?article_id=358

Krizman, J., Skoe, E., & Kraus, N. (2010). Stimulus rate and subcortical auditory processing of speech. *Audiology and Neurotology, 15*(5), 332–342.

Kujala, T., Karma, K., Ceponiene, R., Belitz, S., Turkkila, P., Tervaniemi, M., & Näätänen, R. (2001). Plastic neural changes and reading improvement caused by audiovisual training in reading-impaired children. *Proceedings of the National Academy of Sciences of the United States of America, 98*, 10509–10514.

Lemos, I. C., Jacob, R. T., Gejão, M. G., Bevilacqua, M. C., Feniman, M. R., & Ferrari, D. V. (2009). Frequency modulation (FM) system in auditory processing disorder: An evidence-based practice? *Pro-Fono Revista de Atualizacao Cientifica, 21*(3), 243–248.

Loeb, D. F., Stoke, C., & Fey, M. E. (2001). Language changes associated with Fast ForWord-Language: Evidence from case studies. *American Journal of Speech-Language Pathology, 10*, 216–230.

Loo, J. H. Y., Bamiou, D. E., Campbell, N., & Luxon, L. M. (2010). Computer-based auditory training (CBAT): Benefits for children with language- and reading-related learning difficulties. *Developmental Medicine and Child Neurology, 52*(8), 708–717.

Margolis, R. H., Glasberg, B. R., Creeke, S., & Moore, B. C. J. (2010). AMTAS (R): Automated method for testing auditory sensitivity: Validation studies. *International Journal of Audiology, 49*(3), 185–194.

Marler, J. A., Champlin, C. A., & Gillam, R. B. (2001). Backward and simultaneous masking measured in children with language-learning impairments who received intervention with Fast ForWord or Laureate Learning Systems Software. *American Journal of Speech-Language Pathology, 10*, 258–268.

Massie, R., & Dillon, H. (2006a). The impact of sound-field amplification in mainstream cross-cultural classrooms: Part 1—Educational outcomes. *Australian Journal of Education, 50*(1), 62–77.

Massie, R., & Dillon, H. (2006b). The impact of sound-field amplification in mainstream cross-cultural classrooms: Part 2—Teacher and child opinions. *Australian Journal of Education, 50*(1), 78–94.

Massie, R., Theodoros, D., Byrne, D., McPherson, B., & Smaldino, J. (1999). The effects of sound-field amplification on the communicative interactions of Aboriginal and Torres Strait Islander children. *Australian and New Zealand Journal of Audiology, 21*(2), 93–109.

Massie, R., Theodoros, D., McPherson, B., & Smaldino, J. (2004). Sound-field amplification: Enhancing the classroom listening environment for Aboriginal and Torres Strait Islander children. *Australian Journal of Indigenous Education, 33*, 47–53.

Masters, M. G., Stecker, N. A., & Katz, J. (1998). *Central auditory processing disorders: Mostly management.* Boston, MA: Allyn & Bacon.

McArthur, G. M. (2007). Test-retest effects in treatment studies of reading disability: The devil is in the detail. *Dyslexia, 13*(4), 240–252.

McArthur, G. M. (2009). Auditory processing disorders: Can they be treated? *Current Opinion in Neurology, 22*(2), 137–143.

McArthur, G.M., & Bishop, D.V.M. (2001). Auditory perceptual processing in people with reading and oral language impairments: Current issues and recommendations. *Dyslexia, 7*, 150–170.

McArthur, G. M., Ellis, D., Atkinson, C. M., & Coltheart, M. (2008). Auditory processing deficits in children with reading and language impairments: Can they (and should they) be treated? *Cognition, 107*(3), 946–977.

McFarland, D. J., & Cacace, A. T. (2002). Factor analysis in CAPD and the "unimodal" test battery: Do we have a model that will satisfy? *American Journal of Audiology, 11*(1), 7–9.

McFarland, D. J., & Cacace, A. T. (2009). Models of central auditory processing abilities and disorders. In A. T. Cacace & D. J. McFarland (Eds.), *Controversies in central auditory processing disorder* (pp. 93–108). San Diego, CA: Plural Publishing.

McSporran, E., Butterworth, Y., & Rowson, V. J. (1997). Sound field amplification and listening behaviour in the classroom. *British Educational Research Journal, 23*, 81–96.

Miller, C. A., Uhring, E. A., Brown, J. J. C., Kowalski, E. M., Roberts, B., & Schaefer, B. A. (2005). Case studies of auditory training for children with auditory processing difficulties: A preliminary analysis. *Contemporary Issues in Communication Science and Disorders, 32*, 93–107.

Moore, D. R. (2006). Auditory processing disorder (APD): Definition, diagnosis, neural basis, and intervention. *Audiological Medicine, 4*, 4–11.

Moore, D. R., & Amitay, S. (2007). Auditory training: Rules and applications. *Seminars in Hearing, 28*(2), 99–109.

Moore, D. R., Cowan, J. A., Riley, A., Edmondson-Jones, A. M., & Ferguson, M. A. (2011).

Development of auditory processing in 6- to 11-yr-old children. *Ear and Hearing, 32(3)*, 269–285.

Moore, D. R., Ferguson, M. A., Edmondson-Jones, A. M., Ratib, S., & Riley, A. (2010). Nature of auditory processing disorder in children. *Pediatrics, 126*(2), E382–E390.

Moore, D. R., Halliday, L. F., & Amitay, S. (2009). Use of auditory learning to manage listening problems in children. *Philosophical Transactions of the Royal Society B-Biological Sciences, 364*, 409–420.

Musacchia, G., Sams, M., Skoe, E., & Kraus, N. (2007). Musicians have enhanced subcortical auditory and audiovisual processing of speech and music. *Proceedings of the National Academy of Sciences of the United States of America, 104*(40), 15894–15898.

Musiek, F. E. (1983). Assessment of central auditory dysfunction—The dichotic digit test revisited. *Ear and Hearing, 4*(2), 79–83.

Musiek, F. E., & Chermak, G. D. (1994). Three commonly asked questions about central auditory processing disorders: Assessment. *American Journal of Audiology, 3*, 23–27.

Musiek, F. E., Geurkink, N. A., & Kietel, S. A. (1982). Test battery assessment of auditory perceptual dysfunction in children. *Laryngoscope, 92*(3), 251–257.

National Institute of Child Health and Human Development. (2000). *Report of the National Reading Panel. Teaching children to read: An evidence-based assessment of the scientific research literature on reading and its implications for reading instruction.* Retrieved from http://www.nichd.nih.gov/publications/nrp/smallbook.htm

Needleman, I. (2003). Introduction to evidence based dentistry. In J. Clarkson, J. E. Harrison, A. I. Ismail, I. Needleman & H. Worthington (Eds.), *Evidence-based dentistry for effective practice* (pp. 1–18). London, UK: Martin Dunitz.

Neijenhuis, K. A., Stollman, M. H., Snik, A. F., & van der Broek, P. (2001). Development of a central auditory test battery for adults. *Audiology, 40*, 69–77.

Nilsson, M., Soli, S. D., & Sullivan, J. A. (1994). Development of the Hearing in Noise Test for the measurement of speech reception thresholds in quiet and in noise. *Journal of the Acoustical Society of America, 95*(2), 1085–1099.

Patterson, R. D., & Johnsrude, I. S. (2008). Functional imaging of the auditory processing applied to speech sounds. *Philosophical Transactions of the Royal Society B-Biological Sciences, 363*(1493), 1023–1035.

Phonak. (2006). Ear-level FM receiver stimulates auditory neural plasticity in children with APD. *Field Study News, 44*(March), 1–2. Retrieved from http://www.speechpathology.com/channels/phonak_field_06march.pdf

Pinhiero, M. L. (1977). Tests of central auditory function in children with learning disabilities. In R. W. Keith (Ed.), *Central auditory dysfunction* (pp. 223–256). New York, NY: Grune & Stratton.

Pokorni, J. L., Worthington, C. K., & Jamison, P. J. (2004). Phonological awareness intervention: Comparison of Fast ForWord, Earobics, and LiPS. *Journal of Educational Research, 97*(3), 147–157.

Putter-Katz, H. P. D., Adi-Ben Said, L. M. A., Feldman, I. M. A., Miran, D. B. A., Kushnir, D. M. A., Muchnik, C. P. D., & Hildesheimer, M. (2002). Treatment and evaluation indices of auditory processing disorders. *Seminars in Hearing, 23*(4), 357–364.

Rees, N. S. (1973). Auditory processing factors in language disorders—View from Procrustes bed. *Journal of Speech and Hearing Disorders, 38*(3), 304–315.

Rosenberg, G. G. (2002). Classroom acoustics and personal FM technology in managemet of auditory processing disorder. *Seminars in Hearing, 23*(4), 309–317.

Rouse, C. E., & Krueger, A. B. (2004). Putting computerized instruction to the test: A randomized evaluation of a "scientifically based" reading program. *Economics of Education Review, 23*(4), 323–338.

Russo, N. M., Nicol, T. G., Zecker, S. G., Hayes, E. A., & Kraus, N. (2005). Auditory training improves neural timing in the human brainstem. *Behavioural Brain Research, 156*(1), 95–103.

Schaffler, T., Sonntag, J., Hartnegg, K., & Fischer, B. (2004). The effect of practice on low-level auditory discrimination, phonological skills, and spelling in dyslexia. *Dyslexia, 10*, 119–130.

Schochat, E., Musiek, F. E., Alonso, R., & Ogata, J. (2010). Effect of auditory training on the middle latency resonse in children with (central) auditory processing disorder. *Brazilian Journal of Medical and Biological Research, 43*(8), 777–785.

Schow, R. L., & Seikel, J. A. (2007). Screening for (central) auditory processing disorder. In F. E. Musiek & G. D. Chermak (Eds.), *Handbook of (central) auditory processing disorder: Auditory neuroscience and diagnosis* (Vol. 1, pp. 137–159). San Diego, CA: Plural Publishing.

Schuele, C. M., & Boudreau, D. (2008). Phonological awareness intervention: Beyond the basics. *Language Speech and Hearing Services in Schools, 39*(1), 3–20.

Scientific Learning Corporation. (1998). *Fast ForWord* [Computer software]. Berkeley, CA: Author.

Segers, E., & Verhoeven, L. (2004). Computer-supported phonological awareness intervention for kindergarten children with specific language impairment. *Language Speech and Hearing Services in Schools, 35*(3), 229–239.

Sharma, M., Purdy, S. C., & Kelly, A. S. (2009). Comorbidity of auditory processing, language, and reading disorders. *Journal of Speech Language and Hearing Research, 52*(3), 706–722.

Stevens, C., Fanning, J., Coch, D., Sanders, L., & Neuille, H. (2008). Neural mechanisms of selective auditory attention are enhanced by computerized training: Electrophysiological evidence from language-impaired and typically developing children. *Brain Research, 1205*, 55–69.

Strehlow, U., Haffner, J., Bischof, J., Gratzka, V., Parzer, P., & Resch, F. (2006). Does successful training of temporal processing of sound and phoneme stimuli improve reading and spelling? *European Child & Adolescent Psychiatry, 15*(1), 19–29.

Strong, G. K., Torgerson, C. J., Torgerson, D. & Hulme, C. (2011). A systematic meta-analytic review of the evidence for the effectiveness of the "Fast ForWord" language intervention program. *Journal of Child Psychology and Psychiatry, 52*(3), 224–235.

Troia, G. A., & Whitney, S. D. (2003). A close look at the efficacy of Fast ForWord Language for children with academic weaknesses. *Contemporary Educational Psychology, 28*, 465–494.

Valente, M., Abrams, H. B., Benson, D.E., Hnath-Chisolm, T. E., Citron III, D., Hampton, D., . . . Sweetow, R.W. (2006). Guidelines for the audiolgic management of adult hearing impairment. *Audiology Today, 18*(5), 32–36.

Valentine, D., Hedrick, M. S., & Swanson, L. A. (2006). Effect of an auditory training program on reading, phoneme awareness, and language. *Perceptual and Motor Skills, 103*, 183–196.

Veuillet, E., Magnan, A., Ecalle, J., Thai-Van, H., & Collet, L. (2007). Auditory processing disorder in children with reading disabilities: Effect of audiovisual training. *Brain, 130*, 2915–2928.

Warrier, C. M., Johnson, K. L., Hayes, E. A., Nicol, T., & Kraus, N. (2004). Learning impaired children exhibit timing deficits and training-related improvements in auditory cortical responses to speech in noise. *Experimental Brain Research, 157*(4), 431–441.

World Health Organization. (1980). *International Classification of Impairments, Disabilities and Handicaps*. Geneva: Author.

Willeford, J. (1977). Assessing central auditory behaviour in children: A test battery approach. In R. W. Keith (Ed.), *Central auditory dysfunction* (pp. 43–72). New York, NY: Grune & Stratton.

Wilson, W. J., Heine, C., & Harvey, L. A. (2004). Central auditory processing and Central auditory processing disorder: Fundamental questions and consideration. *Australian and New Zealand Journal of Audiology, 26*(2), 80–93.

Wilson, W. J., Jackson, A., Pender, A., Rose, C., Wilson, J., Heine, C., & Khan, A. (2011). The CHAPS, SIFTER, and TAPS–R as predictors of (C)AP skills and (C)APD. *Journal of Speech, Language, and Hearing Research, 54*, 278–291.

Wilson, W. J., Marinac, J., Pitty, K., & Burrows, C. (2011). The use of soundfield amplification devices in different types of classrooms. *Language Speech and Hearing Services in Schools, 42*, 395–407.

Wright, B. A., & Zhang, Y. X. (2009). A review of the generalization of auditory learning. *Philosophical Transactions of the Royal Society B-Biological Sciences, 364*(1515), 301–311.

Yencer, K. A. (1998). Clinical focus: Grand rounder. The effects of auditory integration training for children with central auditory processing disorders. *American Journal of Audiology, 7*(2), 32–34.

Young, D., McPherson, B., Hickson, L., & Lawson, M. (1997). Preferred FM system listening levels of children with central auditory processing disorders. *Journal of the Academy of Rehabilitative Audiology, 30*, 53–61.

CHAPTER 13

Evaluation and Implementation of EBP in Audiology

Lena Wong and Louise Hickson

INTRODUCTION

This chapter summarizes the evidence related to the various interventions discussed in the book and highlights gaps in the current evidence about the various interventions. The final step in Evidence-Based Practice (EBP) process is also discussed, that is, evaluating the outcomes of EBP. This important step has received much less attention than other aspects of EBP and we present a model, called the Logic Model, to assist with this process. Finally, practical steps for the implementation of EBP in the clinic are suggested.

CURRENT EVIDENCE AND ISSUES

The application of EBP in audiology, as in other health-related professions, is a process. It starts with asking the PICO (Patient, Intervention, Comparison, Outcomes) questions, moves on to identifying and evaluating the best available evidence, then relating the evidence to the client, and, finally, evaluating the EBP process and outcomes. Although emerging evidence may be available for some new technologies (e.g., trainable hearing aids), a larger body of evidence that allows more definitive conclusions is typically only available for more established intervention procedures (e.g., amplification for adults, cochlear implantation). A summary of the evidence on the interventions included in this book is presented in the following section followed by a discussion of factors that might have influenced the overall grade of evidence.

Summary of Evidence and Gaps in Evidence in Audiological Interventions

The chapters in this book have addressed audiological interventions, including conventional amplification, cochlear implantation, aural rehabilitation, as well as treatments for auditory processing disorders and tinnitus. The chapter authors have provided detailed analyses of currently available evidence and pointed out the gaps in research that they consider to be of the highest priority (Table 13–1). The fact that there are a number of gaps in the evidence-base, of course, does not mean that intervention procedures may not be used clinically.

Table 13–1. A Summary of Available Evidences and Gaps for Various Audiological Interventions

Chapter Number/ Type of Intervention	*Evidence*	*Gaps*
4. Amplification for adults	1. Randomized controlled trials are rare (one published), no studies have employed placebo groups as controls, and the use of control groups has also been rare. 2. The overwhelming majority of nonrandomized intervention studies have made use of similar study samples: older adults with mild to severe sloping sensorineural hearing loss fit bilaterally with hearing aids whose frequency-gain characteristics were verified via real-ear measurements. 3. General observations drawn from the analyses of the existing nonrandomized intervention studies demonstrated positive "benefaction," frequent use or wearing of hearing aids, and significantly improved speech understanding.	1. Randomized controlled trials with placebo controls are sorely needed. 2. Existing data on outcomes cannot be easily generalized to young or middle-aged adults, hearing loss other than mild to moderate sloping sensorineural configurations, nonstandard protocols (e.g., without real-ear verification), or monoaural fits. Data on outcomes are needed for each of these common, but unevaluated, conditions.
5. Amplification for children	1. Good quality evidence to support the use of wide-dynamic-range compression and switchable directional microphone technology for children. 2. Fit hearing aids early; verify and evaluate outcomes using objective and subjective methods to optimize performance with amplification.	1. Compression ratio requirements 2. Amplification bandwidth requirements

Table 13–1. *continued*

Chapter Number/ Type of Intervention	*Evidence*	*Gaps*
6. New amplification technologies	Emerging data suggest that: 1. Front/back discrimination can be improved in some listeners by limiting directionality to the high frequencies. 2. Recognition of speech presented behind a listener may be improved by directing the sensitivity of the directional microphones toward the rear. 3. The final self-adjusted response is influenced by the baseline response.	There is a need to understand the real-life implications of having conflicting audio and visual cues (e.g., when the sensitivity of directional microphones is pointing away from the visual scene), and to determine if there is a real-life benefit to sound localization from binaural gain control and extended high-frequency gain.
7. Cochlear implantation in adults	1. Research evidence has demonstrated that modern cochlear implants provide highly significant improvements in auditory skills, particularly for speech perception, for a large proportion of adults with acquired severe and profound hearing loss. 2. Improvements in auditory skills are generally reduced for adults with congenital deafness, those with longer duration of hearing loss, and older adults. 3. Knowledge of outcomes can now provide the basis for evidence-based recommendations for adults considering the cochlear implant procedure.	1. There is a need to gain better understanding of the benefits of binaural hearing for cochlear implant users, including how best to combine acoustic hearing devices with implants and when to recommend bilateral implantation. 2. There is increasing evidence that the surgical procedure may play a significant role in affecting the quality of cochlear implant outcomes. Randomized controlled trials are needed to identify how the surgical procedure (including electrode design) can be optimized. 3. There remains a large proportion of unexplained variance in outcomes, and further work is needed to identify aspects of central auditory function and cognitive skills that affect results.

continues

Table 13–1. *continued*

Chapter Number/ Type of Intervention	*Evidence*	*Gaps*
8. Cochlear implantation in children	1. Young children between the ages of 2 and 12 years who receive a cochlear implant can attain open-set speech perception, sometimes as early as 12 months postimplantation. 2. Pediatric cochlear implant users exhibit great variability in their performance, particularly relative to chronological age at implantation, duration of cochlear implant use, and duration of deafness. However, this variability decreases as the children gain listening experience with the device. 3. Appropriate ongoing assessment is a critical part of patient care.	1. Inconsistent reporting of key demographic variables (i.e., child, auditory history, cochlear implant device, mapping, etc.) and details of test administration limit comparison across studies. 2. Guidelines for performance-appropriate assessment batteries need to be established for consistent monitoring of performance over time and across assessment sites.
9. New developments in cochlear implantation	1. Bilateral stimulation, either via bimodal stimulation or bilateral implantation, is superior to unilateral cochlear implantation. 2. Maximum benefit with bimodal fitting is obtainable if hearing aids are optimized for use with cochlear implants using a validated procedure.	Relative effectiveness of bilateral cochlear implants and bimodal stimulation for children and adults who have residual hearing usable with acoustic amplification.
10. Aural rehabilitation	Individual auditory perceptual training improves speech understanding, and participation in group aural rehabilitation programs improve outcomes in terms of reduced self-perceived participation restriction, at least in the short term.	Long-term outcomes need to be established, and individual differences in needs for and response to interventions need to be determined.
11. Tinnitus treatment	There is consistent evidence, substantiated by two recent meta-analyses, that cognitive behavior therapy reduces distress associated with chronic tinnitus; on the negative side, there is no evidence that any pharmacological agent reliably affects the experience of tinnitus.	There is some evidence of the utility of hearing prosthesis in relieving tinnitus distress, and a systematic study of this factor is warranted; cranial implanting appears promising, and a multicenter study of this would be worthwhile.

Table 13–1. *continued*

Chapter Number/ Type of Intervention	*Evidence*	*Gaps*
12. Rehabilitation of auditory processing disorders	The evidence is suggestive to compelling that direct auditory interventions (using nonspeech and/or simple speech stimuli): 1. Improve AP in school-age children with APD with or without spoken language, reading, or learning difficulties; and 2. Do not improve spoken language and/or reading skills in school-age children with spoken language and/or reading disorders with or without APD. Despite prima facie evidence that the indirect intervention of personal FM systems can improve the signal-to-noise ratio for the listener, the evidence is equivocal regarding their ability to improve AP in school-age children with APD with or without spoken language, reading, or learning difficulties.	There is a critical need for: 1. Universally accepted "gold standards" for defining and diagnosing APD; 2. Greater integration of behavioral and electrophysiological research in AP and APD; and 3. More scientifically rigorous, longitudinal studies of the impact of auditory interventions on AP and cognition, including attention, spoken language, and literacy.

According to the EBP process discussed in this book, the clinician should present the information about the evidence to clients (i.e., what is known and what is unknown) and together make a shared decision about how to proceed. Clients and clinicians may well decide to proceed with a particular "experimental" intervention fully cognizant that it may or may not be successful. It is also important for clients and clinicians to be aware that, although there may be very positive evidence about the efficacy and effectiveness of an intervention, this does not guarantee that it will work for a particular individual. In every case, it is essential therefore, that intervention outcomes are measured for the individual client and it is hoped that such measurement will then contribute to the evidence base about the intervention.

Types and Levels of Evidence in Audiological Intervention

Throughout this book, chapter authors have attempted to identify the highest level of evidence in each area of intervention. Many have performed the most up-to-date systematic or systematized reviews of the literature to arrive at their conclusions. Their efforts have revealed that most studies of audiological interventions are at levels 3 to 4 (e.g., nonrandomized treatment studies, cohort studies, cross-sectional surveys); randomized controlled trials (level 2) occupy only a very small portion of the literature.

Various reasons might have contributed to the lack of higher level evidence about audiological interventions. First, the amount of effort and time required to conduct a randomized controlled trial (RCT) can be daunting and it is not always possible to find the large samples sizes required. Second, although RCTs are held up to be the gold standard for research studies, it can be argued that randomly assigning research participants into groups rids someone of the opportunity to make a choice and also downplays the importance of motivation for a successful outcome. In addition, withholding a treatment may not be ethical in some circumstances. Third, the assumption behind RCTs is that any differences between groups will be random, but this is hardly possible in real life. There are doubts as to whether it is possible to control for all the relevant factors, such as motivation and personality, to ensure the groups are equal; various combinations of factors are often at work (Reilly, 2004).

Finally, another reason for the lack of high level evidence regarding audiological interventions is that, for some technologies, the only studies available are those that have a small sample size, lack appropriate procedures to evaluate outcomes or have been commissioned by the manufacturer. Possible biases cannot be eliminated. This less than ideal evidence is inevitable for new technologies and treatment methods, as discussed in Chapter 6.

When faced with a small number of studies providing low-level evidence or when the overall grade of evidence is low, it may be necessary to consider evidence about intervention options from studies that seem somewhat relevant. For example, while some evidence may be available for new technology in adults, research in children may be scarce. The decision about whether or not to try a technology would have to be based on evidence from adults. Another example is when there is only evidence of efficacy (i.e., in the laboratory) and not of effectiveness (i.e., in the real world). If considering a brand new technology such as trainable hearing aids, a clinician may have to review evidence on related topics or from laboratory measurements or field trials that are documented in non-peer-reviewed journals and present that information to the client about this new type of amplification device (Wong, in press).

Methodological Considerations for Future Research

There are three major issues to be addressed in future research about audiological interventions: (1) more higher level evidence is needed, (2) appropriate sample sizes need to be used to evaluate interventions, and (3) more research about effectiveness is necessary for many interventions. In relation to the first point, RCTs (level 2 evidence) are urgently needed to document effects from many audiological interventions (Reilly, Oates, & Douglas, 2004). However, good quality research that contributes level 3 and 4 evidence should be considered when an RCT is not possible. In all studies, the validity and sensitivity of measurement tools needs to be considered carefully. The Appendix contains a checklist of the major quality indicators that could be used to evaluate most intervention studies.

Second, an appropriate sample size is critical. Sample size should be justified using sample size calculations and effect size estimates should be reported (see examples in Chapter 6 and discussions in Chapter 10). Multicenter studies, such as those reported in Chapter 7 on cochlear implantation, should be considered as they would increase overall sample size and allow findings to be generalized to populations with varying characteristics.

Finally, although many studies report on efficacy, we argue that it is also essential to examine effectiveness using appropriate outcome measures that are reflective of the important functional effects of the intervention (Reilly et al., 2004). For example, efficacy studies may show that a particular form of amplification improves speech perception in noise in the clinic, but does it improve client reports of listening in a noisy restaurant and/or reduce anxiety about such situations and/or encourage the person to participate? Self-reported activity, participation and quality of life need to be measured to determine if the clinical efficacy translates to real-world effectiveness. Outcomes could also be measured in terms of cost-effectiveness.

STEP 5 OF EBP: EVALUATING OUTCOMES OF EBP

Once available research about intervention options has been identified and evaluated and the evidence related to client's concerns, it is time to consider the EBP process itself. The clinician has to ask whether the intervention can be implemented effectively and efficiently in his or her particular service delivery setting. The clinician would have to consider the input process (i.e., resources, procedures, and personnel), short-term outcomes (including indicators and methods to assess these outcomes), long-term outcomes (including indicators and methods to assess these outcomes) and impacts. At this point, how well the other steps of the EBP process have been carried out should also be evaluated. We propose that an appropriate way to do this would be to apply a Logic Model (Chapel, 2004) to describe the relationships between inputs, outputs, outcomes and impacts. Although a new intervention could be evaluated in a clinic as a program, how well the intervention applies to an individual client should also be assessed. In the following section, the Logic Model is described followed by a discussion of how it could be applied to evaluate a whole-of-clinic program as well as the intervention as it applies at the individual level.

What Is a Logic Model?

Logic Models are being promoted at the Centers for Disease Control and Prevention (CDC) in the United States to evaluate health and education programs (Chapel, 2004). The CDC Web site (http://www.cdc.gov/eval/resources/index.htm) provides very comprehensive information on how such programs could be implemented and evaluated, with a special focus on the use of Logic Models to accomplish these tasks. It is, in essence, a visual representation of how the planners of a program think it is going to work in four stages: (1) planning, (2) implementation, (3) evaluation, and (4) reporting. At the planning stage, the model could help with identifying resources required and evaluating whether expected outcomes are reasonable and achievable. At the implementation stage, the model provides a picture of the steps involved. At the evaluation stage, the model allows the clinician or stakeholders to examine whether the steps have been followed and expected outcomes have been achieved. The model could be used as a background against which to explore reasons that could lead to positive or negative outcomes, and identify possible gaps in the EBP process and service provision. At the reporting stage, the issues identified in the other stages could be pointed out using the Logic Model. Information related to each stage could be communicated to stakeholders such as administrators, third-party payers, clients, and their significant others.

Figure 13–1 illustrates the various components of a Logic Model and gives an example related to the evaluation of an audiological intervention program. Another example of how the Logic Model could be used in planning and evaluating rehabilitation in cochlear implant users is illustrated by Tucker et al. (2011). There are slight variations in the components of Logic Models and the one we have adopted here describes: (1) the clinical priorities, (2) the processes that are integral to the implementation of EBP in clinical practice, and (3) expected outcomes and impacts. Readers who are interested may refer to Chapel (2004) for a list of steps used to construct a Logic Model or the CDC Web site for more comprehensive information. A Logic Model is established after the EBP process has been completed and prior to implementation of the new intervention program.

Although the first two chapters have covered the steps related to the establishment of the clinical priorities and the other steps in the EBP process, the clinician will also need to work with administrators to provide the appropriate support for resources and activities, as well as communicate with stakeholders about the desired outcomes and impacts. This planning stage will involve negotiation among many parties and various items in the Logic Model should be clearly stated so that at the evaluation stage, issues, and problems can be identified.

Using the Logic Model for Program-Level Evaluation

At the program level, clinicians are interested in learning whether a new intervention program (e.g., a new APD treatment method) brings benefit in real-life situations and whether the program has been carried out effectively and with cost efficiency. Therefore, a comprehensive review of the EBP process as well as implementation of the program is needed.

Evaluation of the EBP Process

Prior to implementing new interventions, the clinician should examine whether Steps 1 to 4 of the EBP process have resulted in evidence that matches the target clients' needs, values and preferences. Things that need to be considered are highlighted in the first and second columns of Figure 13–1 (clinical priorities, the process). The clinician may want to ask the following questions (Hoffmann, Bennett, & Del Mar, 2010):

- *Step 1:* Have I formulated an appropriate research question? When the research question is too broad, too many sources of evidence would be identified and therefore too much time and effort would be spent on examining evidence. When the research question is too focused, very little evidence may be identified and the evidence may not be applied to clients with varied needs.
- *Step 2:* Did I use the correct search procedures to identify appropriate evidence? Have I identified the appropriate and best evidence for the question? When sufficient evidence could not be found, what other search strategies and/or evidence have I incorporated? Have I searched the database efficiently? Are there ways to improve my search next time?
- *Step 3:* Did I use the hierarchy of evidence appropriately to help me identify the evidence? What were the difficulties in identifying the evidence (e.g., lack of high level evidence, difficulties in reading and understanding the evidence)?
- *Step 4:* How well did the evidence respond to the research question and therefore the needs of target clientele?

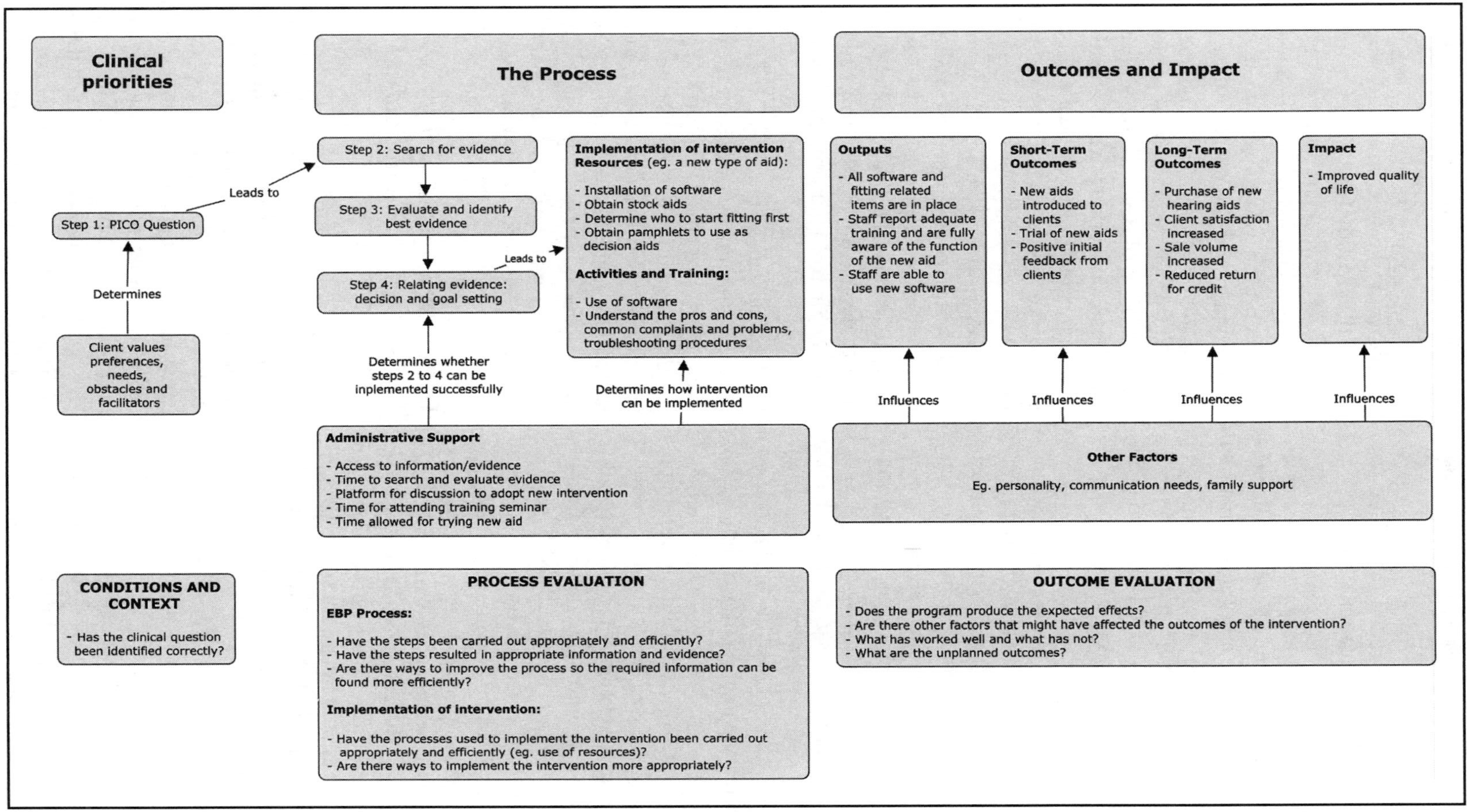

Figure 13–1. *An example of a Logic Model that addresses the incorporation of a audiological intervention in a clinical situation.*

Evaluation of the Procedures Used to Implement New Interventions

There are two process components (resources, activities, and training) to be considered in the implementation of the intervention and four components related to outcomes (outputs, short- and long-term outcomes and impacts). These components are listed below and in the middle and last columns of Figure 13–1.

- *Resources:* the types of resources (e.g., funding, personnel, equipment, and staff time) that are required for successful implementation of the program are listed. It is very likely that these resources represent a compromise between what is ideal and what is currently/realistically available.
- *Activities and Training:* the tasks that are used to achieve the desired outcomes (e.g., training, counseling of clients, communication among staff at a clinic) could be listed here. A realistic schedule should be considered when planning and implementing these activities.
- *Outputs:* immediate and often tangible results that arise from the implementation of the program are listed here (e.g., whether the clinic has been set up properly for initial implementation of the new intervention program).
- *Outcomes:* what we want to achieve are defined as short- or long-term goals (e.g., clients report positive feedback, increased satisfaction). The listed (desired) outcomes could be those defined by the stakeholders or accepted by the professional community.
- *Impacts:* the overall effect of the program (e.g., improved quality of life).

Two issues are essential in determining whether the procedures used to implement a new program were successful. The first question is, "Have the processes used to implement the program been carried out appropriately and efficiently (e.g., use of resources)?" Administrative support importantly influences the decision on how resources and activities can be used to help implement the new program and should be evaluated. The second question is, "Are there ways to implement the program more appropriately and efficiently?" Evaluation of the impact may include an evaluation of cost-effectiveness. Although clinicians should examine whether the program results in positive outcomes at various stages, evaluation should also focus on whether other factors could have influenced outcomes and whether modification of the intervention program is necessary. An example of how the Logic Model could be used to design, implement, and evaluate an EBP training program for professionals in speech pathology and audiology is illustrated by Guo, Bain, and Willer (2011). The authors planned a training program so that clinicians could learn about the EBP process (e.g., how to search for information). Resources and activities involved and desired outcomes were laid out in a Logic Model, prior to the start of the program. The training program was then evaluated to examine whether predefined outcomes had been successfully achieved.

Using the Logic Model for Evaluation at the Individual Level

Although a new intervention program may be evaluated as above in the whole-of-clinic environment, an evaluation at the individual clients' level should not be neglected. Many of the program questions could be applied to the client, however additional questions should be addressed to assess step 4 (relating evidence to the client) of the EBP process. These include, "How well does the evidence match the needs of the individual client? Did I understand the problem from the client's perspective? Was the client able to communicate their goals and preferences? When I related the evidence to the client, was the evidence presented clearly and understood by the client?" In addition, the clinician should also list desired outcomes and impacts as evidence is being related to the client and goals for the intervention are being set.

Advantages in Using the Logic Model

The Logic Model has been proposed here to help design, implement, evaluate and report the outcomes associated with an EBP program. There are many advantages in using the Logic Model. First, it allows an opportunity for various parties to negotiate targets and determine priorities and issues prior to implementation of an intervention program. Second, it encourages relevant parties to discuss expectations, workload, strategies, allocation of resources, timeline and desired outcomes; therefore, enhancing mutual understanding in the team. Issues and potential problems may be identified. Third, it provides an overall picture of the whole EBP process and outcomes. It documents important elements in the process and outcomes and differentiates process from outcomes. Finally, it allows evaluation of outcomes and reporting to be based on these elements. What actually happened when the program was applied is examined and compared to what was planned. In other words, whether the program works is examined.

INCORPORATING EBP IN CLINICAL PRACTICE

Although EBP is a relatively new topic in audiology, it has wide coverage in medicine, nursing and dentistry. Although we recognize the many advantages associated with implementation of EBP in clinical practice, we have learned from other health care colleagues that there is resistance from organizations, stakeholders or other clinicians in implementing changes (Rosenthal, 2004). Clinicians often have difficulties initiating EBP, due to reasons such as a lack of knowledge about the EBP process, the lack of administrative support (Rosenthal, 2004; Upton & Upton, 2005), the poor quality of evidence in some instances, difficulties in translating research findings into clinical practice and misconceptions that EBP should be left to researchers.

Successful Implementation of EBP

Reilly et al. (2004) suggested promoting EBP at various levels, including with professional bodies, university educators, clinical managers and clinicians. They advocated that the profession should set a clear research agenda to further the development of EBP and that the research knowledge thus generated should be readily transferrable to clinical practice. Clinicians should expect that there is evidence for everything and that EBP would enhance service provision and outcomes (Geyman, 2000).

Ways to Engage in EBP

Although chapter authors have provided excellent state-of-the-art reviews of findings for various audiological intervention procedures in this book, clinicians must continue to engage in EBP and in continuous self-learning in order not to be "outdated." Being able to evaluate and interpret the evidence hinges on learning about the research process and about how to critique research papers (Rose & Baldac, 2004). Clinicians should also have a good understanding of the clinical issues, client's values and preferences (Rose & Baldac, 2004) and the ability to make an accurate diagnosis of the case and engage the client in the decision-making process (Guyatt et al., 2000).

Geyman (2000) suggested various ways to introduce and facilitate EBP in clinical practice. These suggestions as well as some additional ideas are as follows:

1. To identify relevant research studies to address the PICO question, the clinicians may want to use some efficient search strategies to facilitate the search and appraisal of evidence. For example, searching could be limited initially to systematic reviews, meta-analysis, and RCTs only (i.e., the highest levels of evidence) and only go beyond this if an initial search is unsuccessful. Palmer (2001) suggested that a good systematic review should produce up to four papers that correspond directly to a specific PICO question (see Chapter 1), which could be manageable in a busy clinician's schedule. Another efficient practice that may be feasible in larger clinical practices or organizations is to identify personnel with the required expertise to carry out the first three steps of the EBP process.
2. It is important to dedicate some time to the reading of resources listed on databases such as MEDLINE and PubMed. Tables 1–2 and 1–3 provide additional lists of resources, and the Web site suggested in Chapter 2 (http://beckerguides.wustl.edu/audiology) contains a collection of links to various resources. One hopes that clinicians will have access to databases via the Internet in their workplace. If so, a meeting with a librarian or attending a workshop to learn how to use search tools such as the MEDLINE could be very helpful. Of course, finding time for reading can be difficult amidst a busy clinic schedule and it would be valuable to establish an evidence-based journal club to encourage more reading and discussion among clinicians.
3. When reading research papers or any type of information that claims evidence to support an intervention, clinicians should be wary of possible biases and question the merits of research methodology, results, analyses and conclusions. The critical appraisal checklist in the Appendix will aid this process.
4. Clinicians could plan continuing education opportunities to include courses on EBP and they could participate in workshops to learn about EBP. ASHA has an updated list of such workshops (http://www.asha.org/Members/ebp/General-EBP-Tutorials/) and workshops are also offered by Critical Appraisal, the Centre for Evidence-Based Medicine (http://www.cebm.net/). Such education is also available online (e.g., http://www.criticalappraisal.com/online-course/online-course-introduction).
5. Knowledge exchange between researchers and clinicians should be increased. It is essential that researchers address relevant clinical questions and guidance about the key issues relevant to clinical practice is available from their clinical colleagues. Clinicians may find ways to facilitate a closer relationship with researchers, for example, by offering to help with participant recruitment through their clinics.

Responsibilities of Professional Organizations

Professional organizations should cultivate and provide a platform for EBP among clinicians. Internet links to position papers and evidence-based clinical or practice guidelines in different areas of audiological interventions could be provided. As discussed in Chapter 1 of this book, the American Speech Language and Hearing Association now has a Compendium of EBP Guidelines and Systematic Reviews to examine the cost-benefit of EBP in audiological intervention (Dollaghan, 2007). Other related organizations also publish guidelines and systematic reviews on their Web sites (see Table 1–4). Such evidence must be made easy to access and read (Law & Baum, 1998).

Workshops on EBP could be held at national and international conferences to facilitate implementation in clinical settings. Continuous professional education credits could also be granted to courses that focus on the application of EBP in the workplace.

Student Education

Students should be prepared for EBP by the inclusion of courses that focus on the skills of effectively searching and critically appraising the research literature. Capstone experiences, student research projects, and/or dissertations have an important role to play here. Reilly et al. (2004) suggested that a problem-based learning curriculum is particularly appropriate for developing the necessary skills to engage future clinicians in the EBP process because the five EBP steps are comparable to the processes involved in problem based learning (Reilly et al., 2004). At present, very few programs have adopted this mode of learning. To our knowledge, the Master of Audiology program in Flinders University in Australia is the only program that has adopted a complete problem-based learning curriculum. Other programs such as the Master of Science in Audiology program at the University of Hong Kong have incorporated this mode of learning in some components.

In a problem-based learning curriculum, students are required to identify learning issues associated with a clinical problem (case). They form hypotheses that guide their search for information and evidence, taking into account other information provided in the case. These procedures are similar to steps 1 to 4 of the EBP process. An example related to audiology would be a case where a child who has bilateral profound hearing impairment and multiple disabilities is being considered for treatment options. Students would search for and evaluate evidence that surrounds various types of treatment options and evidence in relation to outcomes in children with these options, as well as consider how other types of disability could affect the decision and outcomes. A detailed comparison between the processes involved in EBP and problem-based learning can be found in Reilly et al. (2004).

CONCLUSION

EBP has received attention only recently in audiological practice and the process of adopting it will take time, most likely following the steps in Simpson's (2002) model of program change: exposure, adoption, implementation, and practice. In the initial exposure stage, clinicians and/or stakeholders may be learning about EBP from workshops, books or some other forms of training. Books such as this one will be part of this exposure. In the second stage of adoption, relevant parties form an intention to engage in EBP and evaluate the resources that are needed. In the third stage of implementation, clinicians or their stakeholders may trial EBP to inform decisions on what resources are necessary and what exactly is needed to implement the outcomes of EBP, that is, how will changes to practice be achieved? Positive outcomes in the first stages will enhance clinicians' motivation to put EBP into practice in the fourth stage and sustain its use over time.

Although changing one's usual ways of handling evidence and clinical practice is not easy, we hope that this book has at least introduced the reader to what EBP is and how EBP can be applied in clinical practice. Current evidence on audiological interventions has been presented and gaps in research have been identified. The focus of this book is solely on the application of EBP to audiological interventions for children and adults and there is obviously scope to expand this to include diagnostic audiology. We hope that this book will inspire others to take the lead and further develop EBP in audiology.

REFERENCES

Chapel, T. (2004). Constructing and using Logic Models in program evaluation. In A. R. Roberts & K. R. Yeager (Eds.), *Evidence-based practice manual: Research and outcome measures in health and human services* (pp. 636–647). New York, NY: Oxford University Press.

Dollaghan, C. A. (2007). *The handbook for evidence-based pratice in communication disorders.* Baltimore, MD: Paul H. Brookes.

Geyman, J. (2000). Evidence-based medicine in primary care: An overview. In J. Geyman, R. Deyo, & S. Ramsey (Eds.), *Evidence-based clinical practice: Concept and approaches* (pp. 1–12). Woburn, MA: Butterworth-Heinemann.

Guo, R., Bain, B. A., & Willer, J. (2011). Application of a Logic Model to an evidence-based practice training program for speech-language pathologists and audiologists. *Journal of Allied Health, 40*(1), e23–e28.

Guyatt, G. H., Haynes, R. B., Jaeschke, R. Z., Cook, D. J., Green, L., Naylor, C. D., . . . Richardson, W. S. (2000). Users guide to the medical literature XXV. Evidence-based medicine: principles for applying the users guides to patient care. *Journal of the American Medical Association, 284,* 1290–1296.

Hoffmann, T., Bennett, S., & Del Mar, C. (2010). Introduction to evidence-based practice. In T. Hoffmann, S. Bennett & C. Del Mar (Eds.), *Evidence-based practice across the health professions* (pp. 1–15). Chatswood, NSW, Australia: Elsevier.

Law, M., & Baum, C. (1998). Community health: A responsibility, an opportunity, and a fit for occupational therapy. *American Journal of Occupational Therapy, 52*(1), 7–10.

Nutting, P. A., Beasley, J. W., & Werner, J. J. (1999). Practice-based research networks to answer primary care questions. *Journal of the American Medical Association, 281*(8), 686–688.

Palmer, C. V. (2001). An evidence-based approach to applying hearing instrument technology in pediatrics. In R. C. Seewald & J. Gravel (Eds.), *A sound foundation through early amplification (Proceedings of the Second International Conference)* (pp. 121–126). Stafa, Switzerland: Phonak AG.

Reilly, S. (2004). What constitutes evidence? In S. Reilly, J. Douglas, & J. Oates (Eds.), *Evidence-based practice in speech pathology* (pp. 18–34). London, UK: Whurr.

Reilly, S., Oates, J., & Douglas, J. (2004). Evidence-based practice in speech pathology—future directions. In S. Reilly, J. Douglas, & J. Oates (Eds.), *Evidence-based practice in speech pathology* (pp. 330–352). London, UK: Whurr.

Rose, M., & Baldac, S. (2004). Translating evidence into practice. In Reilly, S., Douglas, J., & Oates, J. (Eds.), *Evidence-based practice in speech pathology* (pp. 317–329). London, UK: Whurr.

Rosenthal, R. N. (2004). Overview of evidence-based practice. In A. R. Roberts & K. R. Yeager (Eds.), *Evidence-based practice manual: Research and outcome measures in health and human services* (pp. 20–29). Oxford, UK: Oxford University Press.

Simpson, D. (2002). A conceptual framework for transferring research to practice. *Journal of Substance Abuse Treatment, 22,* 171–182.

Tucker, D., Compton, M. V., Mankoff, L., & Alsalman, O. (2011). Cochlear implant connections: facilitiating the rehabilitation journal with late-deafened adults. *ASHA Leader, 16*(12), 24–27.

Upton, D., & Upton, P. (2005) Nurses' attitudes to evidence-based practice: Impact of a national policy. *British Journal of Nursing, 14*(5), 284–288.

Wong, L. L. N. (in press). Evidence on self-fitting hearing aids. *Trends in Amplification.*

APPENDIX

Critical Appraisal Checklist (CAC) for Individual Intervention Studies[1]

GUIDELINES FOR EACH QUESTION

This checklist could be used to evaluate the quality of each analytic study. Internal validity, external validity and impact are being evaluated (see Chapter 1 for definitions). A brief discussion on how the CAC in this Appendix should be used is given below.

Evaluation of Internal Validity

The Introduction section of a paper should provide information on the aims of the study so that the link to the PICO question can be determined (see Chapter 1 for how to formulate the PICO question).

Question 1. Aims should be clearly stated and readily identifiable.

Question 2. Aims should be plausible, meaning reasonable and credible.

Question 3. The aims should address the clinical PICO question.

When reading the Methods section, it is important to examine how participants were being selected, assessment materials, and procedures used. These methodological details should be documented carefully in the research paper with enough detail to allow for replication of the study.

Question 4. The Methods should be written so that readers can make a judgment on whether the paper is descriptive or analytic (see Chapter 1) and an analytic study could then be evaluated using this CAC.

Question 5. Participant or subject recruitment and selection, including exclusion criteria, should be explained and justified clearly. This is not always the case, as mentioned in Chapter 5 of this book. Biases in participant selection may influence the outcomes. Participants could be selected to optimize the outcomes of an intervention but the findings would not be applicable to the general population. For example, commercially sponsored research may include only participants who are experienced with a particular manufacturer's technology, thus showing optimal benefit; how-

[1] Questions and rating scales adapted from Dollaghan (2007).

ever, when the technology is applied in a general population, the same effects may not be realized. Variations in participant characteristics may or may not be appropriate depending on the purpose of the study. For example, if the study is used to document hearing aid outcomes in the general population, then diversity is necessary. If the study is to assess a technology for a particular type of population, such as frequency transposition hearing aids, then participants should be more homogeneous (i.e., with high-frequency sensorineural hearing loss).

Question 6. Whether and why a control group was used should be stated. If the groups are not randomly assigned, there is a likelihood that the control and experimental groups are not equivalent and therefore, conclusions about treatment effect may not be accurate. In a longitudinal study in pediatrics, the use of a control group would help to tease out improvement in performance due to intervention, in comparison to improved ability as the children become older.

Question 7. What are the similarities and differences between groups? Variations in group characteristics could become confounders. If the groups are not randomly assigned, there is a likelihood that the control and experimental groups are not the same and, therefore, conclusions about intervention effects may not be accurate. Even if randomization is used in a research study, important differences between groups (e.g., age, gender, degree of hearing impairment, amplification experiences) should be checked to ensure that the randomization process has resulted in comparable groups.

Question 8. Do the groups receive the same intervention? How counter-balancing and/or randomization is done should be reported to ensure that the only difference between groups is due to the intervention. To compare outcomes using different interventions, it is important that the participants and/or the researchers are blinded to the interventions and the expected outcomes, so that expectations or biases do not affect the results.

Question 9. The number of participants in the study is particularly important because in order to show intervention effects, sufficient numbers of participants are needed. This is referred to as the power of the study and power analysis should be reported to justify the sample size. Small sample size is often an issue in research on audiological interventions, particularly when new technologies are being evaluated, as discussed in Chapter 6.

Question 10. As participant drop out is quite common in studies that extend over a period of time, the dropout rate should be stated and should not be more than 20%. It is likely that drop out participants may exhibit demographic characteristics or systematic differences in their prognoses that are different from those who remain in the study. Therefore, it is important for research papers to state whether they exhibit similar characteristics. These dropouts may disturb the balance created in the randomization of participants in groups.

Question 11. Details on intervention procedures should be documented so that it is possible to judge whether the intervention was implemented as proposed in a reliable and valid way and whether the intervention could be applied to the client in question. In terms of materials and procedures, authors should state how and when equipment calibration took place, so readers can have confidence that test results are accurate.

Question 12. For outcome measures, authors should provide a rationale for the use of particular measures and these measures should be valid and reliable. Chapters 4 to 9 show that there are a variety of outcome measures for assessing hearing aids and cochlear implants in adults and children. Efficacy studies are normally carried out in a laboratory environment for new technologies such as the feedback management studies discussed in Chapter 2 and new technologies discussed in Chapter 6. To show real-life effectiveness, different outcome measures would be needed. Although tools for verification of hearing aid settings are often used in both efficacy and effectiveness studies; self-report questionnaires are typically used in effectiveness studies.

Question 13. The timing of the study and when outcome measurements are administered should be considered carefully. When the study is planned before the intervention, the study is a prospective one and is classified as a cohort study. When the outcome is measured at the same time as the intervention, a cross-sectional study is being conducted. When a study is not planned before the intervention, it is a retrospective study. A prospective study allows better planning of the study and better control of confounding factors than a retrospective study. In addition, the effects of acclimatization should be accounted for. Chapter 4 further elaborates on this point.

Question 14. Whenever possible, outcomes should be evaluated by a researcher who is blinded to the intervention that the participant has undertaken and, in the case of studies that measure outcomes before and after an intervention, blinded to the preintervention scores.

Question 15. The type of statistics used in the study should be stated carefully and justified. Although this Appendix could not possibly summarize the types of statistics appropriate for each study, readers can refer to statistics textbooks for more information (e.g., Field, 2009).

Evaluation of Impact

The Results and Discussion sections contribute to the evaluation of the impact of an intervention in the study. When reading these sections, it is important to examine the size of the intervention effects. The figures and tables should be examined.

Question 16. The interpretation of statistical findings can be challenging and it is recommended to refer to a brief discussion on evaluation of statistical data from an evidence-based perspective by Cox (2005) or the more detailed discussion by Dollaghan (2007). Other statistics books such as Field (2009) could also serve as guides. Assuming that statistical analyses are done appropriately, it will then be possible to identify whether the intervention has exerted significant effects.

Question 17. The size of intervention effects is very relevant to the clinical applicability of the findings. Effect size is a standardized measure of the measured effects (see Cox, 2005, for a brief review of how effect size could be used to evaluate results from a research study). An increasing number of research publications have adopted this measure to reflect objectively the importance of the effect of an intervention. Effect size could be compared across studies and its use has been mentioned in Chapters 7 and 10.

Question 18. It is important to consider if the findings would have significant impact clinically and how the treatment effects are maintained over time. For example, an intervention may result in a significant improvement in an outcome by 1%, however, this impact may be too small for the clinician to recommend the intervention. The clinician may also want to ask whether the intervention effects are maintained over time and this is an aspect that is frequently missing from intervention studies (see Chapter 10).

Question 19. If the results are not statistically significant, readers should go back to the question on whether statistical power was adequate.

Question 20. The clinician should also evaluate whether possible biases, important data or confounders have been accounted for. Some of the common confounders or sources of bias in hearing aid research include personality, prior exposure to similar technologies, lack of blinding and research studies being funded by a particular company to show benefit of a technology marketed by that company. In pediatric research, improvement in long-term intervention outcomes must be distinguished from maturation.

Question 21. Results should be discussed adequately, related to previous findings and there should be discussion on how results differ or agree with previous findings. In the discussion section, limitations of the study as well as future directions should be identified and discussed.

Question 22. It can be useful to consider whether the benefit justifies the costs (e.g., finances, effort) and risks involved.

Question 23. The final question to ask is whether the research has achieved the study aims and whether the conclusions from the statistical analysis are appropriate.

Evaluation of External Validity

The Results and Discussion sections are most relevant here.

Question 24. To appraise external validity, we must first decide whether the research was designed to evaluate the efficacy or effectiveness of an intervention (Frattali & Colper, 2007). Efficacy reflects the impact of an intervention in a well-specified population under ideal conditions, such as in a laboratory, and the intervention may not have the same effect in the real world. Effectiveness refers to the impact of an intervention applied to an average population under average situations. There are many examples where an intervention has not been found to be as effective as studies of efficacy suggest. Although evidence on effectiveness is desirable, particularly when clinicians are relating the evidence to clients' preferences and values, evidence on efficacy may be the only information available for new intervention techniques. Carefully examining the types of outcomes measured in research studies helps the clinician to determine whether the study evaluated efficacy and/or effectiveness.

Question 25. Whether the study participants are similar to the client who is the focus of the PICO question (see Chapter 1 for how to formulate the PICO question) should be considered.

Question 26. A particular client's preferences, values, goals, and benefits of intervention should be weighed against risks. Questions to ask are: "Will that outcome be meaningful to the particular client being seen in the clinic? Is the evidence relevant to that individual? Is the benefit worth the trouble?" Chapter 3 covers information on how evidence could be related to the client.

Question 27. Whether the intervention is feasible in terms of resources (e.g., cost, time) and clinicians' abilities and expertise and how the intervention could be made feasible should also be considered (Evans, 2003). Chapter 13 contains information on how a Logic Model could be used to plan the implementation of an intervention.

Critical Appraisal Checklist (CAC)

Assessor: ____________________ Date: ____________________

Clinical (PICO) question:

For ______________________________ (Patient/problem)

Does ______________________________ (Intervention)

Result in ______________________________ (Outcome)

In comparison with ______________________________ (Comparing intervention)

Key to Appraisal of Each Question (adapted from Dollaghan, 2007)

Y (yes)	All characteristic criteria are met
Y- (qualified yes)	Some characteristic criteria are met
N (no)	None of the characteristic criteria are met
UR (unable to rate)	Insufficient information has been provided for rating purposes and in this case, the evidence should be considered as not having met the characteristic criteria
NA (not applicable)	The characteristic criteria should not be applied given the type of the study

Key to Making Overall Judgments About Internal Validity, Impact, and External Validity (adapted from Dollaghan, 2007)

Compelling	Impartial experts would consistently determine the evidence to be convincing and significant
Suggestive	Some points are debatable, but impartial experts would most likely concur that the evidence is convincing and significant
Equivocal	The evidence presented is debatable such that impartial experts might come to conflicting conclusions about whether the evidence is convincing and significant.

Internal Validity: Was the Study Carried Out Using Appropriate Methods and Procedures?

In the Introduction Section	
1. What was the aim of the study?	______________________
2. Is the aim plausible?	Y / Y- / N / UR / NA (go to #3 if Y or Y-, otherwise stop, do not use the study)
3. Does the aim address my clinical PICO question?	Y / Y- / N / UR / NA (go to #4 if Y or Y-, otherwise stop, do not use the study)
In the Methods Section	
4. Was the evidence from an analytic study? Descriptive = describe a population Analytic = describe relationships between factors	Descriptive study, stop, do not use this form Analytic study, go to #5
5. What are the participant selection criteria? Can you replicate the study based on this info?	______________________ ______________________ Y / Y- / N / UR / NA
6. Was there a control group or condition?	A control group/condition, go to #7 No control group/condition, skip to #10
7. What are the similarities and differences between groups?	______________________ The groups are similar The groups are different
8. Do the groups receive the same intervention? What are the differences? What procedures were used to randomize participant grouping and the contrasting interventions?	Y / Y- / N / UR / NA ______________________ ______________________ There is randomization → RCT There is no randomization → observational study
9. What is the sample size? Was there a power analysis or justification for the sample size?	Sample size: _________ Sample size calculation/power analysis Other justification

10. How many participants drop out? How do they differ in characteristics from those who remain in the study?	Less than 20% drop out More than 20% drop out ________________________
11. What were the intervention(s)? How were they being implemented? Were they described clearly and implemented as intended? Was the intervention valid and reliable, in principle and as employed?	________________________ ________________________ Y / Y- / N / UR / NA Y / Y- / N / UR / NA
12. What were the outcomes measured? Can you replicate the study based on this info? Are these measures appropriate?	________________________ ________________________ Y / Y- / N / UR / NA Y / Y- / N / UR / NA
13. When was outcome measured? Before the intervention = prospective Same time as the intervention After the intervention = retrospective	Prospectively → cohort study Same time as the intervention → cross-sectional study Retrospectively → case control study
14. Was the outcome (at a minimum) evaluated with blinding?	Y / Y- / N / UR / NA
15. What are the statistical procedures used? Are they justified?	________________________ ________________________ Y / Y- / N / UR / NA

Overall Internal Validity: Compelling _____ Suggestive _____ Equivocal _____

Impact: How Large Were the Intervention Effects?

In the Results and Discussion Sections	
16. Was the intervention statistically significant?	Y / Y- / N / UR / NA
17. How large were the intervention effects? Are the findings reliable?	__________ Y / Y- / N / UR / NA
18. Was the finding important (clinical significance, social validity, maintenance)?	Y / Y- / N / UR / NA
19. If the finding was not statistically significant, was statistical power adequate?	Y / Y- / N / UR / NA
20. Were effects of bias, chance, and confounding variables on results considered? What are they?	Y / Y- / N / UR / NA __________ __________
21. Has important data been ignored or overlooked? What are they? Relationship with previous research—similar or different and why?	Y / Y- / N / UR / NA __________ __________
22. Was there a substantial cost-benefit advantage? How much? In what aspects?	Y / Y- / N / UR / NA __________ __________
23. Have the findings achieved the study aims?	Y / Y- / N / UR / NA

Overall Impact: Compelling _____ Suggestive _____ Equivocal _____

External Validity/Applicability

24. Did the study evaluate effectiveness or efficacy or both?	
25. Is my client comparable to those in the study? What are the differences?	Y / Y- / N / UR / NA __________ __________
26. What are the preferences, values and clinical circumstances of the client? What would be the expected benefit and risks? Would benefit outweigh these?	__________ __________ __________ Y / Y- / N / UR / NA
27. Is the intervention feasible in my setting? What should I do to make this intervention feasible in my setting?	Y / Y- / N / UR / NA __________ __________

Overall External Validity: Compelling _____ Suggestive _____ Equivocal _____

Was conflict of interest declared? Yes _____ No_____

Clinical Bottom Line Based on the Overall Judgments of Internal Validity, Impact, and External Validity: Should the Intervention Be Adopted? (adapted from Dollaghan, 2007)

Overall Judgment	Internal Validity	Impact	External Validity	Clinical Bottom Line
Compelling	Yes	Yes	Yes	Adoption of the intervention should be considered seriously.
Suggestive	One or more "yes" in the *suggestive* category of overall judgment			Clinicians might conscientiously come to different decisions about whether to adopt the intervention.
Equivocal	No	No	No	The intervention should not be adopted.

REFERENCES

Cox, R. M. (2005). Evidence-based practice in provision of amplification. *Journal of the American Academy of Audiology*, *16*(7), 419–438.

Dollaghan, C. A. (2007). *The handbook for evidence-based pratice in communication disorders*. Baltimore, MD: Paul H. Brookes.

Evans, D. (2003). Hierarchy of evidence: A framework for ranking evidence evaluating healthcare interventions. *Journal of Clinical Nursing*, *12*(1), 77–84.

Field, A. P. (2009). *Discovering statistics using SPSS: And sex and drugs and rock 'n' roll* (3rd ed.). London, UK: Sage.

Frattali, C. M., & Colper, L. A. (Eds.). (2007). *Evidence-based pratice and outcome oriented approaches in speech-langauge pathology* (2nd ed.). New York, NY: Thieme.

Index

A

B

C

D

E

G

H

I

L

M

T

V

W